NEXT GENERATION NCLEX-RN® PREP

Preparix

Book formatting and cover design by thiwwy design.

Table Of Contents

CHAPTER 1

Exam Essentials

1.0 NCLEX-RN 2026–2029 Updates

Starting April 1, 2026, the NCLEX-RN follows the updated NCSBN Test Plan 2026–2029. The exam's core structure and Next Generation NCLEX (NGN) format remain the same, continuing to emphasize clinical judgment through case-based and scenario-style questions.

The most visible change is in the Client Needs framework: **"Safety and Infection Control"** is now **"Safety and Infection Prevention and Control."** This reflects a stronger focus on *proactive infection prevention practices* rather than just reactive safety measures.

All other Client Needs categories and their weight ranges remain unchanged. The exam continues to evaluate your ability to apply safe, evidence-based nursing judgment in real-world situations.

This guide fully integrates those updates, including the revised terminology and continued emphasis on the Clinical Judgment Measurement Model (CJMM). Whether you're a first-time test taker or refreshing your knowledge, every strategy, question set, and rationale you'll find here aligns with the expectations of the 2026–2029 test plan.

1.1 How to Use This Guide

This guide is built to train the one thing the NCLEX-RN measures most: safe, repeatable clinical judgment. Everything you do here—practice questions, debriefs, and flashcards—should be aimed at recognizing red flags, choosing the safest RN action, and explaining your choice using the language of the Clinical Judgment Measurement Model (CJMM). Study to perform, not to recite. Your outcome metric is not pages read; it is how consistently you choose safe, prioritized actions across mixed, NGN-style questions under time pressure.

Plan for 6–8 weeks of preparation with a practice-first approach. Each day is mostly doing and analyzing mixed questions. Reading is supplemental and targeted to your misses. Flashcards are not a separate hobby; they are distilled, reusable decisions from your rationales. By the end, you should be able to justify your answers using Client Needs categories and CJMM steps, and you should default automatically to safety rules such as airway/oxygenation, perfusion, mental status, unstable vs. stable, do-not-harm, scope of practice, and infection prevention and control.

A weekly cadence builds endurance and judgment. Aim for daily sets of 40–75 mixed questions that include NGN case sets, done under timed, exam-like conditions without notes. Directly after, spend 15–20 minutes reviewing spaced-repetition cards. The remainder of your study time goes to focused content refresh—but only for the weak areas you uncovered. Once per week, complete one timed, mixed exam-length block with a full debrief that takes as long as the block itself. Guard one rest day every week to protect attention and avoid burnout; the NCLEX is a stamina test as well as a judgment test.

Use a short daily loop—do, debrief, distill, drill—to convert every question into a durable skill. "Do" means creating exam conditions: timed interface, mixed content, no notes, no pausing. Work quickly but safely. If a question includes conflicting data, anchor to what threatens life or limb now, then to what is most reversible with an RN-implementable action.

"Debrief" immediately after each set. This is where you learn. Do not only read why an answer is correct; articulate the answer decision in CJMM steps. Ask yourself: What cues did I recognize? Which did I miss? How did I interpret trends or patterns? Which hypothesis did I prioritize and why? Which safer alternatives did I eliminate? What action did I plan and take, and how would I evaluate it? Document the priority rule you used (for example, airway first; do-not-harm; scope of practice). If you were right, explain why alternatives were less safe. If wrong, label the reason for the miss: content gap, misread cue, framework misuse, or priority error.

"Distill" the rationale you just processed into a short, if→then clinical rule. For example: "If a fresh tracheostomy client has sudden coughing with stridor and low SpO2, then suspect tube displacement and assess airway patency first—prepare to insert a new trach tube or use the obturator; do not remove ties without securing the airway." Capture contraindications and do-not-harm elements.

"Drill" by turning that rule into a flashcard and reviewing it the same day. Cards must be short, specific, and cue-triggered; long essays and trivia do not stick under time pressure.

Make every card do work in three parts: a realistic prompt, a precise action, and a framework tag. The prompt should be cue-rich, similar to a stem: "New tracheostomy with sudden coughing and inspiratory stridor; SpO2 86%—first action?" The answer states the single safest, highest-priority RN action and the reason: "Assess for tube displacement and secure the airway: call for help, use the obturator and spare trach to replace if dislodged; do not remove ties before securing airway. Rationale: airway obstruction is the immediate life threat." Tag the card with the Client Needs category (Safety and Infection Prevention and Control), the CJMM step emphasized (recognize cues → take action), and the safety rule applied (Airway/oxygenation; Do-not-harm). Keep three main card types: red-flag/first action, pharm/med-safety, and delegation/scope. For red flags, build cards around unstable vitals, bleeding, sepsis signs, neuro changes, airway compromise, chest pain, and new confusion. For pharm/med-safety, write cards that prevent harm: high-alert meds, contraindications, infusion rates, antidotes, and monitoring rules (for example, "If a client on heparin has a sudden drop in platelets, then suspect HIT, stop heparin, and notify HCP; do not give warfarin until platelets recover"). For delegation/scope, enforce RN-only tasks and safe assignments (for example, "If the client is unstable, requires initial teaching, or needs nursing judgment, then the RN retains care; LPN may reinforce teaching and perform stable procedures; UAP does standard, predictable tasks without judgment"). Avoid multi-step, multi-concept cards. One rule, one card.

Tag everything you practice. Label each question and each card by Client Needs category and CJMM step. This forces you to think like the exam: Management of Care, Safety and Infection Prevention and Control, Health Promotion and Maintenance, Psychosocial Integrity, and the Physiological Integrity subcategories. For CJMM, be explicit: Recognize cues, Analyze cues, Prioritize hypotheses, Generate solutions, Take actions, Evaluate outcomes. Also note which NGN item type you practiced (for example, case set, matrix multiple response, drag-and-drop, highlight). Maintain a simple error log with four buckets—content gap, misread cue, framework misuse, and priority error. A content gap means you never knew it (e.g., insulin onset/peak durations). A misread cue means you missed or misweighted data (e.g., ignoring a new change in mental status). A framework misuse means you applied the wrong rule (e.g., teaching before stabilizing; assessing when an immediate action is required). A priority error means you recognized the issue but ranked actions incorrectly (e.g., calling the HCP before taking a lifesaving action within your scope). Each logged miss becomes a micro-goal for the next day: five targeted questions and five new cards in that exact category and CJMM step. For example, after a priority error in Safety and Infection Prevention and Control at the Take Action step, your plan might be "Do 10 NGN case items with first-action stems; make 3 red-flag airway cards."

Anchor debriefs to NGN/CJMM thinking. Map the evidence to cues and trends, then state the hypothesis you prioritized and why. For example: hypotension, tachycardia, cool clammy skin, and decreased urine output trend toward hypovolemic shock; airway is intact; perfusion is the critical threat; first action is to position supine with legs elevated if not contraindicated and start or titrate fluids per protocol—before calling the provider—then reassess MAP and urine output. Explicitly justify why other options are unsafe or lower priority. Plan and anticipate next actions: what will you do if the blood pressure does not respond? What labs or diagnostics will you expect? Finally, evaluate outcomes: name the vital cues you would monitor to know whether your action worked (for example, improved mental status, urine output ≥0.5 mL/kg/hr, narrowing heart rate, rising MAP).

Practice partial credit awareness. Many NGN items reward safe thinking across multiple choices. Eliminate the unsafe options first—anything that delays life-saving action, violates scope, increases infection risk, or contradicts data. Then select all safe, indicated actions; do not withhold a safe action because you are unsure if it is the best—partial credit favors accumulating safe decisions. For sequence items, place the immediate safety action before notifications and documentation unless the stem specifies otherwise. For matrix items, let trends guide you: abnormal, new, and worsening cues point to action; stable or baseline cues point to monitoring.

Measure and adjust weekly. Review your accuracy by Client Needs category and CJMM step. If any area falls below roughly 65–70% correct, increase practice volume there and expand your card deck with more specific rules. Shift about 70–80% of your study time toward practice and debriefs and keep reading to the minimum needed to fix a defined gap. Replace aimless content review with targeted card creation. Your goal is not to know everything; it is to reliably recognize danger, act within RN scope, and avoid harm across systems.

Protect a safety mindset in every answer set. When uncertain, default to airway/oxygenation, perfusion, and mental status. Decide quickly whether the client is stable or unstable; unstable clients belong to the RN and require immediate assessment or action, not delegation. Apply do-not-harm rules: verify allergies and identifiers; check compatibilities and infusion rates; anticipate adverse effects; withhold what is unsafe and notify when needed. Keep scope of practice clear: the RN performs initial teaching, assessment, triage, care planning, and clinical judgment; LPNs reinforce teaching and perform focused assessments and stable procedures; UAPs perform standard tasks that do not require clinical judgment. Maintain infection control at all times—hand hygiene, correct isolation precautions, sterile technique for invasive lines, and never reuse single-dose vials. In ambiguous items, choose the action you, as the RN in the room, can implement immediately and safely to prevent deterioration.

Put this workflow into motion on day one. Sit for a timed mixed set. Debrief in CJMM terms. Distill each rationale into an if→then rule. Create three concise cards from your misses and review them before the day ends. Tag and log everything. Repeat tomorrow. By stacking hundreds of small, safe decisions—each tied to cues, priorities, and outcomes—you build the judgment the NCLEX-RN expects and your patients will rely on.

1.2 NCLEX in One Page (Client Needs, NGN/CJMM, Item Types)

At its core, the NCLEX-RN measures whether you can provide safe, entry-level nursing care using sound clinical judgment in real-world scenarios. Every question is ultimately about safety, risk reduction, and applying evidence-based decisions that protect clients and improve outcomes.

The blueprint that drives every exam form is organized by Client Needs. Keep these ranges in mind as you study and as you practice answering questions; they reflect what the exam emphasizes and they sum to 100%, with content integrated across settings, ages, and cultures:

- Safe and Effective Care Environment
    - Management of Care: 15–21%
    - Safety and Infection Prevention and Control: 10–16%
- Health Promotion and Maintenance: 6–12%
- Psychosocial Integrity: 6–12%
- Physiological Integrity
    - Basic Care and Comfort: 6–12%
    - Pharmacological and Parenteral Therapies: 13–19%

    - Reduction of Risk Potential: 9–15%
    - Physiological Adaptation: 11–17%

Next Generation NCLEX (NGN) brings the Clinical Judgment Measurement Model (CJMM) directly into how items are written and scored. Instead of isolated facts, you'll see unfolding scenarios that mirror shift-to-shift thinking. The exam often presents a case, then asks a sequence of linked questions that track the way a nurse reasons at the bedside. Many of these award partial credit, so demonstrating some—though not all—of the correct reasoning can still earn points.

The **CJMM breaks clinical judgment into six skills** that you will use repeatedly as you work through cases. In practical terms, you'll be asked to pick out what matters, figure out what it means, decide what to do, and judge whether it worked:

- **Recognize cues:** Identify relevant findings from patient data.
- **Analyze cues**: Connect those cues to likely problems and risks.
- **Prioritize hypotheses:** Decide what is most urgent or most likely.
- **Generate solutions:** Select safe, evidence-based options.
- **Take action:** Implement the priority intervention(s).
- **Evaluate outcomes:** Determine response and escalate or modify as needed.

Expect multiple case studies built from linked items that progress through these steps, and also expect standalone NGN-enhanced items mixed throughout the exam. In both formats, information may update or expand as you proceed, requiring you to adjust your thinking just as you would in practice.

Scoring on NGN reflects how well you navigate that judgment process. Many NGN items are scored with partial credit, so you can earn points for correct selections even if you do not answer perfectly. Scoring rules vary by item type; some reduce credit when you add incorrect selections to correct ones, and others award points only for critical choices. Your goal is to be accurate and safe; speed does not improve your score, and there is no advantage to guessing hastily.

The one-page takeaway is straightforward: know the Client Needs blueprint, think through each case using the CJMM steps, and be ready for case-based items that often award partial credit. Every selection you make should reflect prioritized, safe nursing judgment aligned to the blueprint's emphasis on outcomes and risk reduction.

1.3 CAT in Practice & Test-Day Checklist

Think of the NCLEX-RN's Computerized Adaptive Testing (CAT) as an exam that is constantly measuring, not counting. Every answer helps the system update an estimate of your nursing ability against a single passing standard. You don't need to "game" the system; you need to give the safest, most defensible answer to the item in front of you, consistently, within time. That's it.

What CAT is doing: The algorithm continuously estimates your ability after each response and selects the next item to maximize information about that ability relative to the passing standard. If you're well above the standard, it tends to serve harder items; if below, it tends to serve easier ones—because those are most informative for determining where you sit.

What you will notice: Item difficulty will feel uneven—that's normal. You cannot go back to change answers. **Next-Generation NCLEX (NGN)** case sets will appear as grouped items tied to the same scenario. Some items are unscored pretest items—you cannot tell which ones, so treat each as real. Partial-credit scoring is used on many NGN items (you can earn some points even if not all parts are correct).

Pass/fail rules, simplified:

- **95% confidence rule:** The exam ends as soon as the system is at least 95% confident your true ability is above (pass) or below (fail) the passing standard.
- **Maximum-length rule:** If you hit the maximum number of items, the decision is made using your final ability estimate relative to the standard (above = pass, below = fail).
- **Run-out-of-time rule:** If time expires before a decision and you've answered fewer than the minimum items, it's an automatic fail. If you've answered at least the minimum, the decision uses how your ability estimates behaved near the end; simplified for you: do not run out of time—keep steady pacing so the exam can make a clean decision.
- **Finishing at minimum or maximum by itself does not indicate pass or fail.** Many passing exams stop early; many failing exams also stop early. Likewise, some pass at maximum length; some fail at maximum. Don't "read the test."
- **Practical behaviors:** Answer each item independently. Avoid trying to interpret item difficulty as a signal of performance. Manage time deliberately. Apply safety-first priorities (airway, breathing, circulation; safety; stable vs. unstable) and run a quick clinical judgment loop on every item: recognize key cues, analyze, prioritize, act, and evaluate the safest option.

Now, anchor all of that to a concrete test-day plan. This checklist is intentionally short so you can actually use it.

Before you go

- Confirm your Authorization to Test and your exact appointment time. If you have approved accommodations, ensure they are tied to this appointment and appear in your confirmation.
- Know the test center's location, parking, and transit options. Build in extra time for traffic and unexpected delays.
- Verify acceptable government-issued ID with a name that exactly matches your registration (no nicknames, check middle initials). Bring the physical ID; photos of ID are not accepted.
- Plan sleep and meals across the 24 hours before the exam. Aim for a steady schedule and a familiar breakfast. Do not experiment with new medications, supplements, or energy drinks.
- Dress in simple, comfortable layers you can easily adjust for room temperature. Avoid bulky jewelry, hats, and devices you'll have to remove. If you normally wear glasses, bring them; if you use contacts, consider bringing spare lenses or glasses in your locker kit.

What to bring and do at the test center

- Bring your valid government ID. Arrive at least 30 minutes early to complete check-in without stress.
- Bring any needed medications, a small snack, and water for your locker. You cannot access food or drink at the computer; you can at breaks.
- Expect security: ID check, photo, signature, palm vein scan, metal detection, and a visual inspection of pockets. You must store your phone, smartwatch, and personal items in your locker. Turn your phone completely off before locking it up.
- Listen carefully to proctor instructions. Ask questions now if something is unclear.

Timing and breaks

- You have up to 5 hours total for the exam, which includes the tutorial, two scheduled optional breaks, and any unscheduled breaks. The clock does not stop for unscheduled breaks.
- Scheduled breaks occur around the 2-hour and 3.5-hour marks. You can take them, shorten them, or skip them. Use breaks strategically to refresh, fuel, and reset.
- Unscheduled breaks are allowed; raise your hand for the proctor. The clock runs—use them only if you must.

Pacing guide

- Aim for an average of about 2 minutes per item if you're trending toward a longer exam. Most items should be answered in 60–120 seconds; NGN case items may take longer but keep the overall average.
- Avoid spending more than about 3 minutes on any single item. If you're stuck after eliminating unsafe or wrong options, choose the best safe answer and move on. Protect yourself against a timeout.
- Glance at the on-screen timer every 10–15 items. If you're behind, gently speed up by tightening reading and focusing on safety cues. If you're ahead, maintain your rhythm—don't overthink.

In-exam conduct

- Read the stem before the answer options, and identify the client type (adult/peds/OB/psych), setting, and the safety-critical cues. For NGN case sets, skim the case quickly, then pull the actionable cues for the current item.
- Apply safety-first thinking: airway and breathing before circulation, unstable before stable, acute before chronic, new-onset before long-standing, systemic before local, and actual risk before potential risk when the situation clearly demands it.
- Eliminate options that are unsafe, violate scope or policy, delay care for unstable clients, or add unnecessary risk. Beware of absolute language that ignores assessment or safety checks.
- Commit to your first well-reasoned answer. Do not backtrack mentally or try to "correct" the algorithm. You cannot change a response once submitted.
- Ignore perceived swings in difficulty. Hard-feeling items do not mean you are failing; easy-feeling items do not mean you are passing. Keep executing the same process.

If something goes wrong

- Raise your hand immediately. The proctor will assist with technical issues (frozen screen, mouse or headphone problems), environmental problems (noise, temperature), or health concerns (illness, urgent bathroom needs before a scheduled break).
- Do not attempt to troubleshoot devices or software yourself. Document the issue with the proctor for proper resolution.

Health and comfort strategy

- At breaks, take a few deep, slow breaths, walk briefly, sip water, and eat a light snack if helpful. Keep it simple—familiar foods that won't spike or crash your energy.
- Avoid heavy caffeine loading. Moderate caffeine is fine if it's part of your usual routine. Excess can worsen anxiety and urgency.
- Use a one-breath reset at the start of each item: exhale fully, inhale quietly through the nose, and on the exhale remind yourself, "Safety first, one question at a time."

After you finish

- You will see a brief survey at the end of your exam; complete it and finish check-out procedures. Do not discuss exam content with others afterward.
- Official results are posted by your nursing regulatory body according to their timeline. If your jurisdiction offers Quick Results via Pearson VUE, those are typically available in about 48 hours for a fee and are unofficial. The only official result is from your board of nursing.

This section's goal is a calm, repeatable execution: answer the item in front of you safely and efficiently, regardless of how it feels. The CAT will do its job. You do yours.

See Appendix: Printable Test-Day Checklist for an expanded, step-by-step version you can print, annotate, and bring to your final review.

1.4 CJMM in Action: The Six Skills With One Running Case

Clinical Judgment on the NCLEX is about turning scattered data into safe, prioritized actions that protect life and prevent deterioration. Here's how to do it the way the exam expects, using one concise, unfolding med–surg case and the six NGN Clinical Judgment Measurement Model (CJMM) skills.

A 68-year-old with COPD is admitted for pneumonia. At shift start you find: SpO2 86% on room air, RR 28/min, HR 118/min, BP 92/54 mm Hg, temperature 38.6°C, new confusion, urine output 20 mL/hr. Lungs have crackles with a productive cough. Labs show WBC 18,000/mm^3 and lactate 3.1 mmol/L.

Begin by thinking in terms of the six skills.

First, recognize cues. Pull out what is immediately dangerous and what might be expected for COPD. The red flags here are clear: hypoxemia (SpO2 86% on room air), hypotension (92/54), tachycardia (118), tachypnea (28), acute change in mental status (new confusion), and oliguria (20 mL/hr). These are not "usual COPD" findings; they signal impaired oxygenation and systemic hypoperfusion. In COPD, chronically low oxygenation is common, but the safe target is typically 88–92% rather than mid-90s. Fever 38.6°C and WBC 18k fit an infectious process; elevated lactate (3.1) suggests tissue hypoperfusion from sepsis. Productive cough and crackles are consistent with pneumonia, but the new confusion and low blood pressure are the dangerous shifts. As you recognize these cues, you also identify exactly what to assess now: mental status and orientation compared with prior baseline, work of breathing and accessory muscle use, ability to speak full sentences, use of pursed-lip breathing, skin color and temperature and capillary refill as perfusion clues, quality of cough and sputum, urine output trend and concentration, patency and location of IV access, and any recent medications already given in the ED or prior unit (antibiotics, antipyretics, bronchodilators), as well as allergies. These observations sharpen your picture before you act.

Second, analyze cues by clustering them into physiologic problems that matter for safety. One cluster points to impaired oxygenation and gas exchange: the pneumonia diagnosis, crackles, cough, tachypnea, and low SpO2. In COPD, ventilation–perfusion mismatch worsens with infection; hypoxemia increases work of breathing and can precipitate confusion. Another cluster points to possible sepsis with poor perfusion: hypotension, tachycardia, fever, leukocytosis, elevated lactate, oliguria, and altered mental status. Systemically, vasodilation and capillary leak reduce effective circulating volume and organ perfusion. This combination places the client at risk for respiratory failure and septic shock. Two high-yield anchors guide you here: COPD oxygen saturation targets are narrower—titrate to 88–92%—and any sign of end-organ hypoperfusion (confusion, low urine output, lactate elevation) demands urgent attention to circulation after the airway and breathing are addressed.

Third, prioritize hypotheses. Decide what could kill the patient first and what you must stabilize right now. Airway and breathing take priority: the client is hypoxemic, tachypneic, and confused. Circulation is close behind: the blood pressure is low enough that mean arterial pressure is borderline, and urine output is low. Using ABCs and stable–unstable thinking, this client is unstable in both breathing and circulation. This means you do not delegate the initial assessment or first interventions; you, the RN, take the lead and prepare to escalate if there is no rapid response to your first actions.

Fourth, generate solutions that are safe, targeted, and likely to be ordered, and prepare to carry them out. Your first nursing actions are noninvasive, quick, and within scope or protocols. Elevate the head of bed to ease breathing and reduce aspiration risk. Apply supplemental oxygen per protocol and titrate to reach a safe COPD target, aiming for 88–92%. If nasal cannula at low flow does not reach target, be prepared to use a Venturi mask for more precise FiO2 control in COPD. Ensure continuous pulse oximetry and frequent respiratory assessment. Verify IV access; if no reliable access is present, obtain it promptly. Initiate a sepsis screen per facility protocol given the fever, hypotension, tachycardia, lactate, and altered mental status. Anticipate and prepare for orders: draw blood cultures before antibiotics if feasible; obtain any additional labs (repeat lactate, BMP) without delay; start broad-spectrum IV antibiotics as soon as they are available; begin isotonic fluids (normal saline or lactated Ringer's) for hypotension if ordered; consider Foley catheter insertion for strict intake and output if ordered. Place fall and aspiration precautions due to confusion and respiratory compromise. Check and verify allergies before administering any new medications, particularly antibiotics. Notify the provider promptly using SBAR with the critical data you have gathered and your immediate interventions and response. This plan touches all three key Client Needs categories: Physiological Integrity (stabilize oxygenation and perfusion), Safe and Effective Care Environment (precautions, delegation limits), and Pharmacological and Parenteral Therapies (oxygen titration, IV fluids, antibiotics, cultures).

Fifth, take action in the right sequence and at the right pace, knowing what you can do now and what needs an order. Immediately raise the head of the bed and apply oxygen per standing order or protocol, starting at a low flow and titrating while watching the saturation and the patient's work of breathing. In COPD you avoid indiscriminate high FiO2; however, you must correct dangerous hypoxemia. Check the effect within a minute or two and adjust; if saturation remains below 88% on nasal cannula or the work of breathing is high, move to a Venturi mask that allows precise FiO2 control. Simultaneously, connect the client to cardiac and blood pressure monitoring if available and reassess mental status. Confirm IV patency and gauge size; if inadequate for fluids and antibiotics, obtain a second peripheral line. Initiate the sepsis screen and draw blood cultures if this is within your protocol or you have the order; if antibiotics have arrived before cultures, you still prioritize giving the first dose promptly and problem-solve to draw cultures from a second site without delaying therapy. Start a crystalloid bolus when the order is received; monitor blood pressure and urine output as you infuse. Institute strict intake and output now by measuring urine; if a Foley is ordered for oliguria in sepsis, insert using sterile technique. Provide fall and aspiration precautions: bed alarm, assist with ambulation, keep suction available, and keep NPO if mental status is impaired and aspiration risk is high until a swallow screen is passed. Deliver an SBAR to the provider with the initial findings, your oxygen titration and response, IV access status, sepsis screen results, and need for antibiotics and fluids. Know when to activate a rapid response: do so for persistent hypoxemia despite oxygen, increasing work of breathing, worsening confusion, or persistent hypotension (mean arterial pressure less than 65) despite fluids, or if you have a gut sense that the patient is failing to respond to initial measures.

Sixth, evaluate outcomes with specific metrics and an immediate timeframe. Within minutes of oxygen application and positioning, you expect SpO2 to reach 88–92% and respiratory rate to trend down toward less than 24. Within the first hour after fluid resuscitation begins, you aim for a mean arterial pressure at or above 65, heart rate trending downward, and mental status improving. Urine output should be monitored hourly, with a target of at least 30 mL/hr; persistently low output suggests ongoing hypoperfusion and the need to escalate care. If the client is not meeting these targets, reassess breath sounds, effort, and oxygen delivery device; obtain arterial blood gases if ordered to quantify oxygenation and ventilation; check for signs of fluid overload in COPD (worsening crackles, hypoxemia that does not improve, increased work of breathing) that might indicate the need to adjust fluids and consider vasopressors if ordered. Anticipate complications: acute hypoxic respiratory failure requiring noninvasive ventilation, septic shock requiring vasopressors, acute kidney injury with worsening oliguria, and delirium. Report trends rather than single numbers: for example, "SpO2 remains 86–87% on 4 L nasal cannula with increased accessory muscle use" or "MAP is 60 after 1 L of fluids and urine output remains 15 mL/hr."

Transfer this process to any scenario by habitually cycling through the six steps: identify the few cues that change safety, cluster them to understand pathophysiology, prioritize what threatens life now, generate targeted, protocol-aligned options, act in sequence within your scope, and evaluate against concrete, time-based goals. Keep ABCs and stable–unstable at the center, and read trends, not single numbers.

1.5 Priority Frameworks Inside CJMM (ABCs, Safety, Stable/Unstable)

Your NCLEX priority is to convert cues into the safest first action using the Clinical Judgment Measurement Model. Think like this: recognize cues, analyze them for threat, prioritize hypotheses (what could kill or harm first), generate solutions that actually remove that threat, take action without delay when appropriate, and evaluate response. The point of frameworks is not to memorize rules in isolation, but to integrate them so that the first action you select is the one that prevents injury and preserves life.

Start with ABCs every time. Airway comes before breathing, which comes before circulation, except during CPR where compressions come first (CAB). On the exam, an oxygen therapy or airway maneuver usually beats "call the provider" because the nurse's immediate action stabilizes the patient and buys time. If ongoing harm is occurring, stop it before assessing further: stop a transfusion in a reaction, stop an infusion that's extravasating, stop a seizure-inducing light stimulus. These are CJMM "take action" moments that do not require additional data because the cue already signals active harm.

Next layer in safety, risk reduction, and infection prevention. Actual problems outrank potential ones. Unexpected changes outrank expected or baseline complaints. New or worsening symptoms outrank unchanged chronic symptoms. Time-sensitive threats rise to the top: anaphylaxis, hypoglycemia with altered mental status, sepsis, stroke, myocardial infarction, postpartum hemorrhage, airway edema after neck surgery. Isolation and source control must occur promptly when indicated—mask a neutropenic patient with fever before moving through a crowded unit, initiate appropriate precautions for airborne pathogens at first suspicion, not after confirmatory testing.

Decide who is unstable. Instability cues include acute change in level of consciousness, airway compromise or stridor, extreme respiratory rates or effort, oxygen saturation below 90% despite oxygen, a suddenly silent chest in asthma, hypotension or MAP under 65 mm Hg, chest pain at rest with hemodynamic compromise, active bleeding (including postpartum hemorrhage), signs of sepsis (fever, tachycardia, hypotension, altered perfusion), uncontrolled labor or late fetal heart rate decelerations, fever in a neonate, and severe electrolyte or ABG derangements such as potassium over 6.0 mEq/L with ECG changes or pH less than 7.25 with rising CO2. These cues demand immediate stabilization before paperwork, calls, or teaching.

After ABC and immediate safety, use least restrictive, least invasive, most effective, and fastest-to-implement to choose among safe options. For example, repositioning and applying oxygen are less invasive and faster than calling for an arterial blood gas; a sitter is less restrictive than restraints; oral glucose is safer and faster than starting an IV in a conscious hypoglycemic patient. Choose the option that achieves the physiologic result quickly without needless invasiveness.

Use the assess-versus-implement rule correctly. If you truly lack data to decide among safe paths, assess first. If there is a life-threatening cue or an intervention that clearly stops ongoing harm and does not delay definitive care, implement immediately. You do not auscultate longer while a patient is cyanotic and apneic—you start ventilation. You do not wait for lab confirmation to begin sepsis bundle steps in a hypotensive, febrile, tachycardic patient—you initiate fluids and cultures per protocol. This is how CJMM prioritizes hypotheses and moves decisively to action.

Keep temporal context clear: acute before chronic, immediate postoperative before stable chronic, new admissions with unstable cues before discharge teaching that can safely occur later. That means a day-one post-op with tachycardia and low urine output beats a stable COPD patient requesting a nicotine patch; a newly febrile neutropenic oncology patient beats routine medications for a stable diabetic; a new chest pain with hypotension beats scheduled PT.

Use this mini priority algorithm on every question:

- Scan for ABC threats.
- Identify instability and severity (actual vs potential, new/worsening, unexpected, time-sensitive).
- Choose the action that removes immediate danger first (least invasive, most effective, fastest).
- Then assess to refine and complete the picture.
- Notify/escalate after initial stabilization or when orders are required for definitive care.
- Evaluate the response and adjust; escalate further if no improvement.

In NGN case sets, you will group cues, create hypotheses, and then prioritize which hypothesis is most dangerous now. For "select the first action" items, pick the single intervention that stabilizes ABCs or stops harm. For "rank actions," put urgent stabilizing steps before assessments that do not change immediate management and before consults or teaching. For matrix/grid items, mark all safety steps that are appropriate now and avoid those that delay stabilization. Watch for traps: prioritizing pain medication over airway or perfusion threats; calling the provider before a nursing safety intervention (apply oxygen, stop the infusion, raise head of bed); ordering labs or tests before stabilizing; choosing invasive actions when a less invasive, effective step is available; documenting or teaching when the patient is unstable.

Use quick mental rehearsal with micro-cues:

- Post-thyroidectomy hoarseness/stridor → prioritize airway; prepare for airway support and notify anesthesia.
- Asthma with wheeze becoming silent → immediate bronchodilator and airway support; call RRT if no response.
- Post-op with SpO2 86% on room air → apply oxygen, reposition, assess breath sounds; then notify if persistent.
- Chest pain + diaphoresis + hypotension → support circulation (O2, IV access, prepare for ECG after stabilization); anticipate MONA per protocol while monitoring BP.
- Urticaria/itching during transfusion → stop transfusion, keep IV with normal saline, assess, then notify provider and send blood back per policy.
- Febrile neutropenia → mask the patient, obtain cultures per protocol, initiate broad-spectrum antibiotics rapidly; place in protective/neutropenic precautions.

Know what not to pick in a priority item. Avoid broad discharge teaching, routine documentation, non-urgent consults and referrals, and reassessments that merely delay life-saving care. Do not choose "notify provider" before you take an immediate nursing safety step that is within RN scope and clearly required to prevent harm. Do not jump to invasive actions when a safer, less invasive intervention would be effective. Do not perform tasks out of sequence, such as drawing lab tests before applying oxygen in hypoxemia or sending a patient to radiology before stabilizing blood pressure.

Finally, always evaluate outcomes. After any intervention, trend vital signs, reassess the primary cues, and look for objective improvement: rising SpO2, eased work of breathing, improved mental status, stabilized blood pressure, reduced bleeding, improved fetal patterns. If the patient does not improve or deteriorates, escalate rapidly—activate the rapid response team, prepare for advanced interventions, and communicate succinctly using SBAR. Anticipate the next best action based on response: if oxygen and positioning fail, consider advanced airway; if fluids fail in sepsis, prepare vasopressors with appropriate access; if chest pain persists, expedite ECG and cardiac interventions. This close-the-loop step is not an afterthought in CJMM—it confirms that your priority choice was effective and guides the next safe move.

CHAPTER 2

Client Needs I — Safe & Effective Care Environment

2.1 Management of Care (Delegation & Prioritization, Legal/Ethical)

Registered nurses coordinate care to prevent harm by allocating resources, setting priorities, and upholding legal and ethical standards. This work is fundamentally cue-based. You will see, assess, and act on stability, predictability, and time-sensitivity—then close the loop by supervising, evaluating, and escalating as needed. That is the Clinical Judgment Measurement Model (CJMM) applied to Management of Care: recognize cues, analyze and prioritize, generate solutions, take action, and evaluate outcomes.

Begin every shift by scanning for cues: which clients are unstable or at risk of becoming unstable; which conditions are predictable versus unexpected; which problems are time-sensitive (airway, perfusion, neurologic compromise, sepsis, hemorrhage). Those cues guide who you should see first, what to delegate, how to assign, and when to escalate. Closed-loop evaluation—returning to the bedside, confirming understanding with team members, read-backs, and reassessment after interventions—keeps clients safe.

A recurring NCLEX distinction is assignment versus delegation versus supervision. An assignment is the distribution of work appropriate to a team member's role and legal scope (for example, assigning a stable post-op client to an LPN, or routine vitals to a UAP). Delegation is transferring a specific task and its performance to a competent person while retaining accountability for the outcome. The RN must verify that the task, person, circumstance, direction/communication, and supervision/evaluation are appropriate. Supervision is the active process of guiding, monitoring, and evaluating the delegate's performance and client outcomes, and intervening as needed. The RN is accountable for the decision to delegate, for assuring appropriate follow-up, and for overall client outcomes; the delegate is responsible for performing the accepted task correctly.

Reasonable assignment hinges on scope and stability. When floating to unfamiliar units, accept clients whose needs match your validated competencies and ask for orientation to unit-specific equipment or protocols. If the assignment appears unsafe—too many high-acuity clients, lack of needed orientation, tasks outside your scope—clarify with the charge nurse, suggest safer alternatives grounded in client safety, and, if unresolved, use the chain of command. Continuity of care matters: keeping the same nurse for complex clients reduces errors; when handing off care, use standardized communication and ensure "who is doing what by when" is clear.

Delegation is governed by five rights: right task, right circumstance, right person, right direction/communication, and right supervision/evaluation. Right task means it is routine, carries minimal risk, and is within the delegate's scope and competency. Right circumstance means the client is stable and the environment supports safe completion. Right person means the individual has demonstrated competence for that task. Right direction/communication requires clear, specific instructions (what, when, parameters for reporting, expected outcomes). Right supervision/evaluation requires follow-up, availability to answer questions, and assessment of the result. Non-delegable RN functions include comprehensive assessment, clinical judgment and care planning, initial teaching and education that requires evaluation of learning, and evaluation of outcomes. Any unstable client, unpredictable response, or task requiring nursing judgment remains with the RN.

Prioritization follows a safety-first logic. Airway comes before breathing, breathing before circulation; life before limb; safety risks before comfort. Unstable trumps stable, acute before chronic, systemic issues before local issues, unexpected findings before expected baseline, and time-critical needs before routine care. For example, a new onset shortness of breath with low oxygen saturation is higher priority than dressing a stable wound. The nursing process helps select the first action: assess before intervene when the picture is unclear, unless immediate life-saving action is obviously required. If you must choose between gathering data that changes immediate decisions (such as checking a pulse, listening to lung sounds, rechecking a critical lab) and doing tasks that can wait, prioritize the assessment that will inform safe action.

Disaster and triage principles assume limited resources. In mass casualty incidents, tags generally follow: red for immediate life-threatening but salvageable, yellow for delayed/major but not immediately life-threatening, green for minor, and black for deceased/unsalvageable. Triage aims for the greatest good for the greatest number; someone with minimal resource needs and high chance of survival may receive priority over someone requiring disproportionate resources with low survival probability. In routine unit-level triage—such as two call lights at once—apply the same logic: threat to life, time sensitivity, and potential to deteriorate dictate your order of response.

Team communication underpins safe coordination. Use SBAR (Situation, Background, Assessment, Recommendation) for handoffs and provider calls to keep messages concise and complete. Ensure read-back of critical values, verbal orders, and high-risk directions to prevent miscommunication. Give instructions in closed loop: state the task, require a repeat-back, and verify completion with outcomes reported back (for example, "Please recheck the blood pressure in five minutes and report if systolic is below 90" followed by "BP now 88/54" prompts immediate RN reassessment). When you encounter unsafe orders or a client who continues to deteriorate despite interventions, escalate using the chain of command: notify the provider, then charge nurse, then house supervisor or rapid response as indicated. Anticipate and initiate interprofessional consults: respiratory therapy for oxygen delivery optimization or weaning, physical/occupational therapy for mobility and ADL planning, social work and case management for discharge barriers, financial/medication access, or abuse concerns. Clear role definition, early consults, and timely documentation reduce delays and near misses.

Legal foundations govern many NCLEX decisions. Informed consent requires that the provider explains the nature, risks, benefits, and alternatives of a procedure; the RN's role is to witness the voluntary signature, verify identity, assess understanding, and clarify using teach-back—without introducing new risks/benefits or coercion—and to notify the provider if the client has questions or lacks understanding. Use a qualified medical interpreter for language barriers; family should not interpret. Capacity is a clinical determination that a person can understand, appreciate consequences, and communicate a choice for a specific decision at a specific time; competence is a legal status determined by a court. If a client lacks capacity and there is no advance directive, follow the legal hierarchy for surrogate decision-makers per state law. Respect advance directives, including durable power of attorney for health care and DNR/AND orders, and clarify ambiguities before procedures.

Clients have the right to refuse treatment and to leave against medical advice if they have capacity; your role is to assess capacity, inform about risks and alternatives, try to address concerns, and document the discussion objectively. If the client lacks capacity and leaving creates imminent danger, follow your facility's policies and legal pathways for holding. The Emergency Medical Treatment and Labor Act (EMTALA) requires EDs to provide a medical screening exam and stabilizing treatment for anyone seeking care, regardless of ability to pay, and restricts inappropriate transfers. Protect privacy under HIPAA by sharing the minimum necessary information with those involved in care, securing records, and obtaining proper authorization for disclosures beyond treatment, payment, and operations. When errors or near misses occur, complete an internal incident report promptly and factually for quality improvement; do not document "incident report filed" in the medical record. Instead, chart the objective facts, assessments, notifications, and client response.

Ethical principles guide choices when rules are insufficient. Autonomy respects the client's right to make informed choices; beneficence promotes good; nonmaleficence avoids harm; justice promotes fairness; fidelity keeps commitments; veracity tells the truth. When ethical tension arises—such as a family request conflicting with a competent client's wishes—clarify values and facts, advocate for the client, seek interprofessional input, and escalate early to the chain of command or ethics consultation. Moral distress is a signal to use formal resources rather than silently acquiescing to unsafe or unethical care.

Quality and safety systems support your clinical judgment. Sentinel events—unexpected events causing death or serious harm—require immediate action, reporting, and root cause analysis focused on processes, not individual blame. Near misses deserve reporting because they reveal system vulnerabilities. Apply a root cause mindset at the bedside: ask what barriers, handoff gaps, equipment, or policy issues contributed, and suggest fixes. Use high-alert safeguards consistently: independent double checks for medications such as insulin, heparin, chemotherapy, and high-dose opioids; standardized concentrations; smart pump libraries; bar code scanning; and clear labeling. Advocate for safe staffing by reporting surges in acuity or unsafe ratios to leadership and documenting objective workload changes; suggest strategies like redistribution, closing admissions temporarily, or calling in additional staff. When resource limits persist and risk remains, escalate.

Coordination extends into community and telehealth settings. In virtual care, protect privacy by confirming identity, using secure platforms, ensuring the client's environment permits private discussion, and verifying contact information for emergencies. The same five rights of delegation apply in home health, but scope varies by state and agency; the RN remains responsible for assessment, care planning, and evaluation, and must ensure adequate supervision and that the client setting supports safe task performance. Resource navigation is part of harm prevention: connect clients with community services for transportation, food, housing, and medication affordability; involve case management early to reduce readmissions. Teach clients how to recognize red flags and when to seek in-person care.

On NGN-style items, let cue-based stability and predictability drive your choices. When the scenario is unclear, choose options that further assess in a way that affects immediate decisions—recheck vitals, assess respiratory effort, review latest labs—before acting, unless there is an obvious life-threatening problem. Prefer actions that maintain safety, scope, and legal/ethical integrity: delegate appropriately and specifically, supervise and reevaluate, use SBAR, read back critical information, obtain needed consent, protect privacy, and escalate early if risks persist. When choosing between equally reasonable tasks, select the one that addresses the greatest risk of harm in the shortest time frame and includes a plan to evaluate the effect.

In summary, Management of Care on the NCLEX expects you to integrate clinical judgment with team leadership. Recognize instability and unpredictability; assign and delegate within scope using the five rights; prioritize with ABCs and risk-based frameworks; communicate clearly with SBAR and closed loop; uphold consent, privacy, and refusal rights; act ethically; engage quality systems; and adapt these principles to every setting. Safety is the throughline, and evaluation is the final step—because care is not complete until you verify the client is safer than before.

2.1.1 Delegation Rules (RN/LPN/UAP) With Quick Scenarios

Delegation on the NCLEX-RN is really a clinical judgment question in disguise. You will be given cues about stability, predictability, and risk of harm, and then asked to decide who should do what, how you will communicate, and how you will supervise. The test rewards safe, role-appropriate delegation that follows the nursing process and the Five Rights of Delegation. Think like the RN who keeps the big picture, assigns the right task, and remains accountable for outcomes.

Start with the core: the Five Rights of Delegation are the right task, right circumstances, right person, right direction/communication, and right supervision/evaluation. These are not just checkboxes; they frame how you match a task to the situation and to the delegate's scope, then give clear instructions and follow up. Never delegate the nursing process. That means the initial assessment, nursing diagnosis and care planning, initial teaching, clinical judgment/decision-making, and evaluation of outcomes stay with the RN. Use the NCSBN criteria as your mental rubric: is the client's outcome predictable, what is the potential for harm, how complex is the task, will it require problem solving or innovation, and what level of therapeutic interaction is involved? Finally, remember accountability: the RN retains accountability for the overall care and the decision to delegate; the delegatee is responsible for performing the task safely within their scope and reporting as instructed.

Scope matters, and NCLEX expects you to know each role's lane. The RN performs all assessments that are initial, on unstable clients, or when there is a change in status; formulates the care plan; triages and prioritizes; makes clinical judgments; administers high-alert medications, IV pushes, titrated drips, chemotherapy; initiates and monitors blood transfusions; manages central lines; and provides comprehensive patient education including discharge teaching. The LPN/VN can collect focused, ongoing data on stable clients and report to the RN; reinforce teaching that has already been initiated by the RN; administer most routine medications except high-risk, chemo, and IV push; perform sterile procedures and technical skills for stable clients such as wound care and catheter insertion; provide ostomy care; perform tracheostomy care and suctioning on stable clients; monitor IV sites, verify flow rates, and report issues but not independently titrate drips; and monitor and report changes promptly. The UAP supports with activities of daily living, hygiene, routine feeding of low-risk clients, standard positioning and ambulation, obtaining routine vital signs and intake/output on stable clients, collecting nonsterile specimens including capillary glucose, performing range-of-motion exercises, postmortem care, and transporting clients. UAPs do not assess, teach, evaluate, or administer medications.

On test day, safe delegation is as much about how you communicate and supervise as it is about who gets the task. Write answers that show you give clear, specific instructions about what to do, when to do it, and exactly what to report, including thresholds that trigger a call to you. Ask for a read-back to confirm understanding, set a time for you to check back, and then actually evaluate the outcome. If the client's status changes or the delegate reports a concerning finding, you intervene and reassess—don't tell them to "keep monitoring."

A few fast heuristics sharpen your choices. Do not delegate care of a new admission, the immediate postoperative assessment, or any client with newly unstable signs, rapidly changing vital signs, or acute changes in neuro, cardiac, or respiratory status. Do not delegate first-time or comprehensive teaching, blood products, IV push medications, titrated drips, chemotherapy, or complex psychosocial care. Delegate to a UAP only when the client is stable, the task is routine and noninvasive, the outcome is predictable, and no assessment or teaching is needed. LPNs are your go-to for stable clients with expected outcomes when the task is technical or involves reinforcement rather than initial judgment or evaluation.

Use scenarios to practice the cue-to-decision chain. For each, ask: Who is the client? What is the risk? Is the outcome predictable? Does the task require nursing judgment, teaching, or evaluation?

1. New admission with pneumonia needs an initial assessment and oxygen started → RN. Rationale: initial assessment and titration of therapy require RN clinical judgment.
2. Stable post-op day 2 hip arthroplasty needs drain output measured and a dressing change with no signs of infection → LPN. Rationale: sterile dressing care and routine monitoring on a stable client fit LPN technical scope.
3. First ambulation 4 hours after surgery with an epidural discontinued 1 hour ago → RN. Rationale: high risk for hypotension and instability during first mobilization demands RN assessment and readiness to intervene.
4. Chronic stroke patient, stable, needs morning hygiene and transfer using an established gait belt plan → UAP. Rationale: predictable ADL with a set safety plan is appropriate for UAP.
5. Type 2 diabetes client needs insulin titration teaching for a new basal-bolus regimen → RN. Rationale: initial teaching and individualized dose adjustment require RN judgment.
6. Client receiving a blood transfusion during the first 15 minutes → RN. Rationale: initiation and early monitoring for transfusion reaction must be performed by the RN.
7. COPD client is stable and needs oral medications and tracheostomy care per established routine → LPN. Rationale: routine med administration and trach care on a stable client are within LPN scope.
8. Client reports new chest pain rated 8/10 → RN. Rationale: acute, unstable cue requires RN assessment and immediate intervention.

9. New mother requires demonstration of newborn bathing and safe sleep for discharge → RN. Rationale: comprehensive discharge teaching and skill demonstration are RN responsibilities.
10. Psychiatric unit: stable client needs daily weight and meal setup → UAP. Rationale: routine measurement and ADL support for a stable client are appropriate; UAP reports intake/weight changes to licensed staff.

Be alert to common NCLEX traps. The word "reinforce" is deliberate; LPNs can reinforce teaching that is already established by the RN but cannot initiate new teaching or change the plan. "Monitor and report" is not "assess and interpret." UAPs can measure vital signs or blood glucose and report numbers, but only licensed nurses interpret those findings and make decisions. "Stable" is not the same as "chronic." A client with a chronic diagnosis (like COPD or heart failure) can be unstable if they have new dyspnea, altered mental status, or changing vital signs—don't let the chronic label fool you. Do not delegate evaluation, such as pain reassessment after an opioid; the RN must determine if the intervention worked and what to do next. Similarly, complex discharge planning and teaching new self-management skills belong to the RN.

When communicating delegated tasks, specify the task, timing, parameters, and what requires immediate reporting, and verify understanding. For example: "Please obtain blood pressure, heart rate, and pulse oximetry on Room 402 now and again in one hour. If systolic blood pressure is under 100 or oxygen saturation less than 92%, call me immediately. Read back the instructions." Then circle back: "I'll be back in 20 minutes to assess pain and review the vitals."

The NGN/CJMM lens ties this all together. Recognize relevant cues (e.g., new chest pain, first post-op ambulation, established plan for a stable transfer). Analyze how those cues affect stability and risk. Prioritize who needs the RN first, then generate and act on a safe plan by matching the task to the role. Finally, evaluate the outcome and adjust. The safest answer choices will highlight this chain and include clear direction and supervision.

As you practice, a brief algorithm keeps you consistent: identify cues → classify stability and risk (predictability, harm, complexity) → match task to scope using the Five Rights → communicate specifics and expected reports → supervise and evaluate outcomes.

Finish each delegation decision with a quick micro-check-in to keep it safe and test-correct:

- Is the client stable with a predictable course?
- Is the task routine and noninvasive with a low risk of harm?
- Does it avoid nursing judgment, initial teaching, and evaluation?
- What will we do if the client's condition changes?
- Have I given clear instructions, asked for read-back, and set a time to follow up?

2.1.2 Prioritization & Triage (ABCs + 6 Red-Flag Cues)

This chapter is about two decisions the NCLEX loves: who to see first and what to do first. Use the Clinical Judgment Measurement Model mindset: recognize cues, analyze stability, prioritize hypotheses, take immediate actions that prevent harm, and evaluate for response. The scope here is narrow and practical—ABCs first, a short list of red-flag cues that always jump to the front, essential ED and disaster triage rules, and the common traps that make safe questions look tricky. When every client looks important, the winner is the one with an actual or impending life threat, a highly unstable trend, or a narrow time window where a quick nursing action prevents deterioration. Leave comfort care, teaching, and routine meds for later unless all are stable and no harm occurs if they wait.

The core prioritization flow is consistent. Start with airway, then breathing, then circulation. Once any ABC threat is addressed, sort by unstable versus stable. Unstable means abnormal vital signs with poor perfusion or mental status, sudden change, or active bleeding—those clients move ahead of stable chronic complaints like longstanding shortness of breath in COPD with unchanged baseline. Next, weigh acute versus chronic; new or worsening wins over baseline. Unexpected findings outrank expected postoperative soreness or predictable pain crises. If everyone is stable, pick the task most likely to prevent deterioration or with a narrow therapeutic window—rechecking a hypoglycemic capillary glucose, starting antibiotics after obtaining cultures in suspected sepsis, performing a 12-lead ECG for new chest pain, or reassessing neuro status after a head injury. Finally, consider infection prevention and source control exposure; a suspected airborne or droplet pathogen may temporarily rise in priority to initiate isolation and prevent system-level harm.

Six red-flag cues reliably bring a client to the top, and each one has an immediate "first nurse action."

Airway threat presents with stridor, choking, facial or neck swelling, anaphylaxis, an inability to speak or complete sentences, gurgling secretions, or a suspected foreign body. Act first to open the airway and optimize patency: reposition with a head tilt–chin lift or jaw thrust if trauma is suspected, apply high-flow oxygen, and prepare to suction secretions. In anaphylaxis, give intramuscular epinephrine per protocol without delay, then add airway adjuncts, high-flow oxygen, and prepare for rapid response. This is a pure A of ABCs; nothing else takes precedence. The why: minutes of hypoxia cause irreversible injury; a quick positioning or epinephrine dose changes the trajectory instantly.

Breathing failure or hypoxia shows up as a respiratory rate less than 8 or greater than 30, oxygen saturation below 90% despite oxygen, cyanosis, accessory muscle use, a silent chest, or a somnolent patient recently given opioids. Elevate the head of the bed, deliver high-flow oxygen, assess breath sounds quickly, and be ready with bag-valve-mask ventilation while you call for help. If opioids are implicated and the patient is not protecting the airway, anticipate naloxone per protocol after oxygenation is underway. The why: inadequate ventilation or oxygenation is an immediate life threat; position and oxygen are nursing actions you do before calls and paperwork.

Circulatory collapse or uncontrolled bleeding is suggested by a systolic blood pressure below 90 or a MAP below 65, heart rate above 130, cool clammy skin, delayed capillary refill, new oliguria, or visible hemorrhage from a surgical site, postpartum, or GI source. Lie the patient flat, start or ensure two large-bore IV lines, and initiate a normal saline or lactated Ringer's bolus per protocol. If bleeding is external, apply direct pressure. Prepare blood products by sending a type and crossmatch; in massive hemorrhage settings, anticipate activation of the transfusion protocol. The why: hypotension and bleeding kill by impaired perfusion; IV access and fluids are nursing priorities you initiate immediately while help is en route.

Acute neurologic compromise often begins with sudden confusion or change in level of consciousness, new focal deficits identified by FAST (facial droop, arm weakness, speech difficulty), a seizure, unequal pupils, or a severe head injury. Protect the airway and breathing first, institute seizure precautions, and obtain a bedside glucose because hypoglycemia can mimic stroke and is immediately reversible. Document last-known-well time and notify for stroke activation and emergent CT. The why: time is brain; checking glucose and protecting ABCs are nursing actions that prevent worsening while the definitive pathway mobilizes.

Cardiac ischemia or pulmonary embolism suspicion surfaces with crushing chest pain, diaphoresis, new ST changes, dyspnea with pleuritic pain, hemoptysis, tachycardia with hypoxia, or a postoperative client with calf pain and sudden shortness of breath. Provide oxygen, place the patient upright if tolerated, obtain vital signs, and acquire a 12-lead ECG immediately; give nitroglycerin if appropriate (no hypotension, no phosphodiesterase-5 inhibitor use, no right ventricular infarct suspected). Expect to give aspirin in suspected myocardial infarction if not contraindicated and anticipate anticoagulation for pulmonary embolism after provider evaluation. The why: early oxygenation and ECG are time-sensitive and change management; nitroglycerin and aspirin reduce ischemic injury but require quick, targeted assessment.

Sepsis or extreme temperature in an unstable or immunosuppressed client is high risk. Look for a temperature above 40°C or below 35°C with hypotension or tachycardia and altered mentation; any fever in a neutropenic client; or a febrile infant under three months. Initiate the sepsis bundle: obtain blood cultures promptly, start broad-spectrum antibiotics after cultures are drawn, and deliver a fluid bolus. In neutropenia, institute reverse isolation immediately to protect the client. The why: every hour of delay in antibiotics worsens outcomes; cultures must come first, and fluids restore perfusion while treatment starts.

Emergency department acuity uses the Emergency Severity Index framework, where Level 1 means the client needs an immediate life-saving intervention such as airway management or emergent electrical therapy, and Level 2 captures those who are high risk, confused or disoriented, or in severe pain with concerning mechanism. Levels 3 to 5 are graded by expected resources. You do not need to memorize the tool; you need to think in its spirit. If a client requires airway repositioning, high-flow oxygen for impending respiratory failure, or rapid fluid resuscitation, they are effectively a one. A high-risk chest pain with concerning history but stable vitals is a two. A stable abdominal pain that will need labs and imaging lands at three. This mindset reinforces that truly life-threatening interventions come before diagnostics.

In a mass-casualty incident, START triage is simple and unforgiving for a reason. If someone is not breathing, open the airway. If they still do not breathe, tag black (expectant). If they begin to breathe, tag red (immediate). Anyone with respirations above 30 per minute, no palpable radial pulse or capillary refill greater than two seconds, or inability to follow simple commands is tagged red. The rest with injuries who are stable enough to wait are tagged yellow (delayed). Those who can walk are tagged green (minor). Do not render prolonged care; your job is to sort rapidly and move on.

When choices are close, use tie-breakers. New or worsening is always higher priority than chronic baseline. Early postoperative day complications, new bleeding, and hypotension outrank routine medications and scheduled treatments. Do not spend time assessing a noncritical system while a clear ABC threat is in front of you. Do not delay giving oxygen, elevating the head of the bed, suctioning, initiating IV access, or starting fluids while waiting for provider orders when protocols allow; NCLEX expects you to act within scope to prevent harm. Infection control can change the order briefly; suspect tuberculosis, measles, varicella, or meningococcemia? Put a mask on the patient as you move them to the correct isolation or close the door and don appropriate PPE to prevent exposure.

NGN items test the same steps you practice. Recognize cues by scanning vitals and trends for instability and the six red flags. Analyze stability versus instability. Prioritize the hypothesis that the airway is threatened before you worry about pain or labs. Generate solutions that are within nursing scope: oxygen, positioning, suction, IV access, ECG, glucose check, cultures before antibiotics, and isolation. Take the action that prevents deterioration right now. Evaluate by repeating vital signs, reassessing symptoms, and watching for response. On bow-tie or drag-and-drop sets, pair each red flag with the highest-yield first action and avoid "notify the provider" when a nursing action prevents deterioration. You can and should notify after immediate stabilization is underway.

A quick practice ranking helps solidify the flow. You are covering four clients on a surgical floor. Which do you assess first, second, third, and fourth?

Client A: Postoperative day 1 after knee arthroplasty; blood pressure 84/52, heart rate 132, cool and clammy; dressing with small serosanguinous stain.

Client B: COPD with productive cough; oxygen saturation 92% on 2 L nasal cannula; requesting albuterol.

Client C: Type 1 diabetes; capillary blood glucose 62 mg/dL; alert, drank 4 ounces of orange juice 10 minutes ago; awaiting recheck.

Client D: Chronic back pain 8/10; requesting scheduled oxycodone in 15 minutes.

The best order is A, C, B, D. Client A shows circulatory collapse—address circulation now with supine positioning, large-bore IVs, and fluid bolus per protocol while reassessing dressing and applying pressure if bleeding increases. Client C has hypoglycemia recently treated; the narrow window task is to recheck glucose promptly and give a snack or dextrose if the value remains low. Client B is stable at baseline saturation and can wait briefly. Client D has pain but is stable and has no time-sensitive risk; pain management follows once instability is addressed.

Now a START triage mini-set at the scene of a bus accident:

Victim 1 is on the ground, not breathing. You open the airway; they begin breathing at 8/min with weak effort. Tag red. Rationale: apnea relieved by airway opening equals immediate.

Victim 2 is ambulatory with superficial lacerations, speaking clearly. Tag green. Rationale: walking wounded.

Victim 3 is sitting, respirations 36/min, no radial pulse, appears anxious. Tag red. Rationale: respiratory rate above 30 and absent radial pulse indicate shock.

Victim 4 is lying down, respirations 22/min, capillary refill under two seconds, obeys commands, closed femur deformity. Tag yellow. Rationale: stable perfusion and mental status with significant injury that can be delayed.

Common pitfalls are worth calling out. Avoid the impulse to collect a full history while a patient is hypoxic or hypotensive; act first, then gather data. Do not choose "notify the provider" when a rapid nursing intervention is available that prevents harm. Do not be distracted by abnormal but expected findings, such as mild postoperative pain or chronic anemia, when new severe symptoms are present elsewhere. Be careful with medications as first actions; nitroglycerin is reasonable only when blood pressure is adequate and there is no contraindication, and insulin is not a first action when the client is NPO and risk of hypoglycemia is high. Avoid choosing teaching, comfort measures, or routine documentation during active instability. Remember exposure risk; placing a surgical mask on a coughing, febrile client with night sweats on arrival to the unit can prevent an outbreak and is a valid near-first action once ABCs are stable.

As you practice, pair each red flag with its first move and a brief rationale in your head. Airway threat equals reposition, suction, high-flow oxygen; anaphylaxis equals epinephrine now because it reverses airway swelling and hypotension. Respiratory failure equals high-flow oxygen and prepare to ventilate, because oxygen first buys time. Shock equals supine, IV access, fluids, and pressure on bleeding, because perfusion is life. Acute neuro changes equal protect airway and check glucose, because hypoglycemia is reversible and time to imaging matters. Chest pain or suspected PE equals oxygen, ECG, vitals, posture, and appropriate meds, because rapid risk stratification changes treatment. Sepsis equals cultures then antibiotics and fluids, because timing changes mortality, and neutropenic fever equals reverse isolation to protect the client.

Finish each vignette with a one-minute mental check. Ask yourself: Is there any airway, breathing, or circulation threat right now? Do any of the six red flags show up? Who is unstable, new, or unexpected? What single action in my scope stops deterioration in the next minute? And what must I reassess after I act—vital signs, oxygen saturation, mental status, pain, bleeding, or glucose? If you can answer those questions quickly and consistently, you will pick the safest "first" on test day and in practice.

2.1.3 Consent, Privacy, Mandatory Reporting (What's Testable)

On NCLEX, legal/ethical items sit inside Management of Care and reward nurses who act on cues quickly and safely. Use what you see, hear, and what's missing to decide your first action. When in doubt, protect the patient's rights, safety, and privacy, verify before proceeding, and escalate through the chain of command.

Informed consent hinges on three elements that must be present and documented: capacity (the patient can make the decision), disclosure/understanding (the risks, benefits, alternatives, and likely outcomes have been explained and understood), and voluntariness (no coercion). The provider—not the RN—obtains consent by explaining the procedure and answering questions. The RN's role is to verify the patient appears to have decision-making capacity, ensure the choice is voluntary, use a certified medical interpreter if needed, witness the signature when appropriate, and document questions and referral back to the provider. Timing matters: consent must occur before any pre-op sedatives or opioids are given; once sedated, capacity is presumed impaired and the process must be delayed or completed by a surrogate if indicated. A patient may refuse or withdraw consent at any time, even after signing—your first action is to stop, assess capacity, clarify understanding, notify the provider, and document refusal and teaching about risks of refusing.

In emergencies, consent is implied when delaying treatment threatens life or limb. Proceed with lifesaving interventions while attempting to reach a surrogate; document the emergent circumstances and attempts to contact decision-makers. For special populations, know who can consent. Minors generally require a parent/guardian, but emancipated minors (court-declared, married, active military, or self-supporting per policy) and mature minors may consent for certain services, especially reproductive/contraception, pregnancy care, STI testing/treatment, substance use, and mental health in many jurisdictions; on NCLEX, protect access for a teen seeking STI care and maintain confidentiality within policy. For adults lacking capacity, a surrogate decision-maker named in a durable power of attorney for health care or a court-appointed guardian provides consent, guided by the patient's known wishes or best interests. When parents refuse lifesaving treatment for a child, the correct action is to seek a court order rather than accept refusal. Telephone or verbal consent is acceptable when permitted by policy: perform a read-back of the consent, ensure the provider has explained and answered questions, obtain two witnesses if required, confirm the identity and relationship of the surrogate, and document the date/time, names/titles, and exact content consented to. The provider remains responsible for the explanation; the RN ensures the process is valid and clearly documented.

Capacity and competence sound similar but differ legally. Nurses assess decision-making capacity at the bedside: is the patient alert and oriented? Can they understand relevant information, appreciate the situation and consequences, reason about options, and communicate a choice? Legal incompetence is a court determination and triggers surrogate decision-making. Many conditions cause fluctuating capacity—delirium, intoxication, hypoxia, severe pain, or acute psychosis. If capacity is questionable and the procedure is non-urgent, delay and re-evaluate, involve the provider, and contact the surrogate if needed. Do not proceed on a "good enough" hunch; NCLEX favors delaying non-urgent care to reassess capacity and ensure valid consent.

Advance directives guide care when capacity is lost. A living will records the patient's wishes about life-sustaining treatments; a durable power of attorney for health care (health care proxy) designates the decision-maker; and DNR/AND orders direct resuscitation status. On admission, the RN asks whether such documents exist, ensures they are in the chart and visible in the plan of care, and clarifies any conflicts. If the family's request contradicts an existing directive or DNR order, the directive controls—honor it and notify the provider and charge nurse to resolve disagreements. Do not initiate CPR when there is a valid, current DNR order; if uncertain whether the order is current, verify immediately and otherwise begin resuscitation while a second nurse checks the record. Always confirm the most recent order—outdated forms do not override new wishes.

Research participation requires consent separate from clinical consent. Participation must be voluntary, with no penalty for refusing or withdrawing. The investigator or provider educates the participant; the RN protects participant rights, monitors for undue influence, ensures questions are answered by the investigator, and stops participation if safety is at risk or consent is withdrawn. Clinical care must not be withheld or conditioned on research participation.

Privacy and HIPAA principles are testable because they are universal. Protected health information (PHI) includes any individually identifiable health information in any form. Apply the minimum necessary standard: share only what is needed for treatment, payment, or operations, and only with those who need to know for care. Verify identity before disclosing information—in person (photo ID or facility wristband), by phone (code word or verification per policy), or via secure messaging systems. Never discuss patients in hallways or elevators, never post any patient content on social media (even de-identified details can be identifiable), and always protect screens, devices, and printouts. Patients have a right to access and receive a copy of their records; route requests per policy. Some information is especially sensitive (psych, HIV, substance use)—handle with heightened discretion and follow specific release rules. Requests from law enforcement, employers, or family members require patient authorization, a valid subpoena/court order, or a mandatory reporting exception. Without one of these, do not disclose; instead, refer to the charge nurse or privacy officer and document the request and your response.

Confidentiality has narrow exceptions when safety or law requires disclosure. Mandatory reporting and the duty to protect override confidentiality for suspected abuse of children, elders, or dependent adults; credible threats of serious harm to self or others (duty to warn per facility policy); certain communicable diseases; gunshot or knife wounds in jurisdictions that require reporting; and impaired coworkers or drug diversion. Your first steps are to ensure immediate safety, document objective facts, notify the chain of command, and follow policy about whom to contact (social services, protective services, public health, security, or law enforcement as applicable). Do not promise secrecy when safety is at stake.

Mandatory reporting on NCLEX focuses on what, when, and to whom. For abuse or neglect of children, elders, or dependent adults, report suspicion, not proof. Clues include inconsistent injury explanations, delays in seeking care, patterned injuries, poor hygiene or malnutrition, caregiver control, or fearfulness. Prioritize the patient's safety, obtain a private history when feasible, preserve forensic evidence (avoid unnecessary bathing or changing clothes after sexual assault; use paper bags, maintain chain of custody), and document the patient's words in quotations and the physical findings objectively. Notify the provider and social services, and file the mandated report immediately per policy; you do not investigate, confront, or delay to "confirm." For communicable diseases like tuberculosis, measles, pertussis, hepatitis, syphilis, and other reportables, notify public health promptly, implement isolation as indicated, and teach exposure precautions. For impaired or unsafe practice by a coworker, your duty is to protect patients first: remove the staff member from assignment if unsafe, notify the charge nurse/manager, secure any controlled substances if diversion is suspected, and complete required reporting to leadership and risk management; do not cover up or confront alone. Sentinel events and incidents require completion of the internal incident report for quality improvement; you still chart the clinical facts of what happened and the patient's assessment and response, but you never mention the incident report in the medical record.

Documentation is where legal protection meets patient safety. Write objective, specific descriptors of findings and actions; include direct quotes when relevant ("My boyfriend hit me with a belt"), body maps or photographs per policy for injuries, and the names/titles and times of all persons notified and consulted. When an interpreter is used, record the interpreter's name or ID number, language, and mode (phone/video/in-person). For verbal or telephone consent, document read-back, witnesses, the decision-maker's identity and relationship, and exactly what was consented to. When a patient refuses treatment, document the education provided about risks and alternatives, the patient's demonstrated understanding, and the decision, then notify the provider and record the response. After safety events, document your assessments and interventions factually and timely; complete the incident report separately.

Tie these rules to NGN/CJMM cues and first actions. If you see a patient prepped for surgery who has already received lorazepam, recognize that capacity may be impaired and consent may be invalid. Your first action is to stop the progression to the OR, assess capacity, notify the provider, and either obtain valid consent when the patient is alert or involve the surrogate if urgent. If a family member at the desk demands results but lacks the code word, do not disclose; verify identity, obtain authorization, or politely decline and offer to involve the patient. When an older adult's injuries do not match the story or a caregiver interrupts and answers all questions, move the patient to a private space, assess for abuse, ensure immediate safety, and file a mandated report—do not wait for proof. If a staff member posts any content about a patient to social media or you overhear hallway discussions about a named patient, intervene to stop the breach, protect PHI, notify the supervisor or privacy officer, and document per policy.

If a teen presents for STI testing, protect confidentiality to the extent allowed by policy and assist with care without requiring parental consent; disclose only as required and support the patient's safety. With fluctuating mentation—say, a delirious patient lucid in the morning but confused in the evening—time non-urgent teaching and consent for when the patient demonstrates capacity; if urgent and capacity is absent, involve the surrogate decision-maker.

Common pitfalls repeatedly tested include attempting to "obtain" consent or explaining risks in place of the provider, using family or friends as interpreters instead of a certified interpreter, proceeding with procedures after sedatives without reassessing capacity, sharing PHI with visitors or law enforcement absent authorization or a legal exception, delaying abuse reports to privately investigate, and documenting that an "incident report was completed" in the medical record. Avoiding these errors is high yield: verify, protect, escalate appropriately, and document precisely.

Do first checklist:

- Verify the patient's identity, decision-making capacity, and need for a certified interpreter; witness consent only after the provider's explanation and before sedation.
- Confirm consent status and any advance directives or DNR/AND orders are current, in the chart, and honored; resolve conflicts quickly by notifying the provider/charge nurse.
- Protect PHI using the minimum necessary standard; verify identity before disclosure and shut down hallway/social media breaches; route outside requests to the privacy officer.
- Report mandated concerns immediately: suspected abuse/neglect, credible threats, reportable diseases, gunshot/knife wounds per policy, and impaired coworkers/diversion; ensure immediate safety first.
- Document objectively and completely: facts, quotes, diagrams/photos per policy, times, names/titles notified, interpreter ID, consent read-backs, teaching on refusal and the patient's response; complete incident reports separately and never write "incident report filed" in the chart.

2.2 Safety & Infection Prevention and Control

On the NCLEX, safety is the first lens for every client scenario. Your goal is to prevent injury and healthcare-associated infections (HAIs) by breaking the chain of infection, controlling hazards, and choosing the first action that stops harm. Think like the Clinical Judgment Measurement Model (CJMM): recognize cues, analyze risk, prioritize the safest immediate action, and evaluate outcomes. If your answer prevents harm now, you're usually on the right track.

Begin by seeing safety cues fast. Fever, new isolation signage, a damp central-line dressing, a wandering older adult, oxygen in use, a fresh post-op with opioids, or a coughing client with uncontrolled secretions all signal risk. Analyze what mode of transmission or hazard is present (airborne, droplet, contact, spore-forming; fall; fire; device-related infection), who is most vulnerable (immunocompromised, older adult, very young, unstable cardio-respiratory status), and what single action most immediately reduces exposure or injury. Typically, that action is hand hygiene, correct PPE selection, securing the environment (bed low, locks on, clutter removed), protecting the airway, removing a contaminated device or restarting a sterile field, or escalating care (rapid response versus routine notify). Evaluate by verifying vitals are stable, no new exposures occurred, skin and device sites remain intact, lines are closed and secure, and the client understands safety instructions.

The chain of infection is your roadmap. Infectious agent, reservoir, portal of exit, mode of transmission, portal of entry, susceptible host—nursing breaks the chain at multiple points. You perform hand hygiene; apply the right PPE; clean and disinfect high-touch surfaces and shared equipment; use safe injections (one needle, one syringe, one patient; avoid reusing single-dose vials); remove unnecessary devices; maintain closed systems; and promote host defenses via immunization, nutrition, and prophylaxis when prescribed. Every break reduces R (risk of spread).

Hand hygiene is the single most important action. Perform it before and after every client contact, before aseptic tasks and after body-fluid exposure, after glove removal, and when moving from dirty to clean tasks. Use alcohol-based rubs unless hands are visibly soiled or caring for spore-formers (C. difficile, norovirus), where soap and water is required. Keep natural nails short; avoid artificial nails and excessive jewelry; gloves never replace hand hygiene and do not excuse skipping it between clients or tasks.

Standard precautions apply to every client. Promote respiratory hygiene and cough etiquette, offer masks and tissues, and place contaminated items in appropriate containers. Practice safe injection at all times and dispose of sharps immediately in puncture-resistant containers; do not recap needles. If exposed to blood or body fluids, immediately wash or flush the area, report, follow facility policy for source testing, obtain post-exposure prophylaxis promptly when indicated, and document.

Transmission-based isolation adds layers based on mode. Airborne diseases (e.g., TB, measles, varicella) require a negative-pressure room and N95 or higher respirator; mask the client for transport and limit movement. Droplet infections (e.g., influenza, meningitis, pertussis) require a surgical mask within 3–6 feet and during transport. Contact organisms (e.g., MRSA, VRE, C. difficile) require gloves and gown; dedicate equipment and clean with appropriate agents; for spore-formers, use soap and water for hand hygiene and sporicidal disinfectants on surfaces. Cohort clients only when organisms are the same and no other high-risk conditions conflict; otherwise, prioritize private rooms for airborne infections and for those who cannot follow hygiene, and separate infectious clients from immunocompromised clients. Protective (neutropenic) isolation is for severely immunocompromised clients; screen visitors for illness, avoid fresh flowers and raw produce as directed, ensure meticulous hand hygiene, and mask the client for transport.

Choose PPE based on anticipated exposure and transmission mode, not habit. Don PPE in the sequence that prevents self-contamination—gown, then mask or respirator, then eye protection, then gloves. Remove PPE in a clean-to-dirty order—gloves first, then eye protection, then gown, then mask or respirator; perform hand hygiene after removal, and step out of negative-pressure rooms before removing a respirator. If a breach occurs (torn glove, touched face shield with contaminated glove), stop, perform hand hygiene, replace PPE, and resume with aseptic technique intact.

Asepsis depends on understanding sterile versus clean. Keep sterile fields above the waist and in view; the outer 1-inch border is contaminated; moisture wicks contamination, so keep the field dry; and never reach across or turn your back on a sterile field. When in doubt, consider it contaminated and start over. During care, work clean-to-dirty: wound to periwound, from catheter port to drainage bag, and from least to most soiled. This simple sequence lowers cross-contamination.

HAI risk falls when you think in bundles and necessity. Use devices only when necessary, review daily whether they are still required, maintain closed systems, and remove promptly. For ventilated clients, elevate the head of the bed 30–45 degrees and provide regular oral care per policy; these two measures alone reduce pneumonia risk. For central lines, use maximal sterile barrier for insertion, chlorhexidine skin prep, secure properly, keep dressings clean and intact, scrub the hub before every access, and evaluate need daily. For urinary catheters, insert aseptically, secure to prevent traction, keep the bag below the bladder without kinks, maintain a closed system, perform perineal hygiene, empty with clean technique, and remove as soon as possible. For surgical sites, prep skin appropriately, clip instead of shave, and ensure prophylactic antibiotics are timed per policy.

Environmental hygiene matters. Disinfect high-touch surfaces and shared equipment between clients, using sporicidal agents for spore-forming organisms. Handle linens away from your uniform, avoid shaking, and bag at the point of use. When collecting specimens, label at the bedside, use the correct container, collect before antibiotics when ordered, and transport promptly to the lab.

Preventing hazards extends beyond infection. Falls are common and preventable with universal precautions: orient the client, keep the call light and personal items within reach, use non-skid footwear, keep the bed low with brakes locked, declutter, and ensure adequate lighting. After a risk assessment, add targeted measures such as placing the client near the nurse's station, using bed/chair alarms, employing sitters for delirium, and teaching safe use of assistive devices; round hourly to address pain, potty, position, and possessions. Remember that raising all four side rails is considered a restraint. For fire and oxygen safety, follow RACE (Rescue, Activate alarm, Contain, Extinguish/Evacuate) and PASS (Pull, Aim, Squeeze, Sweep), enforce no smoking around oxygen, avoid oil-based products near oxygen, keep cylinders secured upright, and use grounded equipment. Restraints are a last resort after alternatives (reorientation, de-escalation, sitter, diversion, environmental modifications) fail. They require a provider order and are time-limited per policy; assess frequently for circulation, skin integrity, comfort, toileting, fluids, and range of motion; use quick-release ties to the bed frame (not side rails), allow two fingers under the restraint, document thoroughly, and discontinue as soon as possible.

Consider special populations. Immunocompromised clients require meticulous infection control and protective isolation principles. Older adults have higher fall and delirium risk; minimize psychoactive medications, optimize hydration, vision and hearing aids, and daytime mobilization. In pediatrics, screen family and visitors for illness, dedicate toys, and ensure age-appropriate environmental safety.

A micro-case illustrates the CJMM sequence. You enter a room posted for C. difficile; the client has watery diarrhea and a soiled gown. Cues: spore-former, high transmission risk, contaminated environment. First action: perform hand hygiene with soap and water, don gown and gloves, contain stool, change linens carefully, and clean high-touch surfaces with a sporicidal agent; do not rely on alcohol gel alone. Evaluate: no further soiling, clean environment, client stable, plan in place for contact precautions and education.

Keep a short list of non-negotiables in mind:

- Always perform hand hygiene before and after contact and after glove removal; use soap and water for C. difficile or visible soil.
- Always dispose of sharps immediately into a puncture-resistant container; never recap.
- Always mask the client for transport when on droplet or airborne precautions.
- Never substitute PPE for hand hygiene, and never ignore a breached sterile field—stop and restart.
- Never raise all four side rails as a "fall prevention" strategy; it is a restraint.

Watch for classic wrong-answer traps:

- "Start antibiotics, then obtain cultures." If cultures are ordered, collect before antibiotics.
- "Put the immunocompromised client with the client who has influenza because they're both on droplet precautions." Do not cohort vulnerable hosts with infectious clients.
- "Tighten restraints when the client fights." Reassess cause, offer toileting/fluids, ensure fit, and consider alternatives; restraints must be the last resort and time-limited.

NGN "do-first" triggers are predictable: correct a sterile or PPE breach immediately with hand hygiene and replacement; isolate based on cues while awaiting orders when transmission risk is high; remove unnecessary devices; place the highest-risk client closest to observation; and escalate care rapidly for acute deterioration (airway, breathing, circulation) rather than merely notifying. Evaluate outcomes by confirming no new HAIs or exposures, stable vital signs, intact device sites and skin, absence of falls or fires, prompt restraint discontinuation, and client understanding of isolation and safety teaching. This is the safety-first mindset the NCLEX expects you to apply—every client, every time.

2.2.1 Isolation & PPE (Airborne/Droplet/Contact One-Pager)

Think Clinical Judgment. On the NCLEX, start by recognizing cues (diagnosis, signage, symptoms), analyze the likely mode of transmission, then prioritize room placement, PPE, and transport. Implement correctly (don and doff in the right order), and evaluate for breaches or exposures. When the stem is ambiguous, choose the higher-protection option.

Begin with what is never optional: standard precautions for every patient, every time. Perform hand hygiene at the five moments—before touching a patient, before clean/aseptic procedures, after body fluid exposure risk, after touching a patient, and after touching patient surroundings. Use an alcohol-based hand rub unless hands are visibly soiled or the pathogen is a spore-former (for Clostridioides difficile and often norovirus, scrub with soap and water). Don clean gloves when you may contact blood, body fluids, secretions/excretions, nonintact skin, or mucous membranes; change gloves between tasks on the same patient and remove promptly after use, then perform hand hygiene. Practice respiratory hygiene/cough etiquette: cover coughs, provide tissues and masks, and post signage. Maintain sharps safety—do not recap needles, activate safety devices, and discard in puncture-resistant containers at the point of use.

Transmission-based precautions add to standard precautions and are selected by matching the disease to its transmission route. Airborne pathogens travel on small particles that remain suspended; droplet pathogens spread via large respiratory droplets; contact pathogens transfer by touch of contaminated people, surfaces, or equipment. Your first actions center on the room and door status, the correct PPE, how the patient moves, and how the environment is managed.

Airborne precautions demand more than a mask at the doorway. Place the patient in a negative-pressure airborne infection isolation room with the door closed at all times; an N95 or higher-level respirator that has been fit tested is required before entry. If the patient must leave the room, put a surgical mask on them and limit movement to only essential tests or procedures. Dedicate equipment to the room whenever possible and perform thorough environmental cleaning. Classic examples include tuberculosis, measles (rubeola), and varicella (chickenpox). Disseminated herpes zoster also requires airborne plus contact precautions. Remember the memory aid "My Chicken Hez TB" to snap into the right choice under time pressure.

Droplet precautions protect within conversational distance. Use a private room or cohort with the same pathogen; a surgical mask is required within approximately 3–6 feet of the patient. Add eye protection when splash or spray of respiratory secretions is possible—e.g., during coughing spasms, suctioning, or nebulization. When transporting, place a surgical mask on the patient and keep movement to essential needs. Dedicate or disinfect equipment between patients and clean high-touch surfaces routinely. High-yield examples include influenza, pertussis, meningococcal disease, mumps, and rubella. A quick memory hook is "SPIDERMAN" for droplet pathogens, but the safer test move is to recognize the named illnesses.

Contact precautions are the backbone for organisms that spread via hands and surfaces. Don gloves and a gown upon entry to the room and before contact with the patient or their environment. Use dedicated equipment such as a stethoscope and blood pressure cuff. Perform meticulous environmental cleaning and disinfect high-touch surfaces with EPA-registered products. Transport only when essential, keep draining wounds well covered, and have the patient perform hand hygiene. Examples include MRSA, VRE, RSV, scabies, and draining wounds. RSV is primarily contact spread in pediatrics; many facilities pair a mask during close care if frequent coughing or suctioning is expected, but the exam core is contact.

Contact Plus (spore-forming) is contact precautions with two critical upgrades: hand hygiene must be soap and water, and the environment requires bleach-based or EPA-registered sporicidal disinfection. C. difficile is the exam-staple pathogen; norovirus is often managed similarly. Alcohol rub is not adequate for spores, and the NCLEX expects you to say "soap and water" when the stem mentions C. diff or a persistent diarrheal outbreak.

Donning and doffing sequences are frequent test targets and must be automatic. Don in this order: hand hygiene, gown, mask or respirator, goggles or face shield, then gloves, ensuring the glove cuffs cover the gown cuffs. Doff in this order: gloves first (they're most contaminated), then goggles or face shield, gown, then mask or respirator, followed by hand hygiene. For airborne rooms, do not remove the respirator until after you have exited the room and closed the door. This small detail is a favorite trap.

Cohorting and room placement hinge on minimizing risk. Cohort only patients with the same organism and ideally the same strain; do not cohort if a roommate is immunocompromised, has open wounds, is post-op, or has uncontrolled secretions. Prioritize single rooms for airborne illnesses, for patients with heavy or uncontrolled secretions or poor hygiene, and whenever an existing patient in a semi-private room is immunocompromised and at risk. If a private room is unavailable, choosing the roommate with the least risk is the safer answer, but do not pair an infectious patient with someone at high risk, even if diagnoses differ.

Patient transport and visitors should be limited to essentials. Mask the patient for airborne or droplet transport, cover all wounds and lesions, and perform hand hygiene before leaving the room. Visitors must be taught hand hygiene and use PPE matching the patient's isolation. Do not allow immunocompromised visitors to enter rooms with airborne or highly infectious patients unless risk is clearly minimized and the scenario indicates physician clearance.

Manage equipment and the environment deliberately. Dedicate noncritical equipment to a single patient when possible; otherwise, clean and disinfect between patients. Use bleach or EPA-registered sporicidal disinfectants for C. diff and suspected norovirus. Handle linen and waste carefully: avoid shaking, bag at the point of use in the room, and double-bag only if the outside is contaminated or leaking. Keep bins from overfilling and close them before removal.

If you breach PPE or are exposed, stop immediately. Remove and replace contaminated PPE, perform hand hygiene, and assess the exposure. For mucous membrane splashes, flush eyes or mucosa with water or normal saline for at least 15 minutes. Report promptly and follow institutional exposure protocols, which may include tuberculosis testing after airborne exposure or bloodborne pathogen assessment with baseline labs and prophylaxis. Document the event. The test wants you to avoid "powering through" a task with torn gloves or a broken face shield.

Certain traps recur on exam day. Alcohol rub alone is not adequate for C. diff; choose soap and water plus bleach cleaning. Do not forget eye protection when there is a splash risk in droplet scenarios or during procedures. Never leave an airborne isolation door open and never remove the respirator in the room. Do not cohort an immunocompromised patient with any infectious patient. Do not reuse single-use PPE. When you are unsure, default to a higher level of protection: a private room, a respirator, or adding eye protection is the exam-safe choice.

Use quick cue-to-action thinking to lock in first steps:

- A patient arrives with cough, weight loss, night sweats, and an abnormal chest X-ray: place in airborne isolation immediately, door closed, staff with N95; the patient wears a surgical mask for transport to imaging.
- A hospitalized patient develops watery diarrhea with C. diff positive stool and stool-soiled environment: initiate Contact Plus; wash hands with soap and water and switch cleaning to bleach-based sporicidal agents.
- On a crowded unit, a patient with fever, sore throat, and positive influenza test needs placement: pick a private room if available or cohort with another influenza patient; wear a surgical mask within 3–6 feet and mask the patient for transport.
- Several residents in a long-term care unit have pruritic papules and burrows; one caregiver has itchy wrists: implement contact precautions for scabies, don gown and gloves on entry, bag linens at point of use, and coordinate treatment for affected patients and close contacts.
- An RSV-positive infant requires suctioning: use contact precautions with gown and gloves, dedicate equipment, and add a face shield or goggles for suctioning due to splash risk.
- A patient with shingles and widespread lesions across multiple dermatomes: airborne plus contact; negative-pressure room, N95, gown, gloves. If shingles are localized and can be fully covered in an immunocompetent patient, use contact precautions; if lesions cannot be covered or the patient is immunocompromised, escalate to airborne plus contact.

Keep the memory aids brief and useful. "My Chicken Hez TB" reminds you that measles, chickenpox (varicella), disseminated herpes zoster, and TB are airborne. "SPIDERMAN" can cue droplet pathogens although naming the disease is faster: think influenza, pertussis, meningococcal disease, mumps, and rubella. "C diff = Contact Plus + soap and water" is the high-yield hand hygiene upgrade.

When analyzing a question, align your steps with clinical judgment: recognize cues like "rule-out TB," "sudden watery diarrhea with antibiotic use," "productive cough with droplet signage," or "weeping lesions;" analyze the transmission route; prioritize by placing the patient in the correct room and putting on the right PPE; implement by donning in the correct order before entry and doffing safely on exit; and evaluate by checking the environment, educating visitors, and correcting any breaches immediately. That approach reliably produces the exam-correct "first action" and keeps you aligned with safety and infection prevention and control.

2.2.2 Sterile Technique & Device Safety (Central Lines, Restraints)

Sterile asepsis is not optional window dressing; it is the primary defense against device-related infection and harm. On the NCLEX, the safe RN recognizes cues that signal contamination, stops the procedure, and restarts correctly—

even if that means delaying a task briefly to prevent a central line–associated bloodstream infection (CLABSI) or other serious complication. Your accountability is twofold: set up and maintain sterility, and detect early problems in high-risk devices such as central lines and restraints, acting immediately to prevent deterioration.

Start with what matters most. Perform hand hygiene every time you enter or re-enter a task, and verify allergies and contraindications before you begin. Chlorhexidine (CHG) allergy, for instance, requires an alternative antiseptic such as povidone-iodine or alcohol, and you must still allow full dry time before proceeding. Latex or adhesive allergies alter product choices and dressing materials. These checks are testable because they directly change the safe plan.

Sterile asepsis hinges on a few nonnegotiable principles. Sterile touches only sterile: once a sterile glove, instrument, or drape touches a nonsterile surface, it becomes contaminated. The outer one-inch border of a sterile field is considered nonsterile, so do not place or retrieve sterile items from that margin. Keep the field above waist level and in your direct line of sight at all times; turning your back or stepping away makes it contaminated. Moisture allows microorganisms to migrate ("strike-through"), which means wet drapes or surfaces are not sterile, and any sterile package that becomes damp is compromised. Opening sterile packages follows a standard sequence—away from you first, then sides, then toward you—so your body and sleeves do not cross the field. When pouring sterile solutions, "lip" a multi-dose bottle by pouring off a small amount to cleanse the rim, hold the label in the palm to prevent it from getting wet, and pour without reaching over the field. Replace caps with the inner surface facing up on a clean surface to avoid contamination. Don sterile gloves using the open method and then protect the field: limit talking and traffic, replace any item that is questionable, and if contamination occurs, stop. Put on clean gloves to remove soiled items and rebuild a new sterile field from scratch.

Central venous devices—CVCs, PICCs, and implanted ports—carry both lifesaving benefits and CLABSI risks. A prevention bundle frames safe care. Hand hygiene precedes any contact with the line. Insertion requires maximal barrier precautions and CHG skin antisepsis; thereafter, all dressing changes and port accesses are sterile procedures. Always scrub the hub before each access using vigorous friction and full dry time; alcohol or CHG/alcohol pads are typical, and the technique matters more than the brand. Use needleless connectors as intended, and never reuse disinfection caps. High-risk infusions such as total parenteral nutrition (TPN) get a dedicated lumen. Prime tubing to eliminate air and replace lines per policy, removing central lines as soon as they are no longer necessary. Securement is with a transparent occlusive dressing; a CHG-impregnated disk at the insertion site is standard. Label the dressing with date, time, and initials so the next nurse can assess dwell time and due dates.

A sterile central-line dressing change follows a concise, repeatable sequence that NCLEX expects you to know. Place a mask on yourself and the patient to limit droplet contamination. Remove the old dressing with clean gloves, stabilizing the catheter to avoid dislodgement, and inspect the site for erythema, tenderness, drainage, and catheter migration. Perform hand hygiene again, then don sterile gloves and set up your sterile field. Cleanse the site with CHG using a back-and-forth friction scrub for a full 30 seconds and allow it to air-dry completely. Apply a CHG disk around the catheter at the insertion point, then cover with a sterile, transparent occlusive dressing. Label with date/time/initials and document site assessment, patient tolerance, and any changes.

Access and flushing are frequent touchpoints for safety. Use a 10 mL syringe or larger to avoid excessive pressure that can damage the catheter. Employ a pulsatile (push–pause) flush to clear the lumen and maintain patency. Finish with positive pressure—clamp as you inject the last 0.5–1 mL or use the connector's neutral/positive displacement—so blood does not reflux into the tip. For intermittent medications, SASH (saline, administer drug, saline, heparin) is a common sequence; follow your facility's heparin concentration and indications for heparin locking, as some systems use saline-only for certain devices.

You must rapidly recognize and act on early complications. Suspected CLABSI presents with fever, local erythema, tenderness, or purulence at the site. The safe first move is to stop any non-essential line use, maintain asepsis, obtain ordered blood cultures (often both peripheral and catheter-drawn) and site cultures if indicated, then notify the provider and anticipate empiric antibiotics. Air embolism is high-stakes: cues include sudden dyspnea, chest pain, tachycardia, hypotension, and sometimes a "mill-wheel" murmur. First clamp the line to stop additional air entry, place the patient in left lateral Trendelenburg to trap air in the right atrium, administer 100% oxygen, and call the provider. For occlusion, stop and assess the system for kinks and closed clamps; reposition the patient (raising the arm or having them cough can help PICC tips move off the vessel wall), and attempt a gentle pulsatile flush. Never force a flush; you can rupture the catheter or dislodge a thrombus. During vesicant extravasation from a central device, stop the infusion immediately, attempt to aspirate residual drug through the existing catheter, leave the catheter in place for possible antidote administration, notify the provider, and follow drug-specific protocols (cold versus warmth varies by agent).

Sometimes removal is within RN scope and ordered. Safety begins with positioning the patient supine or in Trendelenburg to increase venous pressure and reduce air entry. Instruct the patient to perform a Valsalva during removal or exhale as the catheter comes out; apply immediate occlusive pressure and a petroleum-based occlusive dressing to the site, then secure it and monitor for signs of air embolism or bleeding. Inspect the catheter tip to ensure it is intact, and measure the removed length against the documented length to confirm no fragment remains.

Patients with home PICCs or ports need targeted teaching. Emphasize meticulous hand hygiene before any handling, keeping the dressing clean, dry, and intact, and protecting the site during bathing. No blood pressures or venipunctures are permitted in the PICC arm. Report fever, swelling, warmth, drainage, pain, or visible catheter migration promptly. For ports, teach that access is by a sterile noncoring needle only; once accessed, the dressing must remain occlusive.

Restraints and seclusion are as much about legality and dignity as they are about safety, and the exam tests that balance. Use restraints only when there is an immediate risk of harm and when less restrictive alternatives have failed: reorientation, sitter, de-escalation, providing glasses or hearing aids, pain control, toileting, diversional activities, and bed or chair alarms are all reasonable first attempts. Restraints are never for staff convenience or punishment. A provider order is required, time-limited, and no PRN orders are allowed. Reassess frequently and discontinue as soon as the patient is safe without them. For seclusion, applicable to violent or self-destructive behavior with imminent risk, continuous monitoring is required.

Application must protect circulation, skin, airway, and devices. Choose the least restrictive device; for a patient pulling at a central line, start with mitts and close supervision instead of bilateral wrist restraints when feasible. Pad bony prominences, and apply restraints so two fingers fit between the device and the patient's skin. Tie with a quick-release knot to a bed frame, never to side rails, and position the call light within reach. Continuous care involves regular neurovascular checks of restrained extremities (color, warmth, sensation, movement, capillary refill), skin care and hygiene, range-of-motion exercises, and offering fluids, nutrition, and toileting at frequent intervals. Document the behaviors that necessitated restraints, alternatives attempted, assessments, care provided, patient response, and the ongoing need. Always consider how restraint placement interacts with lines and tubes; do not place a device in a way that kinks a central line, compresses a dialysis access, or restricts chest wall expansion. Avoid vest or full-coverage designs that risk asphyxiation.

To integrate this with clinical judgment, practice reading cues and moving to the first safest action with rationale.

Mini-scenario 1: You are preparing to access an implanted port. After opening sterile supplies, your nonsterile sleeve brushes the edge of the sterile field, and you notice the CHG prep pad touched the table. Cues: potential contamination of field and prep, high infection-risk device. First action: stop the procedure, don clean gloves to remove contaminated items, and rebuild a new sterile field with new supplies. Rationale: sterile-to-sterile only; contaminated items must be replaced to prevent CLABSI.

Mini-scenario 2: Immediately after changing the needleless cap on a PICC, the patient becomes acutely short of breath and tachycardic. You hear a new, harsh cardiac sound. Cues: sudden dyspnea and "mill-wheel" murmur after line manipulation suggest air embolism. First action: clamp the line, place the patient in left lateral Trendelenburg, administer 100% oxygen, and notify the provider. Rationale: this position traps air in the right atrium and reduces right ventricular outflow obstruction while oxygen treats hypoxemia.

Mini-scenario 3: A patient in bilateral soft wrist restraints for line safety has cool, pale fingers with sluggish capillary refill. Cues: neurovascular compromise from too-tight restraints. First action: release the restraints immediately on the affected side(s), assess circulation and sensation, provide skin care, and notify the provider. Rationale: airway and circulation threats override the restraint order; least restraint and frequent checks are required.

Be mindful of frequent test traps that undermine safety. Do not touch the one-inch border and then treat it as sterile. Do not apply antiseptic and immediately cover; CHG and alcohol require complete air dry time to be effective and to avoid chemical burns. Do not reuse needleless caps or disinfection caps. Do not tie restraints to movable side rails. Do not force a flush against resistance; doing so risks catheter rupture or embolization. If a step feels expedient but violates a sterile or safety principle, the NCLEX answer is to pause and correct, not to push through.

Sterile technique, central line care, and restraint use converge on a single theme: prevent harm through discipline and early action. When you recognize cues of contamination or complication, your first move is to halt the risk, stabilize the patient's physiology, and restart with correct technique. That is the clinical judgment the exam expects.

Sterile field do/don't quick list:

- Do perform hand hygiene, verify allergies (including CHG, latex, adhesives), and gather all supplies before opening.
- Do open sterile packages away from you first, keep items above waist and in sight, and allow antiseptics to fully air-dry.
- Do "lip" multi-dose solution bottles, pour without reaching over the field, and label solutions and dressings with date/time/initials.
- Don't consider the one-inch border sterile; don't turn your back or leave the field; don't use wet or questionable items.
- Don't continue after contamination; stop, remove soiled items with clean gloves, and rebuild a new sterile field.

CLABSI prevention bundle (at-a-glance):

- Hand hygiene every access; maximal barrier and CHG skin prep at insertion; sterile technique for dressing changes and port access.
- Scrub the hub with friction and allow full dry time before every access; use needleless connectors correctly and replace per policy.
- Use a dedicated lumen for high-risk infusions (e.g., TPN); prime tubing and remove central lines as soon as no longer needed.
- Apply CHG-impregnated disk and transparent occlusive dressing; label dressings and document assessments; avoid unnecessary line entries.

Restraint application and monitoring quick steps:

- Confirm immediate safety indication and failure of less restrictive alternatives; obtain a time-limited provider order (no PRN).
- Choose the least restrictive device; pad, apply with two-finger slack; tie quick-release knots to bed frame; ensure call light access.
- Perform frequent neurovascular checks, skin care, ROM, fluids/nutrition, and toileting; reassess need continuously; discontinue ASAP.
- For seclusion (violent/self-destructive risk), maintain continuous monitoring and document behavior, interventions, and patient response.

2.3 Knowledge Check

Clinical Vignette 1

A 72-year-old man presents to the emergency department with progressive shortness of breath for 24 hours, worse when lying flat and associated with a cough that produced frothy sputum; his wife drove him in. Past medical history includes chronic systolic heart failure, hypertension, and atrial fibrillation; home medications are furosemide 40 mg daily, lisinopril, metoprolol, and warfarin; he has no known drug allergies. He is a former smoker, lives with his spouse, and is anxious about breathing. On exam he is tachypneic (RR 28), tachycardic (irregularly irregular HR 110), BP 160/88, and oxygen saturation 88% on room air; auscultation reveals bilateral coarse crackles to the mid-lungs, jugular venous distention, and 2+ pitting edema to the ankles. Portable chest x-ray shows cardiomegaly with pulmonary vascular congestion and interstitial/alveolar infiltrates; BNP is 1,200 pg/mL; 12-lead ECG shows atrial fibrillation with rapid ventricular response. INR is 2.5. While triage staff are obtaining vitals, the patient tells the nurse he does not want to be intubated or placed "on a breathing machine," and his wife says he has not discussed advance directives with the family. The RN must prioritize care, coordinate immediate interventions, and address the patient's statement about life-sustaining treatment.

Question 1: Based on the vignette, which condition is the most likely cause of the patient's acute dyspnea?

[A] Community-acquired pneumonia
[B] Acute decompensated heart failure with pulmonary edema
[C] Acute pulmonary embolism
[D] Exacerbation of chronic obstructive pulmonary disease

Qestion 2: While awaiting the provider, what is the RN's most appropriate immediate action for this patient referenced in the vignette?

[A] Obtain a CT pulmonary angiogram to rule out embolism before treating.
[B] Place the patient upright, administer supplemental oxygen, and notify the provider for urgent treatment.
[C] Withhold oxygen because the patient is on warfarin and may mask bleeding.
[D] Send the patient to the medical floor for routine observation since INR is therapeutic.

Question 3: Which pathophysiologic process best explains the pulmonary findings described in the vignette (frothy sputum, crackles, pulmonary vascular congestion)?

[A] Increased plasma oncotic pressure from hypoalbuminemia causing fluid shift into alveoli.
[B] Loss of alveolar surfactant leading to alveolar collapse and diffusion impairment.
[C] Pulmonary capillary endothelial injury with increased permeability causing protein-rich edema.
[D] Elevated pulmonary venous hydrostatic pressure from left ventricular dysfunction causing transudation of fluid into the interstitium and alveoli.

Question 4: Which medication should the RN anticipate as the most appropriate immediate pharmacologic treatment to reduce pulmonary congestion in this patient?

[A] IV loop diuretic (e.g., IV furosemide)
[B] Oral warfarin loading dose to prevent thromboembolism
[C] Subcutaneous low-molecular-weight heparin for deep vein thrombosis prophylaxis
[D] IV beta-blocker bolus to slow ventricular rate before addressing pulmonary edema

Question 5: The patient tells the nurse he does not want to be intubated. What is the RN's best next action regarding the patient's statement about life-sustaining treatment?

[A] Ask the spouse to sign a do-not-resuscitate order immediately to honor the statement.
[B] Document "refused intubation" and discharge the patient to home per his wishes.
[C] Assess the patient's decision-making capacity, clarify understanding and risks using teach-back, document the discussion, notify the provider, and involve advance-care planning resources as needed.
[D] Ignore the statement now because emergent treatment takes precedence and revisit the discussion later.

ANSWERS

1. Correct Answer: B
Rationale: The vignette shows acute decompensated HF: systolic HF history, orthopnea, weight gain/edema, bibasilar crackles, JVD, cardiomegaly, and high BNP—all pointing to pulmonary edema from HF. A is less likely (pneumonia usually has fever, focal consolidation, leukocytosis). C (PE) causes acute dyspnea/hypoxia but not cardiomegaly, high BNP, or bilateral crackles. D (COPD) is less consistent since findings indicate cardiac rather than obstructive disease.

2. Correct Answer: B
Rationale: Priority actions follow cue-based assessment and ABCs: the patient is hypoxemic (SpO2 88%) and tachypneic; placing him upright and giving supplemental oxygen are immediate, time-sensitive interventions that improve oxygenation and reduce preload, and notifying the provider initiates definitive therapy (diuretics, vasodilators if indicated). A is inappropriate to delay oxygenation for imaging when the patient is unstable. C is incorrect—warfarin use is not a contraindication to oxygen and withholding oxygen would risk further hypoxia. D is unsafe because the patient is unstable and requires urgent intervention, not routine observation.

3. Correct Answer: D
Rationale: In left ventricular failure, decreased forward output raises left-sided filling pressures → increased pulmonary venous hydrostatic pressure → fluid transudates into interstitium and alveoli, producing crackles, frothy sputum, and radiographic congestion. A is incorrect because hypoalbuminemia causes decreased oncotic pressure and generalized edema, not this acute cardiogenic pulmonary edema pattern. B (surfactant loss) is related to neonatal RDS or diffuse alveolar collapse, not typical HF presentation. C (increased permeability from endothelial injury) describes noncardiogenic pulmonary edema (e.g., ARDS), which is not supported by the cardiac signs and elevated BNP.

4. Correct Answer: A
Rationale: IV loop diuretics (furosemide) are first-line pharmacologic therapy for acute pulmonary edema to remove intravascular volume, reduce preload, and improve oxygenation; anticipate rapid IV dosing in symptomatic patients. B (warfarin loading) is irrelevant to acute pulmonary congestion and risks bleeding. C (LMWH prophylaxis) is for thrombosis prevention and not the immediate treatment for pulmonary edema. D (IV beta-blocker bolus) could worsen cardiac output or precipitate hypotension in acute decompensation and is not the priority; rate control may be addressed later after stabilization.

5. Correct Answer: C
Rationale: The RN must assess the patient's decision-making capacity (understand, appreciate, reason, communicate), use teach-back to confirm understanding, document the refusal, notify the provider, and involve ethics or advance-care planning if needed—protecting autonomy and ensuring legal/ethical compliance. A is wrong since only authorized clinicians can establish DNRs; a spouse's signature alone is insufficient. B is unsafe because documenting refusal is essential, but discharging an unstable patient is inappropriate. D is incorrect since patient wishes on life-sustaining treatment require prompt assessment and documentation, even in emergencies.

Clinical Vignette 2

A 67-year-old man presents to the medical-surgical unit for treatment of an acute exacerbation of chronic obstructive pulmonary disease with a history of heart failure with reduced ejection fraction, hypertension, and a 45 pack-year tobacco history; current home meds include tiotropium, albuterol PRN, lisinopril, and metoprolol, and he has no known drug allergies. He reports increased shortness of breath for 48 hours but is alert and oriented, speaking in short sentences and resting comfortably on 2 L oxygen by nasal cannula. Vital signs: T 37.1°C, HR 98/min, BP 138/82 mm Hg, RR 20/min, SpO_2 92% on 2 L NC. Focused exam shows mild bilateral wheezes and trace bibasilar crackles without new focal deficits. A portable chest x-ray shows chronic hyperinflation with mild cardiomegaly; ECG shows sinus rhythm without acute ST changes. An arterial blood gas on 2 L NC: pH 7.33, $PaCO_2$ 56 mm Hg, PaO_2 68 mm Hg. The physician orders scheduled nebulized albuterol treatments and IV furosemide 40 mg; nursing assigns routine vital signs every 4 hours. Shortly after admission he reports new chest tightness rated 6/10. He lives with his wife and is motivated to return home.

Question 1: Based on the vignette ABG results, which acid-base disturbance is most consistent with the values provided?

[A] Metabolic acidosis with respiratory compensation
[B] Respiratory alkalosis with hypoxemia
[C] Respiratory acidosis with hypoxemia (acute on chronic CO_2 retention)
[D] Metabolic alkalosis with hypoventilation

Question 2: The RN needs to assign a team member to obtain routine vital signs and assist the patient with morning hygiene. Which assignment is most appropriate given the vignette?

[A] UAP (unlicensed assistive personnel) to obtain vitals and assist with hygiene per established plan
[B] LPN to obtain vitals and perform hygiene because of the patient's cardiac history
[C] RN only; no delegation is appropriate for any ADL or vitals for this patient
[D] Nursing student to obtain vitals and assist with hygiene without supervision

Question 3: The elevated $PaCO_2$ in the ABG is most likely due to which physiologic mechanism in this patient?

[A] Increased metabolic acid production from heart failure
[B] Hyperventilation from anxiety causing CO_2 retention
[C] Alveolar hypoventilation from airflow obstruction and decreased CO_2 elimination
[D] Renal retention of bicarbonate leading to secondary hypercapnia

Question 4: When the patient reports new chest tightness rated 6/10, what is the nurse's best immediate action?

[A] RN to perform an immediate focused assessment and obtain a 12-lead ECG and notify the provider as indicated
[B] LPN to administer sublingual nitroglycerin per routine post-op chest pain protocol
[C] Ask the UAP to continue routine monitoring and report if pain worsens
[D] Call the physician immediately without additional bedside assessment

Question 5: Which of the following tasks should NOT be delegated to the unit's UAP for this patient?

[A] Obtain and record pulse oximetry and report values to the RN
[B] Assist the patient from bed to chair using an established transfer plan and gait belt
[C] Provide routine oral care and morning hygiene assistance per the patient's plan of care
[D] Teach the patient how to use and troubleshoot his new home oxygen prescription for discharge

ANSWERS

1. Correct Answer: C

Rationale: The ABG shows pH 7.33 (acidotic) with an elevated $PaCO_2$ of 56 mm Hg, indicating a primary respiratory acidosis; PaO_2 68 mm Hg indicates hypoxemia. In a patient with chronic COPD, this represents acute on chronic CO_2 retention. Option A is incorrect because a metabolic acidosis would show low HCO_3^- and a low CO_2 as compensation; Option B is incorrect because respiratory alkalosis has low $PaCO_2$ and high pH; Option D is incorrect because metabolic alkalosis would show elevated pH, not the acidemia seen here.

2. Correct Answer: A

Rationale: The patient is alert and hemodynamically stable with routine orders; UAPs may obtain routine vital signs and assist with ADLs/hygiene for a stable patient using an established plan and clear reporting instructions. Option B is less correct because LPNs can perform many tasks but routine vitals and hygiene assistance are within UAP scope and free LPN/RN time for skill-based tasks; Option C is incorrect because not all ADLs and routine vitals require RN-level care when the client is stable and predictable; Option D is incorrect because an unsupervised student should not be relied on for independent care without appropriate supervision.

3. Correct Answer: C

Rationale: In COPD, airflow obstruction and reduced alveolar ventilation impair CO_2 elimination, causing alveolar hypoventilation and elevated $PaCO_2$. Option A is incorrect because metabolic acid production from HF does not directly raise $PaCO_2$; Option B is incorrect because hyperventilation lowers $PaCO_2$ rather than raising it; Option D is incorrect because renal bicarbonate retention would affect HCO_3^- and pH chronically and does not explain an elevated $PaCO_2$ as the primary mechanism.

4. Correct Answer: A

Rationale: New chest tightness is an acute change in status requiring RN assessment, immediate focused evaluation (including vital signs and 12-lead ECG) and prompt notification of the provider; the RN retains responsibility for initial assessment and clinical judgment. Option B is incorrect because LPNs should not independently initiate treatments for new acute chest pain without RN assessment and orders; Option C is incorrect because UAPs do not assess or triage new acute symptoms; Option D is incorrect because calling the physician without bedside RN assessment and objective data is not appropriate—RN must assess and provide information.

5. Correct Answer: D

Rationale: Initial teaching about a new home oxygen prescription is a comprehensive teaching task requiring RN assessment, individualized education, and evaluation and therefore cannot be delegated to a UAP. Option A is incorrect as a rationale because UAPs may obtain and record pulse oximetry and must report abnormal values per instruction; Option B is incorrect because UAPs may assist with transfers using an established plan/gait belt for stable patients; Option C is incorrect because routine oral care and hygiene assistance are within the UAP scope when the plan of care is established.

Clinical Vignette 3

A 45-year-old woman presents to the emergency department with sudden onset of left-sided pleuritic chest pain and shortness of breath that began one hour ago during a flight home. She is alert but anxious; past medical history is notable for recent total knee arthroplasty two weeks ago, current oral contraceptive use, and a 20-pack-year smoking history; she takes no anticoagulants and has no known drug allergies. Initial vital signs: temperature 37.1°C, heart rate 126/min, respiratory rate 28/min, blood pressure 110/70 mmHg, and pulse oximetry 88% on room air. Focused exam reveals clear lung sounds, tachycardia without murmurs, and mild swelling of the left calf compared with the right. A 12-lead ECG shows sinus tachycardia with no acute ST changes; portable chest x-ray is unremarkable. D-dimer is elevated; arterial blood gas on room air: pH 7.48, PaCO2 30 mmHg, PaO2 60 mmHg, HCO3- 22 mEq/L. The patient asks if she can wait to be seen because she is worried about missing work, and she appears fearful but oriented to person, place, and time.

Question 1: Based on the vignette, which is the most likely diagnosis?

[A] Acute myocardial infarction
[B] Pulmonary embolism
[C] Community-acquired pneumonia
[D] Panic attack

Question 2: While awaiting definitive imaging, what is the nurse's highest-priority immediate action for this patient?

[A] Apply high-flow oxygen and establish IV access while notifying the provider about suspected pulmonary vascular obstruction.
[B] Obtain a thorough past medical and family history before any interventions.
[C] Administer chewable aspirin and sublingual nitroglycerin.
[D] Draw blood cultures and start broad-spectrum antibiotics.

Question 3: Which pathophysiologic mechanism best explains the patient's hypoxemia and normal chest x-ray?

[A] Airway bronchospasm causing diffuse small-airway obstruction.
[B] Alveolar consolidation producing a right-to-left intrapulmonary shunt.
[C] Left ventricular failure causing cardiogenic pulmonary edema.
[D] Ventilation–perfusion mismatch due to pulmonary arterial obstruction increasing dead space.

Question 4: How should the arterial blood gas (pH 7.48, PaCO2 30 mmHg, PaO2 60 mmHg, HCO3- 22 mEq/L) be interpreted in this clinical context?

[A] Primary metabolic alkalosis without respiratory compensation.
[B] Acute respiratory acidosis with hypoxemia indicating ventilatory failure.
[C] Acute respiratory alkalosis with hypoxemia, consistent with hyperventilation from pulmonary vascular compromise.
[D] Normal gas exchange for age and activity level.

Question 5: If the provider orders an intravenous unfractionated heparin bolus and infusion for suspected massive pulmonary embolism, which laboratory test should the nurse monitor to titrate the infusion?

[A] International normalized ratio (INR)
[B] Platelet count
[C] Activated partial thromboplastin time (aPTT)
[D] Serum creatinine

ANSWERS

1. Correct Answer: B
Rationale: Sudden pleuritic chest pain, acute dyspnea, hypoxemia (SpO2 88%), tachycardia, recent prolonged immobilization/orthopedic surgery, oral contraceptive use, and unilateral calf swelling are classic clues for pulmonary embolism in the vignette. A: Acute MI can present with chest pain and tachycardia but typically has ischemic ECG changes or crushing central pain and less commonly isolated hypoxemia with clear CXR and unilateral calf swelling. C: Pneumonia usually produces fever, focal crackles, and radiographic consolidation, which are absent here. D: Panic attack can cause tachycardia and hyperventilation but would not explain the objective hypoxemia, elevated D-dimer, recent surgery, and calf swelling.

2. Correct Answer: A
Rationale: The chapter emphasizes ABCs and time-sensitive actions: apply high-flow oxygen to treat hypoxemia and establish IV access while notifying the provider when pulmonary embolism is suspected; these nursing actions prevent deterioration and enable rapid treatment. B: Obtaining a full history is important but should not delay immediate oxygenation and IV access in a hypoxemic, tachycardic patient. C: Aspirin and nitroglycerin are for ischemic chest pain and are inappropriate first actions for suspected pulmonary embolism without provider assessment. D: Blood cultures and antibiotics address infection/sepsis and are not the priority for suspected PE withhypoxemia.

3. Correct Answer: D
Rationale: Pulmonary arterial obstruction from emboli creates areas of lung that are ventilated but not perfused (increased physiologic dead space), producing hypoxemia with a normal chest x-ray—consistent with this vignette. A: Bronchospasm causes airflow limitation and wheezing; exam notes clear lung sounds without wheeze. B: Alveolar consolidation (pneumonia) causes shunt physiology with radiographic opacities, not a normal CXR. C: Left ventricular failure leads to pulmonary edema with crackles and chest x-ray changes, which are not present.

4. Correct Answer: C
Rationale: The ABG shows alkalemia with low PaCO2 and normal-ish HCO3, indicating an acute respiratory alkalosis from hyperventilation; the low PaO2 indicates hypoxemia, which in context of sudden dyspnea supports pulmonary vascular compromise causing tachypnea and respiratory alkalosis. A: Metabolic alkalosis would have elevated HCO3; here HCO3 is near normal. B: Respiratory acidosis would show elevated PaCO2, not low. D: The values are not normal—PaO2 is low and acid–base status shows a primary respiratory alkalosis related to acute hyperventilation.

5. Correct Answer: C
Rationale: Unfractionated heparin is titrated using the activated partial thromboplastin time (aPTT); the nurse should monitor aPTT to achieve and maintain therapeutic anticoagulation. A: INR is used to monitor warfarin therapy, not unfractionated heparin titration. B: Platelet count is monitored for heparin-induced thrombocytopenia risk but not for dose titration. D: Serum creatinine guides dosing of some anticoagulants (e.g., LMWH or direct oral agents) but is not the primary test to titrate IV unfractionated heparin.

Clinical Vignette 4

A 17-year-old female presents to urgent care with 3 days of increasing lower abdominal pain and purulent vaginal discharge after a new sexual partner 6 weeks ago; she is sexually active and uses condoms inconsistently. She speaks Spanish at home and says her mother came with her; the mother remains in the room and interrupts answers. Vital signs show T 38.1°C, HR 96, BP 110/68. Pelvic exam reveals cervical motion tenderness and mucopurulent cervical discharge; a urine pregnancy test is negative. A nucleic acid amplification test (NAAT) for sexually transmitted infections is obtained. The patient appears alert, oriented, and able to answer questions coherently; she tells the nurse privately that she does not want her mother informed and requests treatment today. The mother asks to see the test results and offers to sign consent for antibiotics. The patient asks for Spanish language help but the mother offers to interpret; the nurse's computer shows no documented advance directive or power of attorney. No allergies are recorded.

Question 1: Based on the vignette, which condition is most likely causing this patient's symptoms?

- [A] Acute cystitis from a urinary tract infection
- [B] Pelvic inflammatory disease from an ascending sexually transmitted infection
- [C] Bacterial vaginosis causing malodorous discharge only
- [D] Ectopic pregnancy presenting with lower abdominal pain

Question 2: The mother demands to see the NAAT results and sign consent for treatment. Which is the nurse's best action, referencing the vignette?

- [A] Honor the patient's request for confidentiality, arrange treatment for the patient, and decline to disclose results to the mother without the patient's permission.
- [B] Share the results with the mother and obtain her written consent before treating the patient.
- [C] Refuse to treat because the patient is a minor and insist on parental consent before any antibiotics are given.
- [D] Ask the mother to step out and then withhold treatment until the provider explains the risks to both the patient and parent together.

Question 3: What pathophysiologic process most directly explains this patient's risk for future infertility if her condition is untreated?

- [A] Bacterial toxin–mediated destruction of ovarian follicles
- [B] Chronic endometrial hyperplasia preventing implantation
- [C] Reduced cervical mucus production leading to ascending infection
- [D] Inflammatory scarring and adhesions of the fallopian tubes impairing ovum transport

Question 4: Assuming the NAAT later returns positive for Chlamydia trachomatis and the patient is not pregnant, which antibiotic regimen is most appropriate for outpatient treatment?

- [A] Single-dose oral azithromycin 1 g
- [B] Intramuscular ceftriaxone alone
- [C] Oral doxycycline 100 mg twice daily for the recommended course
- [D] Oral metronidazole for bacterial vaginosis coverage

Question 5: The patient asks that her mother interpret for her in Spanish during counseling. According to best practice and the vignette details, what should the nurse do?

- [A] Allow the mother to interpret since she is present and fluent.
- [B] Arrange for a certified medical interpreter (in-person or phone/video) and document the interpreter's name/ID and mode.
- [C] Proceed in English because medical interpreters are not required for minors.
- [D] Use a smartphone translation app to save time and protect privacy.

ANSWERS

1. Correct Answer: B
Rationale: Cervical motion tenderness, mucopurulent discharge, fever, and recent new sexual partner are classic for an ascending STI causing pelvic inflammatory disease (PID). A. Acute cystitis usually causes dysuria and urinary frequency rather than cervical motion tenderness and mucopurulent discharge. C. Bacterial vaginosis typically causes homogenous discharge without fever or cervical motion tenderness. D. Ectopic pregnancy would have a positive pregnancy test and may present with unilateral pain or bleeding; the urine pregnancy test here is negative.

2. Correct Answer: A
Rationale: Many jurisdictions allow minors to consent to STI testing and treatment and confidentiality should be preserved; the vignette notes the patient is alert, requests privacy, and requests treatment—so the nurse should honor confidentiality and facilitate care. B. Disclosing without authorization breaches privacy/HIPAA principles and undermines access to care. C. Insisting on parental consent ignores minors' allowed consent for STI care and could delay needed treatment. D. Withholding treatment until a joint explanation occurs delays care and could harm the patient; the RN should escalate to the provider if clarification is needed but protect the patient's rights.

3. Correct Answer: D
Rationale: Untreated PID causes inflammatory damage with scarring and adhesions of the fallopian tubes, which impairs ovum transport and increases infertility and ectopic pregnancy risk. A. Bacterial toxins destroying ovarian follicles is not the primary mechanism of infertility in PID. B. Endometrial hyperplasia is unrelated to acute PID. C. Reduced cervical mucus is not the main pathophysiologic pathway leading to tubal infertility from ascending infection.

4. Correct Answer: C
Rationale: For nonpregnant patients with Chlamydia trachomatis, doxycycline 100 mg PO twice daily for the recommended course is an appropriate outpatient regimen. A. Single-dose azithromycin was used historically but doxycycline is now preferred in many guidelines for chlamydial infection. B. Ceftriaxone IM treats gonorrhea and is not sufficient alone for chlamydia. D. Metronidazole treats anaerobic infections/bacterial vaginosis, not chlamydia.

5. Correct Answer: B
Rationale: Use of a certified medical interpreter protects confidentiality, ensures accurate communication, and complies with best practice; the nurse should arrange an interpreter and document the interpreter's name/ID and mode per policy (vignette notes the patient requested Spanish help and the mother offered to interpret). A. Using the mother as interpreter risks breaches of confidentiality and is discouraged by standards of care. C. Proceeding in English when the patient needs interpretation is inappropriate and may impair informed decision-making. D. Smartphone apps are not an acceptable substitute for a certified medical interpreter for sensitive medical information.

Clinical Vignette 5

A 72-year-old man presents to the medical unit with a 2-day history of profuse watery diarrhea (about 6 stools/day), lower abdominal cramping, and low-grade fever; his family reports increasing fatigue and two episodes of brief confusion today. He was treated for a lower-extremity cellulitis with a 7-day course of clindamycin that finished 5 days ago; current medications include lisinopril and an albuterol inhaler, and he has no drug allergies. On exam he is alert but intermittently disoriented, T 38.1°C, HR 98, BP 132/78, and his abdomen is diffusely tender without rebound; perianal skin excoriation and a soiled gown are noted. Laboratory studies show WBC 14,200/mm3 with a left shift; basic metabolic panel is within baseline. The nurse reports visible loose stool on the bed linens and that hand sanitizer dispensers are available at the doorway. A stool specimen for testing has been ordered. There is no cough, vomiting, or recent travel; his wife, who cares for him at home, is currently well.

Question 1: Based on the vignette, which is the most likely cause of this patient's current symptoms?

- [A] Norovirus infection
- [B] Clostridioides difficile infection
- [C] Loperamide-induced ileus
- [D] Mesenteric ischemia

Question 2: Referencing the vignette, what is the nurse's single most important immediate action to reduce harm to other patients and staff?

- [A] Perform hand washing with soap and water, don gown and gloves, and place the patient on contact precautions in a private room.
- [B] Begin oral vancomycin empirically while awaiting stool test results.
- [C] Collect the ordered stool specimen first, then implement contact precautions.
- [D] Use alcohol-based hand rub and continue routine care, documenting the diarrhea.

Question 3: Which statement best explains why alcohol-based hand rubs are inadequate alone in preventing transmission in this scenario?

- [A] The organism produces a capsule that prevents alcohol penetration and requires heat inactivation.
- [B] The pathogen forms spores that are resistant to alcohol and can persist on surfaces, so soap and water plus sporicidal cleaning are required.
- [C] The infection is transmitted by large respiratory droplets that alcohol rubs do not neutralize on surfaces.
- [D] The causative organism is intracellular, requiring systemic antibiotics rather than surface disinfection.

Question 4: Which pharmacologic choice is most appropriate for initial treatment of this patient's likely infection, assuming a non-severe first episode?

- [A] Intravenous vancomycin
- [B] Oral metronidazole
- [C] Intravenous broad-spectrum cephalosporin
- [D] Oral vancomycin

Question 5: Considering ethics and infection-control priorities from the vignette, which action is most appropriate regarding room assignment and visitors?

- [A] Cohort the patient with another patient who is colonized with MRSA to conserve single rooms.
- [B] Place this patient in a room with an immunocompromised (neutropenic) patient to allow nursing visibility.
- [C] Permit all visitors, including those with mild respiratory symptoms, if they wear masks.
- [D] Place the patient in a private room on contact precautions and ask symptomatic visitors (diarrhea or vomiting)

ANSWERS

1. Correct Answer: B

Rationale: Recent clindamycin exposure, profuse watery diarrhea, fever, leukocytosis, and perianal excoriation are classic for C. difficile infection. A (norovirus) typically causes vomiting and rapid outbreaks and is less strongly associated with recent antibiotic exposure. C (loperamide-induced ileus) would present with decreased bowel sounds and constipation/abdominal distention rather than watery stools. D (mesenteric ischemia) causes severe pain out of proportion to exam and bloody stools, not this pattern following antibiotics.

2. Correct Answer: A

Rationale: The highest-priority immediate action is to stop further spread: perform soap-and-water hand hygiene (alcohol is insufficient for spores), don gown and gloves, and implement contact precautions in a private room while handling soiled linens appropriately. B (start oral vancomycin) is important for treatment but not the first immediate safety action to prevent transmission. C (collect stool first) is reasonable for diagnostics, but containment and hand hygiene should occur immediately to prevent exposure. D (use alcohol rub and continue routine care) is incorrect because alcohol does not reliably remove C. difficile spores.

3. Correct Answer: B

Rationale: C. difficile forms spores that resist alcohol and persist on surfaces; therefore soap and water for hand hygiene and sporicidal environmental cleaning are required. A is incorrect—resistance is due to spores, not a capsule or heat requirement. C is incorrect because transmission is contact with spores, not respiratory droplets. D is incorrect because the organism is not primarily an intracellular pathogen; infection prevention focuses on breaking contact transmission.

4. Correct Answer: D

Rationale: For an initial, non-severe episode of C. difficile, oral vancomycin is appropriate because it achieves therapeutic concentrations in the gut lumen. A (IV vancomycin) does not reach adequate intestinal levels. B (oral metronidazole) is no longer first-line for initial C. difficile in most guidelines. C (IV broad-spectrum cephalosporin) could worsen C. difficile and is not a treatment.

5. Correct Answer: D

Rationale: The ethical and infection-control priority is to prevent exposing others—place the patient in a private room with contact precautions and restrict symptomatic visitors, especially those with diarrhea or vomiting. A (cohorting with MRSA) is inappropriate because organisms differ and cohorting is only for the same organism with no conflicting risks. B (rooming with an immunocompromised patient) is dangerous because immunocompromised patients are highly susceptible to harm. C (allow symptomatic visitors with masks) is inappropriate—visitors with gastroenteritis symptoms should be excluded to prevent spread.

Clinical Vignette 6

A 45-year-old man presents with 3 months of progressive cough, nightly drenching sweats, 20-lb unintentional weight loss, and 2 episodes of blood-tinged sputum; history includes recent homelessness, prior incarceration, and smoking ½ pack/day. He lives in a crowded shelter, takes no chronic medications, and has no drug allergies. Exam: T 38.2°C, HR 96, RR 22, SpO_2 95% RA; decreased breath sounds and coarse crackles in the right upper lung. CXR shows a cavitary right upper lobe lesion. In the ED he was initially placed in a curtained bay with staff wearing surgical masks only; sputum AFB is ordered, and CT chest is planned. He is anxious about infecting others and asks how staff will protect themselves and other patients.

Question 1: Based on the vignette, which is the most likely diagnosis for this patient's pulmonary process?

[A] Community-acquired lobar pneumonia from Streptococcus pneumoniae
[B] Pulmonary tuberculosis (Mycobacterium tuberculosis)
[C] Primary lung malignancy with cavitation
[D] Pulmonary embolism with infarction

Question 2: You are the RN who first encounters this patient in the ED. What is the most appropriate immediate infection-control action?

[A] Place a surgical mask on the patient and continue current staff use of surgical masks at the doorway.
[B] Don gown and gloves only and place a sign for contact precautions.
[C] Keep the door open for observation but post droplet precaution signage.
[D] Immediately place the patient in an airborne infection isolation room (negative pressure) with the door closed and staff use fit-tested N95 or higher respirators; mask the patient if transport is necessary.

Question 3: Which statement best describes the primary mode of transmission for the suspected organism in this vignette?

[A] Transmission occurs mainly by large respiratory droplets that fall out within 3 feet of the source and require surgical masks only.
[B] Transmission is primarily via direct contact with contaminated surfaces and hands, requiring gown and gloves.
[C] Transmission occurs via small droplet nuclei that remain suspended in the air and can be inhaled at a distance, requiring airborne precautions and respirators.
[D] Transmission is vector-borne via arthropods and not impacted by respiratory PPE.

Question 4: If the patient is confirmed to have active pulmonary tuberculosis, which first-line antitubercular medication is most associated with peripheral neuropathy that is prevented by prescribing pyridoxine (vitamin B6)?

[A] Rifampin
[B] Ethambutol
[C] Pyrazinamide
[D] Isoniazid

Question 5: During initial triage you discover the ED nurse briefly entered the open bay without an N95 and had a torn glove while drawing blood; she remained in the area for 10 minutes before a supervisor moved the patient to airborne isolation. What is the nurse's best next action regarding the potential exposure?

[A] Stop the exposure activity, perform hand hygiene, report the exposure to occupational health immediately, and follow institutional protocols for baseline testing and follow-up.
[B] Continue working without reporting since no visible mucus splashed onto mucous membranes and she feels well.
[C] Self-quarantine at home for 2 weeks without notifying the employer unless symptoms develop.
[D] Dispose of the torn glove, finish the shift, and advise the patient to inform his shelter contacts instead of reporting the staff exposure.

ANSWERS

1. Correct Answer: B

Rationale: The vignette gives classic TB cues: chronic cough, night sweats, significant weight loss, hemoptysis, history of homelessness/incarceration (risk factors), and a right upper lobe cavitary lesion on chest x-ray—these strongly suggest pulmonary tuberculosis. A (community-acquired lobar pneumonia) typically presents more acutely, often with lobar consolidation rather than a chronic course and cavitation over months. C (lung malignancy) can cavitate but is less likely with systemic night sweats and the social/epidemiologic risk factors; imaging and biopsy would be needed to differentiate. D (pulmonary embolism) usually presents acutely with pleuritic chest pain, sudden dyspnea, and may show wedge infarct—not a months-long history with cavitation and night sweats.

2. Correct Answer: D

Rationale: For suspected pulmonary TB the chapter directs immediate airborne precautions: place the patient in a negative-pressure airborne infection isolation room with the door closed and staff must use fit-tested N95 or higher respirators; mask the patient if they must be transported. A (surgical mask only) is inadequate for airborne organisms. B (gown and gloves/contact) addresses contact spread but misses the airborne route. C (keeping the door open and droplet signage) violates airborne-room requirements and under-protects staff; doors must remain closed and respirators used.

3. Correct Answer: C

Rationale: Mycobacterium tuberculosis spreads via small droplet nuclei that can remain suspended in the air and be inhaled at a distance; this is the definition of airborne transmission, requiring respirators and negative-pressure rooms. A describes droplet transmission (large droplets)—not correct for TB. B describes contact transmission and is more relevant to MRSA, VRE, or B. difficile (with contact plus). D is unrelated.

4. Correct Answer: D

Rationale: Isoniazid commonly causes peripheral neuropathy by interfering with pyridoxine metabolism; prophylactic pyridoxine (vitamin B6) is given to reduce this risk. A (rifampin) causes hepatotoxicity and orange discoloration of bodily fluids but is not the classic neuropathy drug. B (ethambutol) is associated with optic neuritis and color-vision changes. C (pyrazinamide) can cause hyperuricemia and hepatotoxicity.

5. Correct Answer: A

Rationale: The chapter emphasizes stopping immediately after a PPE breach, performing hand hygiene, and promptly reporting exposures to occupational health for assessment, baseline testing, and follow-up (e.g., TB testing and possible chest x-ray). B (doing nothing) is unsafe and contrary to exposure protocols. C (self-quarantine without notifying employer) is inappropriate and defeats institutional reporting and follow-up processes. D (finishing the shift and shifting responsibility to the patient) neglects staff safety procedures and proper documentation/reporting.

CHAPTER 3

Client Needs II — Health Promotion & Maintenance

3.1 Growth & Development (Milestones + Red Flags)

Know how normal development unfolds so you can spot when it doesn't. Skills build cephalocaudally (head to toe) and proximodistally (center to periphery) and progress from simple reflexes to complex, purposeful actions. Normal has wide ranges, but loss of any previously gained skill (regression) is always concerning and requires prompt evaluation. Use the age bands below to compare what you observe to what's expected, surface red flags fast, and choose safe next steps.

Newborn–2 months:

Must-know: strong rooting/suck; brief head lift when prone; tracks to midline; coos; social smile emerges by 6–8 weeks.
Red flags: absent startle; no visual tracking; no social smile by 2 months; absent or asymmetric Moro.

4 months:

Must-know: rolls front to back; brings hands to midline; laughs; good head control without lag.
Red flags: persistent head lag; not rolling by 6 months.

6 months:

Must-know: rolls both ways; sits with support; reaches and transfers objects hand-to-hand; babbles (reduplicative sounds); emerging stranger anxiety.
Red flags: no babbling; not reaching/transferring; hypotonia or "floppy" infant.

9 months:

Must-know: sits without support; crawls/creeps; pulls to stand; immature (raking) pincer; object permanence; responds to name; waves bye-bye.
Red flags: not sitting independently; no consonant sounds; no back-and-forth sounds/gestures (poor social reciprocity).

12 months:

Must-know: cruises or walks; mature pincer grasp; 1–3 single words with meaning; follows 1-step command with gesture; drinks from a cup.
Red flags: not pulling to stand; not bearing weight; no pincer grasp; no single words or pointing to request.

15 months:

Must-know: walks well; scribbles spontaneously; 3–5 words; identifies/points to one body part.
Red flags: not walking by 18 months; persistent hand fisting beyond infancy (tone/neuromotor concern).

18 months:

Must-know: runs; stacks 3–4 blocks; uses spoon with some spill; 10–25+ words; parallel play; begins pretend (feeding doll).
Red flags: no purposeful words; no imitation or pretend play; persistent toe-walking.

24 months (2 years):

Must-know: stairs up/down with two feet per step; jumps; 2-word phrases; ≥50 words; 50% intelligible speech; 6-block tower; early toilet readiness signs.
Red flags: no two-word phrases; <50 words; not following simple commands; no interest in other children.

3 years:

Must-know: pedals tricycle; stairs with alternating feet; 3-word sentences; 75% intelligible; copies circle; daytime toilet trained (most).
Red flags: speech largely unintelligible; frequent falls/clumsiness; no pretend play.

4 years:

Must-know: hops on one foot; balances briefly; 100% intelligible speech; tells stories; copies cross/square; cooperative play with peers.
Red flags: cannot hop or draw simple shapes; lack of peer interaction.

5 years:

Must-know: skips; ties basic knots; copies triangle; prints some letters/numbers; understands and follows rules/games.
Red flags: persistent day-and-night enuresis; severe speech articulation issues.

Growth and dentition benchmarks you must be able to recall on test day include weight doubling by 4–6 months, tripling by 12 months, and quadrupling by 24–30 months. Length increases by about 50% by 12 months and doubles (from birth) by around 4 years. Head growth is fastest in the first year; the posterior fontanel closes by about 2 months and the anterior fontanel by 12–18 months. The first tooth usually erupts around 6 months, and all 20 primary teeth are present by about 30 months. When presented with vignettes about feeding, teething discomfort, or fontanel status, these numbers guide safe counseling and recognition of abnormal patterns such as macrocephaly or microcephaly or delayed dentition.

Pubertal timing also shows up in screening and anticipatory guidance items. For girls, breast budding (thelarche) typically begins between 8 and 13 years; menarche follows about 2–3 years later (average ~12.5 years). Red flags are breast development before age 8 (precocious) or no breast development by 13 (delayed). For boys, testicular enlargement (first sign of puberty) normally occurs between 9 and 14 years; <9 suggests precocious puberty and no testicular enlargement by 14 suggests delayed puberty. On the NCLEX, the safe response is to recognize out-of-range onset, provide neutral anticipatory guidance, and refer for endocrine evaluation when indicated.

Social development and play evolve in predictable stages that also inform safety counseling. Infants engage in solitary play and are at risk for rolling off surfaces as early as 4 months; new mobility (rolling, sitting, crawling) dramatically increases fall and aspiration risk, so crib and surface safety is essential. Toddlers practice parallel play and explore autonomously; with the pincer grasp emerging around 9–12 months, choking risk peaks as they pick up small objects, and childproofing (outlets, cabinets, stairs) becomes critical. Preschoolers shift to associative and then cooperative play; they share, follow rules, and use wheeled toys—helmet use and supervision around streets and water are high-yield anticipatory guidance points. School-age children fully engage in team-based cooperative play and organized sports, raising the need for sport-specific safety.

High-yield cues for autism spectrum and developmental disorders should trigger immediate standardized screening and referral. Concerning signs include lack of babbling, pointing, or other gestures by 12 months; no single words by 15 months; no two-word spontaneous phrases by 24 months; poor eye contact, lack of joint attention, or absence of back-and-forth social interaction; and any regression in language or social skills at any age. Also note no response to name by 9–12 months can suggest hearing loss or social communication issues and warrants audiology evaluation. Your safe action is to avoid "watchful waiting" when these are present: document specific behaviors and initiate screening and referral to early intervention.

Some physical findings are normal variants and should not be pathologized on exam questions. Bowlegs (genu varum) are common until about 2 years, and knock-knees (genu valgum) peak around 3–4 years; infants and toddlers naturally have a wide-based gait as they learn to walk. In contrast, early hand dominance before 18 months, persistent toe-walking, asymmetric limb use or movement, and loss of milestones are concerning and should prompt neurologic evaluation for conditions like cerebral palsy or hemiparesis.

NGN-ready nursing actions tie observation to priority and response. Recognize by comparing observed skills to the age-band anchors above and noting red flags, growth deviations, and any regression. Always consider safety linked to new skills, such as falls with rolling or stairs use, or choking with the pincer grasp. Prioritize conditions that can harm quickly: regression, focal neurologic signs or abnormal tone, failure to thrive or crossing down growth percentiles, suspected abuse/neglect, and dehydration in infants with vomiting/diarrhea. Respond by notifying the provider of specific, objective findings; initiating or completing developmental screening tools as appropriate for age; arranging or encouraging early intervention and audiology/vision assessments when cues point to communication or sensory deficits; reinforcing targeted anticipatory guidance such as anchoring furniture for climbers, using rear-facing car seats per current safety guidelines, advancing textures appropriately with new oral-motor skills, and supervising near water; and documenting concrete behaviors (e.g., "no response to name," "no words," "does not point") rather than judgments.

Quick recall pearls consolidate what you'll most often retrieve under time pressure:

- One year is for one-word sentences and one-step commands; two years for two-word phrases and two-step commands; three years for tricycle and three-word sentences.
- Think "pincer at 1," "stairs alternate at 3," "hop at 4," "skip at 5."
- Weight doubles by 4–6 months, triples by 12 months, and quadruples by 24–30 months; length is up 50% at 12 months and doubles by about 4 years.
- Posterior fontanel closes around 2 months; anterior by 12–18 months.
- First tooth at about 6 months; full primary dentition by 30 months.

Use the age bands below as your rapid scan for normal vs concerning patterns and the safest next action.

- Newborn–2 months: rooting/suck; brief head lift; midline tracking; coos; social smile by 6–8 weeks. Red flags: no startle or tracking; no smile by 2 months; absent/asymmetric Moro.
- 4 months: rolls front to back; hands to midline; laughs; good head control. Red flags: head lag; not rolling by 6 months.
- 6 months: rolls both ways; sits with support; transfers objects; babbles; stranger anxiety begins. Red flags: no babbling; no reaching/transferring; hypotonia.
- 9 months: sits without support; crawls/creeps; pulls to stand; immature pincer; object permanence; responds to name. Red flags: not sitting; no consonants; no reciprocal sounds/gestures.
- 12 months: cruises/walks; mature pincer; 1–3 words; follows 1-step command with gesture; drinks from cup. Red flags: not pulling to stand; not bearing weight; no pincer; no single words or pointing.
- 15 months: walks well; scribbles; 3–5 words; points to body parts. Red flags: not walking by 18 months; persistent hand fisting.
- 18 months: runs; 3–4 block tower; 10–25+ words; parallel play; uses spoon. Red flags: no purposeful words; no imitation/pretend; persistent toe-walking.
- 24 months: stairs two feet/step; jumps; 2-word phrases; 50+ words; 50% intelligible; 6-block tower; toilet readiness starts. Red flags: no two-word phrases; <50 words; not following simple commands; no interest in others.
- 3 years: tricycle; stairs alternating feet; 3-word sentences; 75% intelligible; copies circle; daytime toilet trained. Red flags: speech mostly unintelligible; frequent falls; no pretend play.

- 4 years: hops; balances; 100% intelligible; tells stories; copies cross/square; cooperative play. Red flags: cannot hop/draw simple shapes; lacks peer interaction.
- 5 years: skips; ties basic knots; copies triangle; prints some letters; understands rules/games. Red flags: persistent day/night enuresis; severe articulation problems.

When a test item presents a child who is outside these anchors, select responses that safeguard the child now and initiate the right evaluation. For instance, a 9-month-old who is not sitting independently or not babbling needs developmental screening and further assessment rather than reassurance alone. A new pincer grasp calls for revised feeding guidance to reduce choking, and a toddler climbing and using stairs calls for environmental safety and supervision counseling. Combine milestone mastery with growth trajectories and pubertal timing to recognize normal variation while catching what cannot be missed.

3.1.1 Infant to Adolescent Highlights

Think in age bands, know what should be happening, and be ready to teach safety while spotting what needs action. Use developmental cues to decide if reassurance, teaching, screening, or referral is the first safe RN move.

From birth through 12 months, the newborn/infant period is characterized by rapid physical and neurologic growth. Primitive reflexes are present and then integrate in predictable windows: the Moro startle and rooting typically disappear by about 4 months; palmar grasp by 5–6 months; tonic neck ("fencer") by around 6 months; plantar grasp by 9–12 months. A Babinski response (dorsiflex of big toe, fanning) can be normal up to about 12–24 months; persistence beyond toddlerhood or asymmetry at any time warrants evaluation. Weight should double by 6 months and triple by 12 months; length increases about 50% by the end of the first year, and head growth is brisk early on. The posterior fontanel closes by 2–3 months; the anterior fontanel closes by 12–18 months. The first tooth usually erupts around 6 months (commonly lower central incisors), and several incisors are often present by the end of the first year.

Motor development proceeds cephalocaudally and proximodistally. Expect good head control by 3–4 months, rolling front-to-back by about 4–5 months and back-to-front by 5–6 months, sitting unsupported by 8–9 months, crawling/creeping around 6–9 months, pulling to stand by 9–10 months, cruising by 10–12 months, and a first independent step near 12 months. Fine motor work evolves from hands fisted in the newborn to purposeful reaching by 4 months, transferring objects hand-to-hand by around 6 months, raking grasp at about 6–7 months, and immature to mature pincer grasp between 9–12 months. Language moves from cooing around 2 months to babbling consonant-vowel strings by 6 months. By 9 months, many infants say "mama/dada" nonspecifically and understand "no"; by 12 months, expect a first meaningful word and simple gestures like waving or pointing. Socially, a social smile emerges around 6 weeks–2 months, stranger anxiety commonly appears between 6–9 months, and separation anxiety emerges around 9–18 months as object permanence (realizing that people and things still exist when out of sight) develops around 8–12 months.

Anticipatory guidance for infants prioritizes safety and nutrition. Teach safe sleep every time: on the back, in a firm, empty crib; no blankets, bumpers, or bed-sharing. Car seats are rear-facing in the back seat as long as possible per seat limits, at least through age 2. Prevent choking by avoiding small hard foods (whole nuts, popcorn, whole grapes, hot dog coins) and by supervising feeds and play; keep small objects, batteries, and magnets out of reach. Bathe with constant touch supervision; set water heaters to around 49°C/120°F to prevent scald burns. Introduce solids when developmentally ready, typically near 6 months: sits with support, good head control, diminished tongue-thrust, shows interest. Offer iron-rich options; introduce common allergens (peanut, egg) during infancy if no contraindications and as culturally practiced. Breastfed infants need 400 IU/day vitamin D; consider iron supplementation for exclusively breastfed infants beyond 4 months if intake is insufficient. Avoid cow's milk until 12 months; avoid honey until 12 months to prevent botulism.

Toddlers (1–3 years) consolidate mobility and language and assert autonomy. Most walk by 12–15 months, run around 18 months, climb furniture, and manage stairs with a hand or railing by about 18–24 months; they jump with both feet around age 2 and kick or throw a ball overhead near 18–24 months. Fine motor skills refine the pincer;

they scribble by 15 months, stack 2–3 blocks at 15 months and 6 or more by 2 years, turn pages, and use a spoon with less spilling by 2 years. Language shows a burst: 10–25 words by 18 months, 50+ words and two-word phrases by age 2; receptive language outpaces expressive. Socially, toddlers engage in parallel play and display ritualism and negativism as they develop autonomy. Toilet-training readiness (often 18–24+ months) includes awareness of wet vs dry, ability to follow simple commands, staying dry for about 2 hours, pulling pants up/down, and interest in the toilet; readiness drives success more than age. Night dryness often lags behind day.

Toddler anticipatory guidance focuses on hazards and boundaries. Prevent poisoning by locking up medications and chemicals and using child-resistant packaging; never call medicine "candy." Be alert for lead exposure in older housing; teach wet-mopping for dust, handwashing, and not to let children chew painted surfaces; refer for screening per risk. Drowning risk is high—constant, arm's-length supervision around tubs, buckets, and any water; use toilet and door locks and pool barriers. Car seats transition to forward-facing with a harness in the back seat after outgrowing the rear-facing limits; keep harnessed as long as possible. Childproof the home: secure furniture, use stair gates and outlet covers, and keep hot liquids and cords out of reach. Guide tantrums with calm consistency, clear limits, and brief time-outs; reinforce positive behaviors. Limit milk to about 16–24 oz/day to prevent iron deficiency, and limit juice (if given at all) to 4 oz/day; brush teeth twice daily with a smear/pea-sized fluoride toothpaste depending on age.

Preschoolers (3–5 years) show improved coordination, imagination, and language. Gross motor abilities include pedaling a tricycle around age 3, jumping and hopping, and later skipping by 5. They can balance briefly on one foot, throw and catch a ball, and climb well. Fine motor advances include copying a circle at 3, a cross around 4, and more complex shapes by 5; by 4–5, they can draw a person with several parts and use scissors with supervision. Language jumps to 3–4 word sentences, and speech becomes increasingly intelligible to strangers—about 75% at age 3 and near-complete by 4. Magical thinking, imaginary friends, and vivid fears are developmentally normal; play becomes more cooperative with sharing and turn-taking. Encourage routines, choices, and simple responsibilities to bolster initiative.

Preschooler health teaching includes continuing proper car restraint—remain in a forward-facing harness until outgrown, then use a booster; always ride in the back seat. Helmets are required for bikes, scooters, and skateboards; teach safe street-crossing and driveway safety. Begin body safety rules: correct anatomical terms, private parts, safe vs unsafe touch, and the rule that secrets about bodies are never kept. Review "stranger safety" with nuance: focus on safe adults and using code words for pickups. Guide screen time to high-quality content and about an hour per day, and keep screens out of bedrooms. Continue water safety, firearm safety (lock, separate firearm and ammunition), and supervision at playgrounds.

School-age children (6–12 years) grow steadily (about 2–3 inches/year, 4–7 lb/year), lose primary teeth starting around 6 years, and improve strength and coordination, making organized sports appropriate with correct protective gear. Cognitively they enter concrete operations: understand conservation, categories, and cause-effect; socially, peers and rules matter, and they thrive on mastery and industry. Encourage reading, chores, and goal-setting; watch for bullying and school difficulties early.

For school-age anticipatory guidance, emphasize 60 minutes of daily physical activity, balanced nutrition with family meals, and adequate sleep (often 9–12 hours). Screen time should be balanced and supervised with family media plans and internet safety (privacy, cyberbullying awareness). Support dental care with fluoride, sealants, and mouthguards for sports. Reinforce booster seats until seat belts fit properly—usually until 4'9" and 8–12 years—and continue teaching road, bike, and sports safety. Teach about pubertal changes before they happen to reduce anxiety.

Adolescence (12–18 years) brings puberty, rapid growth, abstract thought, and identity formation. Puberty begins earlier for girls (often 8–13 years) than boys (9–14 years). In girls, the usual sequence is thelarche (breast budding) first, then pubic/axillary hair, a growth spurt, and menarche about 2–2.5 years after thelarche. In boys, testicular enlargement is first, followed by pubic hair, penile enlargement, voice change, and later a peak growth spurt. Cognitively, formal operations emerge with improved reasoning but variable risk assessment; peers and autonomy are powerful drivers of behavior. The RN should normalize pubertal changes, support healthy identity development, and screen for risk behaviors and mental health concerns with confidential, respectful questioning and clear safety limits.

Adolescent anticipatory guidance includes layered safety: driving (seat belts always, no impaired or distracted driving, graduated license rules), sports and concussion awareness, substance use prevention and brief intervention, safe sex basics with condoms and STI information, and informed discussions about consent and healthy relationships. Address sleep (8–10 hours), nutrition and activity, and media/social media hygiene. Respect privacy; in many jurisdictions, adolescents can consent to STI services, contraception, and certain mental health or substance use care. Clarify confidentiality limits up front: safety concerns like suicidal ideation or abuse require disclosure to protect the teen.

Across all ages, red flags signal the need to recognize, prioritize, and act. No social smile by about 2 months, persistent or asymmetric primitive reflexes past their expected integration, not rolling by around 6 months, not sitting by 8–9 months, no babbling by 6–9 months, no gesturing or pointing by 12 months, no pincer grasp by 12 months, not walking by 18 months, no single words by 15 months, no two-word phrases by 2 years, speech that is less than 50% intelligible at age 2, or any loss of previously acquired skills should prompt further assessment. Other cues include extreme or persistent behavioral dysregulation, lack of joint attention, growth faltering, feeding problems, signs of neglect or abuse, and for adolescents, suicidal ideation, self-harm, significant weight loss or bradycardia suggestive of an eating disorder, substance use, or traumatic stress. First actions include validating caregiver concerns, collecting more cues (developmental history, growth chart, family/medical history), screening (vision, hearing, lead risk, developmental tools), ensuring immediate safety, and notifying the provider for evaluation and referral (early intervention, audiology, speech-language pathology, behavioral health) as indicated.

Integrating clinical judgment at the bedside often means distinguishing normal variants from urgent findings. Consider a 10-month-old who pulls to stand and cruises along furniture but does not crawl. Cue collection shows standing and cruising, transferring objects, babbling, and pointing to request. Analysis: gross motor is progressing; some infants skip crawling. Recognize that the child is mobile by another route and meeting other milestones. The priority is parent education and environmental safety (gates, furniture anchoring, fall prevention), not referral. The first action is to reassure and teach childproofing. Evaluation is met when caregivers verbalize safety steps and routine follow-up confirms continued progress, such as independent steps around 12 months.

Contrast that with a 24-month-old with fewer than 10 spoken words and no two-word phrases. Cues include limited expressive vocabulary, poor speech intelligibility, and lack of pointing or joint attention. Analysis: this exceeds a normal variation; by age 2, children typically use two-word phrases and have at least 50 words, with speech about 50% intelligible. Priority is developmental and hearing evaluation. The first action is to screen hearing formally and refer to the provider for early intervention and speech-language pathology; provide communication strategies (read daily, expand the child's attempts, limit passive screen time). Evaluation is met when audiology is completed and therapy initiated, with monitored gains over time.

A preschool case can test judgment around imaginative play. A 4-year-old has an imaginary friend and fears of monsters, sleeps with a night-light, and draws a person with four parts. These are normal for magical thinking. The appropriate response is reassurance and guidance: validate fears, use routines, and avoid punitive dismissal. However, the same age child with persistent, frightening voices commanding harm, regression in toileting, and disclosures suggestive of trauma shifts priority to safety and urgent mental health referral; the first action is to ensure the child is safe, follow mandatory reporting laws if abuse is suspected, and notify the provider.

For adolescents, assess risk with concrete safety steps. A 16-year-old reports low mood, social withdrawal, and "sometimes I wish I wouldn't wake up." This is a red flag for suicidal ideation. Priority is immediate safety: stay with the patient, conduct a brief suicide risk assessment per policy, remove lethal means if present, notify the provider, and arrange urgent mental health evaluation. Confidentiality is maintained within safety limits; tell the teen what must be shared and why.

In testing scenarios, keep high-yield pearls at hand. Infant weight typically doubles by 6 months and triples by 12 months; stranger anxiety commonly appears at 6–9 months; separation anxiety follows as object permanence emerges. The social smile by about 2 months is expected; absence prompts screening. Primitive reflexes should integrate on time; persistence suggests neurologic issues. For language, the "speech intelligibility rule of fours" helps: at age 2, speech is about 50% intelligible to strangers; at 3, about 75%; by 4, nearly 100%. Toilet training hinges on readiness signs rather than age; night continence may not be reliable until about 5–7 years, so nocturnal enuresis in early school years can be normal. Imaginary friends and magical thinking are normal in preschoolers and are not psychosis. Car seat safety is strict: rear-facing as long as possible, then forward-facing with a harness, then booster until the seat belt fits properly—always in the back seat. For infants, teach safe sleep and choking prevention; for toddlers, emphasize poisoning, lead, drowning prevention, and consistent discipline; for preschoolers, continue restraints and helmets and introduce body-safety rules; for school-age children, add sports safety, bullying, internet privacy, sleep, and nutrition; and for adolescents, ensure conversations about driving, substances, sexual health with condoms, mental health, and confidentiality.

When you see developmental concerns on the NCLEX, think like a safety-first RN using the clinical judgment model: recognize the cue set (age, milestone gaps, concerning behaviors), analyze whether it's within normal variance, set the priority (urgent safety vs teaching vs routine referral), take the first safe action (teach, screen, notify, refer), and evaluate by confirming understanding and follow-up.

3.1.2 Older Adult Changes (What's Tested)

On the NCLEX, older adult content centers on distinguishing expected age-related changes from signs of illness, then acting early to prevent complications. Read each cue for "sudden change," consider common geriatric syndromes (delirium, falls, functional decline, weight loss), review medications and hydration, and implement low-risk, safety-first interventions while you investigate reversible causes. Normal aging happens; it is not synonymous with disease. Your job is to know which findings are benign and which require immediate assessment or escalation.

Starting with neurocognition, expect slower processing speed and mild forgetfulness that does not impair social or occupational function. That is not the same as dementia, a chronic, progressive decline with impairment in complex tasks and memory that unfolds over months to years. Depression can masquerade as cognitive decline; look for anergia, anhedonia, sleep/appetite changes, and depressive affect, and remember that older adults may emphasize somatic complaints. Delirium, by contrast, is acute, fluctuating inattention and altered cognition that often follows infection, pain, constipation, urinary retention, hypoxia, dehydration, or medication effects (especially anticholinergics, benzodiazepines, opioids, and polypharmacy). First actions when cognition changes: obtain vital signs with oxygen saturation; ensure airway and oxygenation; check blood glucose if available; screen for delirium using a tool such as the CAM; review the medication list including OTC and herbals; assess for UTI, constipation, urinary retention, pain, hypoxia, and dehydration; and institute safety measures (supervision, low bed, frequent reorientation, ensure glasses and hearing aids are in place). Escalate promptly if there is fever or hypothermia, hypotension, hypoxia, focal neurologic deficit, or new-onset agitation with threats to safety.

Age-related sensory changes commonly include presbycusis (loss of high-frequency hearing) and presbyopia (near-vision difficulty), along with reduced contrast sensitivity and glare tolerance. Communicate in a lower-pitched voice, face the patient so they can read lips/facial cues, reduce background noise, and ensure adequate lighting without glare. Offer large-print materials and verify understanding with teach-back. Sudden vision loss or a curtain-like shadow suggests retinal detachment; acute eye pain with halos around lights suggests acute angle-closure glaucoma—both are time-sensitive emergencies. Unilateral sudden hearing loss can indicate cerumen impaction or, more rarely, a neurologic event; assess promptly and do not assume it is "just aging."

Cardiovascular changes include reduced baroreflex sensitivity and vascular stiffness. Orthostatic hypotension is common and increases fall risk; many older adults also have isolated systolic hypertension. Assess orthostatics correctly (after 5 minutes supine, then standing at 1 and 3 minutes) and interpret a drop of at least 20 mm Hg systolic or 10 mm Hg diastolic, or symptomatic lightheadedness, as abnormal. Intervene with slow position changes, hydration if not contraindicated, compressive stockings if ordered, medication review (antihypertensives, diuretics, alpha blockers, nitrates, psychoactive agents), and fall precautions. Recognize atypical myocardial infarction presentations: dyspnea, fatigue, syncope, new confusion, nausea/epigastric pain, or a vague "not feeling right" may be more common than crushing chest pain. Treat syncope, chest discomfort, hypotension with new confusion, or new arrhythmias as red flags; obtain vital signs, oxygen, a 12-lead ECG if available, and notify the provider.

Respiratory aging features decreased chest wall compliance, diminished cough and gag reflexes, and weaker respiratory muscles, all of which increase the risk of infection and aspiration. Preventive nursing actions make a difference: encourage incentive spirometry and coughing/deep breathing postoperatively, mobilize early, keep the head of bed elevated especially during and after meals, and perform meticulous oral care to reduce aspiration pneumonia risk. Be alert to atypical presentations; fever may be absent in sepsis, and the first clue may be tachypnea, hypoxia, or confusion. Treat respiratory rate over 30, oxygen saturation below 90% on room air, new-onset confusion, or a productive cough with systemic symptoms as urgent; apply oxygen per protocol, obtain vitals and lung assessment, and notify the provider.

With renal and hepatic function, the key test concept is that creatinine alone can look deceptively "normal" due to lower muscle mass; use estimated GFR to judge clearance. Hepatic metabolism also slows, raising the risk for drug accumulation and adverse effects. Conduct routine polypharmacy reviews, remove duplications and high-risk agents from the Beers Criteria when possible (benzodiazepines, anticholinergics like diphenhydramine, certain hypnotics, meperidine, some antipsychotics), and apply "start low, go slow" dosing. Monitor high-alert medications closely: bradyarrhythmias or visual changes with digoxin, bleeding with anticoagulants, oversedation with opioids or benzodiazepines, and delirium with anticholinergic burden. Any new delirium, a fall, bradycardia, or unexplained bleeding are red flags that warrant immediate reassessment of medications and labs.

Endocrine and thermoregulation changes include impaired glucose tolerance and blunted febrile responses. Hypoglycemia often presents with confusion rather than adrenergic symptoms; prioritize blood glucose checks with altered mental status. Maintain a warm environment and layered clothing, as older adults are more susceptible to hypothermia, which can be a manifestation of infection or endocrine dysfunction. Do not rule out infection in the absence of fever; look for functional decline, tachypnea, tachycardia, hypotension, or leukocytosis.

Musculoskeletal and skin changes include sarcopenia, decreased joint flexibility, kyphosis, and osteopenia/osteoporosis. Skin becomes thinner and more fragile with reduced subcutaneous fat and perfusion, elevating pressure-injury risk. Nursing priorities are fall prevention and skin protection. Encourage weight-bearing exercise as tolerated, adequate dietary calcium and vitamin D, safe footwear with non-slip soles, proper use of assistive devices, and home/environment modifications. Reposition at least every two hours for immobile patients, use pressure-redistributing surfaces, and inspect bony prominences daily. Device-related pressure points (nasal cannula, masks, splints) deserve special attention. Suspect a hip fracture when a patient reports hip pain with the leg shortened and externally rotated—this is an urgent situation requiring immobilization and prompt provider notification. Stageable pressure injuries, especially stage 2 or greater, are red flags and require a comprehensive plan including pressure relief, moisture management, nutritional optimization, and wound care consultation.

Gastrointestinal, nutrition, and oral health changes include slower GI motility, reduced taste and smell, dentition problems, and a diminished thirst drive. These contribute to constipation, poor intake, dehydration, and weight loss. Address modifiable causes: add fiber and fluids if not contraindicated, increase physical activity, review and rationalize constipating medications (opioids, anticholinergics, iron), and implement prophylactic bowel regimens with opioids (stimulant plus stool softener, not stool softener alone). Provide oral care and ensure well-fitting dentures to improve intake. Screen for dysphagia—coughing or choking with meals, wet/gurgly voice, or recurrent pneumonia are warning signs; keep the patient upright during meals and 30–60 minutes after, consider a speech-language pathology referral, and modify diet/liquids as recommended. Unintended weight loss is a red flag for malignancy, depression, social determinants (food insecurity), or dysphagia; assess promptly and involve a dietitian.

Genitourinary changes include benign prostatic hyperplasia in men and pelvic floor weakness in women, leading to urinary symptoms and varied incontinence types. Differentiate urge incontinence (overactive detrusor with sudden urge), stress incontinence (leakage with cough/sneeze/lifting), overflow (retention with dribbling from obstruction or weak detrusor), and functional incontinence (mobility or cognitive barriers). First-line management is nonpharmacologic: bladder training, pelvic floor (Kegel) exercises, scheduled toileting, and timing fluids earlier in the day while avoiding dehydration. Avoid indwelling catheters unless there is acute retention, urinary obstruction, strict monitoring of output in critical illness, or for end-of-life comfort; use the least invasive option, such as external catheters, when appropriate. Acute urinary retention and delirium from UTI or dehydration are red flags; assess bladder volume, obtain a urinalysis according to symptoms and facility policy, relieve retention per protocol, and hydrate as indicated.

Sleep, pain, and sexual health require age-aware approaches. Deep sleep diminishes with age; promote sleep hygiene rather than sedatives: consistent schedule, daytime light and activity, limit caffeine and naps, and reduce nighttime noise. Avoid benzodiazepines and sedative-hypnotics when possible due to falls and delirium risk. Pain may present atypically, and undertreatment is common; use validated pain scales suitable for cognition level and select safer regimens. For chronic osteoarthritis, acetaminophen can be first-line if liver function allows; use NSAIDs cautiously due to renal, GI, and cardiovascular risks. Opioids, if needed, require low starting doses, bowel regimens, and close monitoring. Sexual activity remains important for many older adults; normalize the conversation, address vaginal dryness or erectile dysfunction, and reinforce STI prevention—risk persists. Teach that phosphodiesterase-5 inhibitors (e.g., sildenafil) are contraindicated with nitrates due to the risk of severe hypotension.

Functional and safety assessment is central to preventing injury and preserving independence. Evaluate basic ADLs (bathing, dressing, toileting, transferring, continence, feeding) and instrumental ADLs (medication management, finances, shopping, transportation, meal prep, housekeeping). Observe gait and balance; a Timed Up and Go test longer than about 12 seconds indicates increased fall risk and warrants targeted interventions. Inspect footwear for fit and non-slip soles, ensure assistive devices are appropriately sized and used correctly, and verify that glasses and hearing aids are clean, functional, and available. Consider home hazards such as poor lighting, clutter, loose rugs, cords across walkways, and lack of grab bars or handrails; even in inpatient settings, simulate these principles by keeping call lights within reach, decluttering, and ensuring adequate lighting. Plan timely referrals: physical therapy for gait/balance and strength, occupational therapy for ADL training and home safety strategies, dietitian for weight loss or special diets, and social work for resources, caregiver support, transportation, or financial barriers.

Always attend to psychosocial context and possible abuse. Isolation, caregiver strain, unexplained injuries, poor hygiene, frequent ED visits, fearful behavior, or inconsistent histories warrant a deeper look. Screen for depression with a brief tool such as the PHQ-2 ("little interest or pleasure," "feeling down/depressed") and follow up positives appropriately. Assess caregiver capacity and burnout; offer respite and community resources. Ensure privacy for sensitive questions, honor autonomy and consent, and use shared decision-making. Know your jurisdiction's mandatory reporting: any suspicion of elder abuse or neglect must be reported per law and facility policy, even if proof is not certain.

High-yield do-first actions to anchor your decisions on exam day include:

- Check orthostatic vital signs when falls, dizziness, or hypotension are possible.
- Review all medications, including over-the-counter drugs and herbals, looking for high-risk agents and interactions.
- Hydrate unless contraindicated; assess intake and output and signs of dehydration.
- Search for reversible causes of delirium (infection, hypoxia, hypoglycemia, pain, constipation, urinary retention, medications).
- Implement fall and pressure-injury prevention immediately while you continue assessment.

- Ensure sensory supports are in place (glasses, hearing aids) and adapt communication (lighting, low-pitched voice, minimize noise).
- Verify understanding with teach-back, adjusting for sensory or cognitive barriers.

Just as important are the pitfalls to avoid:

- Do not label confusion as "normal aging"; treat acute mental status changes as delirium until proven otherwise.
- Do not use physical or chemical restraints as first-line for agitation; try reorientation, pain treatment, family presence, toileting, sleep, and sensory aids first.
- Do not place indwelling urinary catheters for convenience; use noninvasive strategies and remove catheters promptly.
- Do not withhold analgesia solely because of age; dose carefully and monitor.

Through the lens of the clinical judgment model, sudden changes such as falls, new confusion, functional decline, or weight loss are critical cues. Hypothesize common, reversible causes—medication effects and interactions, infection without fever, dehydration or electrolyte imbalance, hypoxia, pain, constipation, urinary retention—and test your hypotheses with focused assessments and low-risk interventions. Prioritize immediate safety (fall precautions, oxygen if indicated, supervision), obtain targeted vitals and bedside tests (orthostatics, SpO_2, blood glucose), review medications, and apply supportive measures while arranging definitive evaluation. Evaluate the response: improved mentation after oxygen or fluids supports hypoxia or dehydration; persistent delirium despite these actions prompts further diagnostics and escalation. This is the essence of safe, age-competent nursing care and exactly how the exam expects you to think.

3.2 Immunizations & Screening (What to Do/Teach)

On immunization and screening items, think like the Clinical Judgment nurse: recognize cues (age, pregnancy, immune status, allergies, prior disease, medications, exposures, travel/occupation), analyze risk/benefit, prioritize safe actions, implement correctly, and teach what happens next. Most wrong answers ignore one key cue (e.g., "pregnant" + "live vaccine") or break a spacing/timing rule.

Start with vaccine fundamentals you can apply to any client. Live vaccines (MMR, varicella, live-attenuated influenza [intranasal], yellow fever) are contraindicated in pregnancy and severe immunodeficiency. Inactivated or recombinant vaccines (influenza injection, Tdap/Td, HPV, hepatitis A and B, pneumococcal, meningococcal, polio [IPV], COVID-19, recombinant zoster) are safe for immunocompetent and typically safe in pregnancy. Co-administration is allowed: give all needed vaccines on the same day at different sites; do not mix in the same syringe. Spacing matters for live vaccines given on different days: if not given the same day, separate by at least four weeks. If a series is delayed, never restart; resume and honor minimum intervals.

Know absolute contraindications versus precautions. Absolute contraindications include anaphylaxis to a previous dose or a vaccine component (for example, gelatin or neomycin with MMR/varicella; yeast with hepatitis B), and pregnancy or severe immunodeficiency for live vaccines. A history of encephalopathy within seven days after a previous pertussis-containing vaccine is a contraindication to further DTaP/Tdap. Moderate or severe acute illness with or without fever is a precaution—defer until improved. Mild illness (low-grade fever, otitis media, mild URI) is not a reason to defer. Latex allergy is a product-specific precaution (check packaging). For special timing interactions, antibody-containing blood products can neutralize live vaccines: delay MMR/varicella for several months after immune globulin or transfusion (interval varies by product; do not memorize exact durations—know that a delay is needed). If a live vaccine is given first, wait at least two weeks before administering an antibody-containing product. With tuberculosis testing, give TST/IGRA the same day as a live vaccine or delay TST/IGRA until at least four weeks after; doing the TST first is fine if you administer the live vaccine after the test is read.

Certain populations trigger automatic actions. In pregnancy, give Tdap during each pregnancy (optimally 27–36 weeks), and inactivated influenza during any trimester; avoid live vaccines. If nonimmune postpartum, give MMR (and varicella if indicated) before discharge—safe with breastfeeding—and advise to avoid conception for one month after live vaccines. In immunocompromised clients, avoid live vaccines; give inactivated vaccines on schedule (recombinant zoster is not live and is recommended for many immunocompromised adults). Healthcare workers need proof of immunity to measles, mumps, rubella, and varicella; hepatitis B series with post-vaccination serology; annual influenza; Tdap; and COVID-19 per current guidance. Older adults need annual influenza (high-dose or adjuvanted preferred ≥65), pneumococcal vaccination (either a single PCV20, or PCV15 followed by PPSV23 one year later; earlier and shorter intervals for select high-risk groups), and recombinant zoster vaccine (two doses starting at age 50, including for immunocompromised adults ≥19).

Safe administration begins with screening and consent. Review for acute illness, pregnancy, immunosuppression, prior reactions, allergies to vaccine components, recent blood products, and TB testing plans. Provide and review the Vaccine Information Statement (VIS), answer questions, and obtain consent. Choose the correct route and site by age: intramuscular injections go into the vastus lateralis for infants and young toddlers; the deltoid is used for older children and adults. Subcutaneous injections go into fatty tissue of the anterolateral thigh in infants and the triceps area in older children/adults. Rotavirus is oral; live-attenuated influenza is intranasal. Use general needle-length guidance: IM 1 inch for most infants; 1–1.25 inches for toddlers; 1–1.5 inches for older children/adults (1.5 inches for larger/obese adults); SubQ 5/8 inch. Avoid the gluteal muscle for routine immunization. When giving multiple injections, separate sites by at least one inch and administer the most painful last to minimize distress (pertussis-containing and pneumococcal vaccines tend to be more painful). Use pain-minimizing strategies: sucrose or breastfeeding for infants, topical anesthetics when appropriate, distraction and comfort positioning, and keep clients seated or supine—adolescents in particular can faint.

Prepare for and respond to adverse events. Observe all clients for at least 15 minutes after vaccination (consider 30 minutes for those with a history of anaphylaxis to any cause). Have epinephrine and airway equipment immediately available. Treat anaphylaxis with epinephrine 1 mg/mL (1:1000) intramuscularly into the mid-anterolateral thigh: adults 0.3–0.5 mg; children 0.01 mg/kg up to 0.3 mg; repeat every 5–15 minutes as needed. Position supine with legs elevated, give oxygen, call for emergency support, and monitor closely. Document thoroughly: vaccine name, lot number, manufacturer, expiration date, dose, site and route, date, VIS edition date and date provided, and client response.

Teaching drives adherence. Set expectations for common, self-limited reactions such as local soreness, mild fever, irritability, or fatigue; advise cool compresses, acetaminophen if needed, and hydration. Instruct clients to seek care for danger signs: signs of anaphylaxis, high or persistent fever, wheeze or stridor, severe or rapidly enlarging local swelling, or neurologic symptoms. Reinforce the catch-up principle: if a dose was missed, continue the series without restarting; maintain minimum intervals. Highlight a few age-specific rules that often appear on exams: do not initiate rotavirus after 14 weeks 6 days, and complete the series by eight months of age; administer MMR and varicella starting at 12 months (two doses); give HPV at ages 11–12 with a two-dose schedule if started before age 15 (three doses if 15 or older or immunocompromised). For tetanus-containing vaccines, give one Tdap in adulthood, then Td or Tdap every 10 years; use Tdap for wound management if never received before or if five or more years have passed for a dirty wound. In pregnancy-related teaching, emphasize Tdap each pregnancy, inactivated influenza, avoidance of live vaccines, and the one-month contraception window after a live vaccine. Explain herd immunity simply: vaccines reduce community transmission and protect vulnerable people; offer respectful, evidence-based responses to hesitancy, invite questions, acknowledge concerns, and correct myths without confrontation. If a client declines, document refusal and continue the conversation at future visits.

Screening is different from diagnostic testing; it looks for disease in asymptomatic people to enable early intervention. Do not "screen" clients with symptoms—evaluate and treat. Anchor to a few high-yield, lifespan screens and what the nurse teaches. Newborns receive metabolic screening via heel stick (timed after adequate feeding), hearing screening, and critical congenital heart disease screening with pre- and post-ductal pulse oximetry. In early childhood, vision screening transitions from observation/referral to chart-based screening around ages 3–5; hearing screening is periodic and whenever there are language delays or recurrent otitis media. Lead screening occurs at

12 and 24 months in high-prevalence areas or for at-risk children; iron-deficiency anemia screening is common at 12 months in risk groups. Scoliosis screening typically occurs during early adolescence; be prepared to teach about posture, backpack weight, and referral if asymmetry is observed.

In adolescents and adults, integrate mental health and safety screens into routine care: screen for depression (PHQ-2/9), intimate partner violence in women of reproductive age, and substance use with brief interventions as indicated. Measure blood pressure starting in adulthood at routine visits, and track BMI. Lipid screening is performed at least once in young adulthood and periodically thereafter based on risk; recent guidance supports broader adult screening beginning by midlife—teach that fasting is not required for most lipid panels. Diabetes screening is recommended for adults with overweight/obesity beginning in midlife (commonly age 35–70) and earlier for high-risk groups; in pregnancy, screen for gestational diabetes at 24–28 weeks. Cancer screening timelines to know conceptually: cervical cancer screening begins at age 21 with cytology alone every three years through 29; from ages 30–65, acceptable strategies include cytology every three years, high-risk HPV testing every five years, or cotesting every five years; stop after 65 with adequate prior normal results and no high-risk history, and do not screen after total hysterectomy for benign disease. Breast cancer screening generally begins between ages 40 and 50 at regular intervals; clients should follow clinician guidance based on risk and current recommendations. Colorectal cancer screening now begins at 45 for average-risk adults with options such as annual FIT, stool DNA every 1–3 years, flexible sigmoidoscopy every five years, or colonoscopy every 10 years; teach bowel prep and need for an escort if sedated. Prostate cancer screening is shared decision-making for average-risk men beginning around age 50 (earlier for higher-risk groups such as African American men or those with a strong family history); discuss PSA benefits and harms. Infectious disease screening highlights include HIV at least once for all adolescents and adults (and in every pregnancy), with repeat testing based on risk; hepatitis C one-time testing for most adults and periodic for ongoing risk; syphilis and other STIs for pregnant clients and at-risk populations; TB screening for those with exposure or risk factors. In older adults, screen women for osteoporosis with DXA at 65 (earlier if high risk) and consider men who are at risk; reduce fall risk through multifactorial assessment. Screen for abdominal aortic aneurysm once via ultrasound in men ages 65–75 who have ever smoked.

Provide practical preparation and follow-up teaching. For Pap tests, avoid intercourse, douching, vaginal medications, or tampons for 24–48 hours before the test, and schedule when not menstruating if possible. For mammography, avoid deodorant or powders on the day of the test. For colonoscopy, emphasize completing bowel prep and arranging a driver due to sedation; clarify that stool-based tests do not require bowel prep and are done at home. Most lipid panels do not require fasting; fasting may still be used in select circumstances. Explain what results mean, the plan for abnormal findings, and confidentiality—especially for adolescent sexual health, mental health, and substance use screenings, which often allow minor consent and require careful privacy practices.

Expect NGN-style items to embed cues you must surface and act on. If you see pregnancy or severe immunosuppression, eliminate live vaccines and choose inactivated options; if postpartum and rubella nonimmune, give MMR now and instruct contraception for one month. If a client recently received immune globulin, postpone live vaccines; if they need TST and a live vaccine, schedule both today or delay TST four weeks. If an adolescent is receiving multiple shots, choose deltoid sites, give the most painful last, have the client seated to prevent syncope, and monitor for 15 minutes. If a healthcare worker lacks hepatitis B surface antibody after the series, follow post-vaccination testing protocols and revaccinate per guidance. For screening, never choose "screen" when the stem describes symptoms; arrange diagnostic evaluation. Select age-appropriate screens and teach prep succinctly. Escalate for red flags: suspected anaphylaxis after vaccination, markedly abnormal screening results, or intimate partner violence disclosures that threaten immediate safety.

Finally, remember a few high-yield pearls that often decide the question. The rotavirus series has hard age cutoffs. Live vaccines can be given together, but otherwise must be separated by four weeks. Mild illness is not a reason to defer. Tdap is given in every pregnancy. Recombinant zoster is not live and is indicated at 50 and older. Pneumococcal vaccination in older adults can be completed with a single PCV20 dose. Screening is preventative; symptoms trigger diagnostics. If you consistently recognize these cues and apply these rules, you will select the safe, test-correct action.

3.2.1 Routine + Catch-Up Principles

Immunizations are a prevention-and-safety domain where the NCLEX expects you to apply clinical judgment, not memorize every footnote. Think CJMM: recognize cues (age, prior doses, risks), apply rules (routine schedule and minimum intervals), deliver safely (right vaccine, dose, route, site), teach (what to expect and what not to fear), document, then evaluate/report adverse events. On exam day, the "do first" move is to protect the child today without breaking minimum age/interval rules or exposing them to a true contraindication. Everything below is organized to help you do exactly that.

Start with a few high-yield anchors for the routine pediatric/adolescent schedule. These let you quickly decide what's due today:

- Birth: HepB.
- 2, 4, 6 months: DTaP, IPV, Hib, PCV, Rotavirus (RV1 at 2,4; RV5 at 2,4,6); HepB appears at birth and again at 1–2 months; many children get the third HepB around 6 months.
- 12–15 months: MMR, Varicella, Hib booster, PCV booster, HepA dose 1.
- 15–18 months: DTaP booster.
- 4–6 years (pre–school entry): DTaP, IPV, MMR, Varicella.
- Influenza: annually starting at 6 months; during the first flu season if younger than 9 years and vaccine-naïve, give 2 doses at least 4 weeks apart.
- 11–12 years: Tdap; HPV series (2-dose if started before 15th birthday, otherwise 3-dose; immunocompromised adolescents need 3-dose); MenACWY with a booster at 16 years.
- MenB: 16–23 years via shared clinical decision-making; give earlier if high risk (e.g., asplenia, complement deficiency, outbreak exposure).

A few memory anchors make the details stick: "2-4-6 does the tricks" for infant series; "live at one year" for MMR and Varicella; "boost at school entry" for 4–6 years; "Tdap + HPV + MenACWY at 11–12, MenACWY boost at 16." For rotavirus, remember two hard deadlines: start no later than 14 weeks 6 days, and finish by 8 months 0 days—there is no late catch-up for rotavirus.

Catch-up questions require rule-based thinking. The single most important rule is that you never restart a vaccine series, no matter how much time has elapsed; you simply continue, observing minimum ages and minimum intervals. For NCLEX, the following intervals are the ones you must recognize and apply safely:

- HepB: dose 2 at least 4 weeks after dose 1; dose 3 at least 8 weeks after dose 2 and at least 16 weeks after dose 1; minimum age for the final dose is 24 weeks. A quick "4–8/16/24" memory chain helps: 4 weeks to dose 2, 8 more weeks and 16 from start to final, not before 24 weeks of age.
- DTaP: minimum 4 weeks between dose 1→2 and 2→3; minimum 6 months between 3→4 and 4→5. The fifth dose isn't needed if the fourth was given at 4 years or older and at least 6 months after dose 3.
- IPV: 4 weeks between early doses; the final dose must be at least 6 months after the previous one and given at age 4 years or older.
- MMR (live): space doses by at least 4 weeks.
- Varicella (live): if younger than 13 years, space doses by 3 months; if 13 years or older, space by at least 4 weeks.
- HepA: 2 doses at least 6 months apart.
- Hib and PCV: the number of doses depends on the age at start. Healthy children who begin the series in in-

fancy need primary doses and a booster around 12–15 months. If starting late, give only the age-appropriate catch-up doses; healthy children generally do not begin Hib after 5 years of age, but do give indicated boosters if they started earlier and are incomplete. PCV catch-up is recommended for children under 5 who are behind; risk-based PCV (and sometimes PPSV23) applies to some older children with specific conditions.

- Rotavirus: must start by 14 weeks 6 days and finish by 8 months 0 days; do not initiate catch-up after the start maximum age.

Live-vaccine timing questions are frequent traps. When two live parenteral or intranasal vaccines are being given (e.g., MMR, Varicella, live-attenuated influenza nasal spray), either administer them on the same day or separate by at least 4 weeks; this avoids interference in antibody response. This rule intersects with TB screening: TST/IGRA can be placed the same day as a live vaccine, or you delay the TB test at least 4 weeks after a live vaccine. If you give a live vaccine today and the TST was scheduled for tomorrow, you should reschedule the TB test 4 weeks out unless you can give both today.

Recent immune globulin or blood product can blunt live-virus vaccine response. On exam questions, the safe move is to delay MMR and Varicella after IG/blood products per guidance intervals (which vary by product); you don't need to recall the exact number of months to pass, only that you shouldn't give live vaccines immediately after IG/blood unless benefits outweigh risks and follow-up serology is planned.

Next, sort contraindications from precautions—NCLEX loves these distinctions. True contraindications are absolute: a severe anaphylaxis to a prior dose or a vaccine component means you don't give that vaccine again; severe immunosuppression (e.g., chemotherapy, congenital immunodeficiency, high-dose systemic steroids) or pregnancy is a contraindication to live vaccines like MMR, Varicella, and LAIV; and encephalopathy within 7 days of a pertussis-containing vaccine is a contraindication to any further pertussis-containing vaccines. Precautions are conditions where you weigh risks and benefits or defer until safer: moderate or severe acute illness (fever and systemic symptoms) is a reason to defer; Guillain–Barré syndrome within 6 weeks of a tetanus-toxoid or influenza vaccine is a precaution; and a progressive or unstable neurologic disorder calls for holding pertussis-containing vaccines until stabilized. Several "not contraindications" are test favorites: mild illness or low-grade fever does not warrant delaying vaccines; breastfeeding is fine; and egg allergy is not a reason to avoid influenza vaccination—use any licensed influenza vaccine unless the person had a severe reaction to a previous influenza vaccine product itself.

Certain populations have predictable twists. Preterm infants are immunized by chronological age, not corrected age, with one HepB nuance: if the infant weighs less than 2 kg at birth and the mother is HBsAg negative, the birth dose of HepB may be delayed until age 1 month or hospital discharge. If the mother is HBsAg positive or her status is unknown, give HepB plus HBIG within 12 hours of birth regardless of infant weight; then follow the recommended schedule. During pregnancy, avoid live vaccines; give inactivated influenza in any trimester and Tdap at 27–36 weeks every pregnancy to protect the newborn via passive antibody. Children and adolescents with asplenia or complement deficiencies need MenACWY and MenB on an accelerated or risk-based schedule, and many risk conditions call for pneumococcal beyond routine PCV—PPSV23 may be given after PCV depending on the condition. Children with cochlear implants or CSF leak fall into risk-based pneumococcal categories as well.

Routine administration safety is where the RN earns full credit. Before you inject anything, verify the order and the child's age, screen for contraindications and precautions, check that minimum ages and intervals are met, and confirm the correct route and site for each vaccine. Maintain the cold chain. Inspect expiration dates. If a vaccine requires reconstitution, use the manufacturer's diluent and administer within the time window after mixing.

Use the correct route/site: DTaP, Tdap, HepB, Hib, PCV, and inactivated influenza are given intramuscularly; IPV can be IM or subcutaneous; MMR and Varicella (and MMRV if used) are subcutaneous; LAIV is intranasal. In infants, the vastus lateralis (anterolateral thigh) is the preferred IM site; in older children and adolescents, use the deltoid if muscle mass allows. Simultaneous administration of all indicated vaccines at separate sites is safe and recommended; separate injection sites by at least 1 inch so you can identify any local reaction to the correct product. If several vaccines are due in the same limb, space them appropriately and note which went where.

Adverse reactions are usually mild—local soreness, low-grade fever, and, for live vaccines, a mild rash 1–2 weeks later. Teach comfort measures such as cool compresses and adequate fluids; avoid prophylactic antipyretics before vaccination because they may slightly reduce immune response. The emergency you must recognize is anaphylaxis: act on ABCs immediately and give IM epinephrine 1 mg/mL at 0.01 mg/kg up to a maximum of 0.5 mg into the mid-anterolateral thigh, repeating at 5–15 minute intervals as needed while you activate emergency response, maintain airway, and prepare for transfer. To mitigate fainting risk in adolescents, have them seated or supine during injection and observe everyone for at least 15 minutes afterward (longer if they have syncope risk or a concerning history). Report severe or unexpected events to VAERS.

Documentation and teaching close the loop. Provide the current Vaccine Information Statement (VIS) for each vaccine before administration and answer questions. Document the date, vaccine name, lot number, manufacturer, dose, route, site, and the VIS edition date; obtain and record consent per facility policy. Schedule the next dose before they leave and reinforce that vaccine series are not restarted—the next dose will count as long as minimum intervals are met. Teach that mild illness is not a reason to delay vaccination, that pregnancy should be avoided for 1 month after live vaccines (e.g., MMR, Varicella), and that TB testing timing and live vaccines may necessitate rescheduling.

Finally, tie it back to CJMM and what to do first when cues conflict. If a 2-year-old has missed visits and shows up with a mild cold and low-grade fever, the safe decision is to vaccinate today with indicated inactivated and live vaccines (mild illness is not a contraindication), making sure live vaccines are either both given today or spaced by 4 weeks. If an adolescent starting HPV at 14 years 10 months asks about the schedule, choose the 2-dose series with doses separated by 6–12 months (minimum 5 months), but if they start at 15 years 0 months or are immunocompromised, plan a 3-dose series at 0, 1–2, and 6 months. If the mother of a newborn is HBsAg positive and the infant is 1.8 kg, prioritize giving HepB and HBIG within 12 hours of birth and coordinate follow-up. If a patient received IVIG last week and is scheduled for MMR today, defer the live vaccine and reschedule according to guidance. If a teen has a history suggestive of Guillain–Barré within 6 weeks of a tetanus-containing vaccine, treat tetanus toxoid as a precaution and discuss risks/benefits; for influenza, consider non-egg issues and the same GBS timing principle.

In short, use the anchors to identify what's due, apply the minimum interval rules to catch up without restarting, respect true contraindications, choose inactivated options when necessary, and execute safe administration with proper teaching and documentation. That is the NCLEX-friendly path from recognition to action to evaluation in immunization items.

3.2.2 High-Yield Screenings

On exam day, think like a safety-forward RN who knows when to screen, when to stop, who counts as high-risk, and what to do immediately when a screen is positive. Anchor to average-risk schedules, identify cues that suggest high-risk exceptions, use shared decision-making for preference-sensitive tests (like PSA), and protect confidentiality for adolescents and anyone disclosing intimate partner violence. Do not over-screen: avoid Pap tests before age 21, HPV cotesting before 30, PSA without discussion, or TB testing in low-risk, asymptomatic people. Stop screening when prior results are adequate and life expectancy would not benefit from detection.

For infants and children, the very first screen is the newborn panel, which is state-specific but always includes metabolic disorders such as phenylketonuria and congenital hypothyroidism. The nurse's role is to confirm it is drawn before hospital discharge, educate caregivers about possible repeat testing if early or borderline results occur, and ensure follow-up if abnormal. Two other universal newborn screens occur before discharge: hearing (otoacoustic emissions or automated auditory brainstem response) and pulse oximetry to detect critical congenital heart disease. A failed hearing screen demands a timely repeat and audiology referral; a low oxygen saturation or a right/left or hand/foot differential suggests heart disease and triggers immediate recheck, provider notification, and possible echocardiography. As children grow, emphasize exposure-based tests. Lead screening is required at 12 and 24 months for children on Medicaid and recommended for those living in or frequently visiting homes built before 1978, with renovations, or with siblings with elevated levels. If a capillary lead test is elevated, the next safe action is to obtain confirmatory venous levels and institute environmental controls and nutrition counseling. Anemia screening with hemoglobin at 12 months is universal; if low, prioritize iron-deficiency evaluation (diet history, cow's milk excess, pica) and start iron therapy with plan to recheck. Vision screening moves from observation in infancy to instrument-based screening once children can cooperate (commonly beginning at ages 3 to 5), with periodic checks thereafter; refer promptly for strabismus, amblyopia risk, or failed screening. Hearing is screened at birth and again when concerns arise (recurrent otitis media, speech delay). Autism-specific screening should be standardized at 18 and 24 months; a positive screen requires referral for diagnostic evaluation and early intervention therapies without delay—do not "wait and see."

Adolescents require the nurse to blend confidentiality, rapport, and risk detection. Screen for depression annually (a quick PHQ-2 followed by PHQ-9 if positive). A teen who affirms suicidal ideation requires the RN to remain with the patient, perform a suicide risk assessment, remove hazards, and notify the provider while ensuring immediate safety planning; confidentiality yields to safety and mandated reporting when imminent risk is present. Screen for sexually transmitted infections based on sexual behavior rather than age alone: sexually active females under 25 need annual chlamydia and gonorrhea testing, and those 25 and older require testing if at risk. HIV should be offered at least once to all between 15 and 65, with more frequent testing if risk is ongoing. Add syphilis screening for adolescents with high-risk behaviors or pregnant teens. Substance use, vaping and tobacco, and alcohol misuse screening should occur routinely; a positive screen triggers brief intervention, counseling, and referral when indicated. Throughout, ensure privacy for discussions and clarify limits of confidentiality up front; this is critical when assessing intimate partner violence, sexual activity, and mental health.

In adults, build a default prevention rhythm and then adjust based on cues. Blood pressure should be checked at every encounter or at least annually. Elevated readings must be confirmed with proper cuff size and technique, repeated after rest, and preferably corroborated with home or ambulatory monitoring. Red flags such as headache, chest pain, dyspnea, neurologic deficits, or acute kidney injury suggest hypertensive urgency or emergency and move the nurse toward emergent evaluation. Body mass index and obesity counseling occur at each visit; pair screening with behavioral interventions. For type 2 diabetes, screen adults aged 35 to 70 with overweight or obesity every three years, earlier and more often if there is a strong family history, gestational diabetes, polycystic ovary syndrome, or high-risk ethnicity. If an A1C or fasting glucose is elevated, confirm with a repeat test or an alternative diagnostic test, provide lifestyle counseling, and coordinate follow-up. In pregnancy, screen for gestational diabetes between 24 and 28 weeks (earlier if high-risk); a positive 1-hour glucose challenge leads to the diagnostic 3-hour test or a 2-step strategy per protocol.

Lipid screening supports cardiovascular risk reduction. Obtain a baseline lipid panel in adults aged 40 to 75, earlier if they have diabetes, familial hypercholesterolemia, or other risk factors, and repeat approximately every five years if normal. An abnormal result prompts counseling, calculation of cardiovascular risk, and discussion of statin therapy with the prescriber.

Colorectal cancer screening now starts at age 45 for average-risk adults and continues to age 75. Offer a stool-based test like FIT annually, or structural exams like colonoscopy every 10 years, among other options. The NCLEX-critical action is to schedule a diagnostic colonoscopy if any noninvasive stool test is positive; do not repeat the stool test as a "double check." Screen individuals aged 76 to 85 based on overall health, prior screening history, and preferences; stop screening if life expectancy is limited or after age 85. For cervical cancer, start screening at age 21 with cytology alone every three years through age 29. From 30 to 65, choose either cytology every three years, high-risk HPV testing every five years, or cotesting every five years. Do not screen before age 21 regardless of sexual activity. Stop at 65 if the individual has adequate prior negative tests and no high-risk conditions. Do not screen after a total hysterectomy for benign disease. High-risk exceptions—such as immunocompromised status, HIV infection, or in utero DES exposure—require earlier and more frequent screening and should trigger a consult to specifics, but the RN must recognize the exception and avoid stopping inappropriately.

Breast cancer screening for average-risk patients is biennial mammography for ages 50 to 74, with a discussion about starting at 40 based on values and risk. Those at high risk, including carriers of BRCA mutations, those with a strong family history, or those who had chest radiation at a young age, often need earlier and sometimes annual imaging and MRI adjuncts; the nurse's task is to cue into family history and prior radiation. Do not recommend routine clinical breast exams on exam day; teach breast self-awareness rather than formal self-exams.

Prostate cancer screening with PSA is preference-sensitive. Offer shared decision-making for men aged 55 to 69 after discussing benefits and harms, and generally avoid screening after age 70. If the patient chooses screening and a PSA is elevated, the next step is not immediate biopsy; instead, arrange confirmatory testing, possible repeat PSA, and urology referral.

Lung cancer screening is one of the highest-yield interventions to remember. Patients between 50 and 80 years old with a 20 pack-year history who currently smoke or quit within the last 15 years need annual low-dose CT scanning. Stop screening if it has been more than 15 years since quitting, if the patient develops a health problem that substantially limits life expectancy, or if they cannot undergo treatment. The nurse should pair LDCT with smoking cessation counseling at every visit.

Osteoporosis screening with DEXA is recommended for women aged 65 and older and for younger postmenopausal women whose fracture risk is similar to or exceeds that of a 65-year-old based on clinical risk calculators. Consider screening in men aged 70 and older or earlier in men with major risk factors, such as chronic glucocorticoid use, hypogonadism, or prior fragility fracture. If DEXA shows osteoporosis, anticipate fall-prevention measures, calcium/vitamin D counseling, weight-bearing exercise, home safety assessment, and pharmacotherapy discussion.

For abdominal aortic aneurysm, one-time ultrasound is indicated for men aged 65 to 75 who have ever smoked. It is not routinely recommended for women without risk factors. A positive finding requires blood pressure control, vascular surgery referral, smoking cessation, and size-based surveillance.

Infectious disease screening is a cornerstone. Offer HIV testing at least once to all between ages 15 and 65 (earlier and more often with risk, and during each pregnancy at the first prenatal visit, with repeat in the third trimester if high-risk). Hepatitis C screening is recommended once for adults aged 18 to 79, with repeat testing for ongoing risk, such as injection drug use or hemodialysis. In pregnancy, screen early for hepatitis B surface antigen and syphilis; add chlamydia, gonorrhea, and HIV as appropriate. TB screening is not for low-risk asymptomatic patients; reserve TST or IGRA for those with risk factors such as exposure, immunosuppression, or occupational risk, and move promptly to chest radiography and symptom evaluation if the test is positive.

Screen women of reproductive age for intimate partner violence, but only in a private setting; document in the health record using the patient's words when possible, and offer a warm handoff to resources. Know your state's mandatory reporting rules while ensuring the patient's immediate safety and confidentiality.

As patients age, incorporate functional screening. Periodic vision and hearing checks reduce falls and isolation. Assess falls risk routinely by asking about recent falls, balance, gait, and medications; institute fall precautions, home safety modifications, vitamin D assessment when appropriate, and physical therapy referral if risk is identified. Cognitive screening is not universal, but if caregivers or the patient express concerns, a brief screen such as MoCA or Mini-Cog is appropriate; abnormal findings should lead to a fuller evaluation and safety planning for driving, medication management, and home support.

Patients need simple preparation instructions to complete screens accurately. The day of a mammogram, avoid deodorants and powders that can mimic microcalcifications on the image. Before a Pap test, advise avoiding intercourse, douching, and vaginal medications for 24 to 48 hours, and schedule when not menstruating when possible. For colonoscopy, explain the clear-liquid diet and bowel preparation; anticoagulants should be held only if prescribed by the provider with risk-benefit assessment. Low-dose CT is painless and quick, but every encounter is a chance to reinforce smoking cessation. DEXA scanning does not require day-of changes in calcium intake.

Know the first nurse actions when a screen is abnormal. A positive depression screen or suicidal ideation requires that you stay with the patient, assess risk and intent, remove accessible hazards, and escalate to the provider immediately; document and initiate a safety plan. A positive FIT or other stool-based colorectal test moves directly to diagnostic colonoscopy; repeating FIT is not appropriate. An abnormal Pap smear or positive high-risk HPV test should lead to timely colposcopy scheduling per age and result category; teach that HPV positivity is common and often transient, but reinforce the need for follow-up. An HIV antigen/antibody screen that is positive needs confirmatory testing (differentiation immunoassay), nonjudgmental counseling, linkage to care, and discussion of PrEP for partners. Elevated blood pressure on screening requires a repeat measurement with correct technique, a brief symptom check for headache, chest pain, dyspnea, or neurologic signs, and escalation if features of hypertensive urgency or emergency appear. A positive IPV screen should trigger safety planning, privacy, and connection to community resources; follow reporting laws without compromising the patient's safety.

Micro-scenarios sharpen decision-making. A 52-year-old with a 30 pack-year smoking history who quit eight years ago presents for an annual visit. Recognize the cue set—age, pack-years, quit within 15 years—prompting annual low-dose CT; add smoking cessation counseling and verify readiness to quit. A 23-year-old sexually active female at a college clinic has dysuria and a new partner; she requests a Pap test. Identify the cue—age under 21 is too young, but she is 23, so Pap is appropriate by age; however, do not HPV cotest at this age. Screen for chlamydia and gonorrhea; if positive, arrange treatment and partner therapy. A 67-year-old with multiple prior normal Pap tests, no high-risk conditions, and a total hysterectomy for fibroids asks if she still needs Pap smears. Prior adequate negative results and benign hysterectomy are cues to stop cervical screening; reinforce that no further Paps are needed. A 46-year-old asymptomatic man with a BMI of 32 comes for a work physical. This is the time to screen for type 2 diabetes based on age and BMI, check lipid profile, confirm blood pressure on repeat, and introduce colorectal screening starting at 45 with choice of FIT or colonoscopy.

Avoid common traps that cost points. Start colorectal cancer screening at 45, not 50. Do not perform Pap smears in people under 21 regardless of sexual activity, and do not order HPV cotesting before age 30. Mammography for average risk is biennial from 50 to 74; clinical breast exam is not recommended and breast self-exams are not required—teach awareness instead. PSA screening occurs only after shared decision-making in men 55 to 69; it is generally avoided beyond 70. Do not test for TB in low-risk, asymptomatic individuals. Do not repeat stool tests after a positive result; escalate to colonoscopy. For lead, a positive capillary screen must be confirmed with a venous sample. For smoking-related lung cancer screening, remember to stop when it has been more than 15 years since quitting or if the patient could not tolerate curative therapy. For cervical cancer, screening continues only if age criteria are met; first sexual activity does not move the start earlier than 21. Across all modalities, stop screening when age, prior negative results, and limited life expectancy mean that harms outweigh benefits.

Thinking like the NCLEX favors cue recognition, risk prioritization, and the next safe action. When you see age plus risk factors, match them to the correct screen and timing; when you see a positive result, know which escalation pathway is required and which reflex tests to avoid. Pair every screening moment with education that improves adherence and safety.

3.3 Knowledge Check

Clinical Vignette 1

A 24-month-old boy is brought to the pediatric clinic by his mother for concerns about speech and social skills. He was born full term via uncomplicated vaginal delivery, has no chronic medical conditions, takes no medications, and has no known allergies; immunizations are up to date. The mother reports he uses about 6–8 single words but does not combine words into two-word phrases, rarely points to request or show objects, and often does not respond when his name is called; she also notes limited eye contact and minimal interest in other children at playgrounds. He ambulates independently and runs, but his play is mostly solitary rather than interactive; he stacks only 3 small blocks when asked. Growth parameters are at the 50th percentile for weight, height, and head circumference; neurologic and cardiac exams are unremarkable. A parent-completed M-CHAT screening in the office was flagged as positive; otoacoustic emissions testing performed in clinic returned present bilaterally. There is a family history of an older sibling diagnosed with autism spectrum disorder. The mother requests guidance about next steps and is worried about long-term outcomes.

Question 1: Based on the vignette, which is the most likely primary concern explaining this child's presentation?

[A] Bilateral sensorineural hearing loss
[B] Autism spectrum disorder (social communication disorder)
[C] Global developmental delay due to intellectual disability
[D] Selective mutism related to anxiety

Question 2: What is the nurse's best next action for this child after the clinic visit?

[A] Reassure the parents that language often varies and schedule routine follow-up in 6 months
[B] Begin speech therapy only and defer other evaluations until therapy progress is seen
[C] Order an immediate brain MRI to evaluate for structural causes of delay
[D] Arrange comprehensive audiology testing, initiate referral to early intervention/developmental services, and document specific observed behaviors

Question 3: The otoacoustic emissions (OAE) test in clinic were present bilaterally. Which statement best interprets this result in the context of the vignette?

[A] A present OAE rules out any auditory pathway disorder beyond the cochlea, so hearing is definitively normal
[B] Present OAEs indicate middle ear effusion as the likely cause of poor speech and social engagement
[C] Present OAEs show cochlear outer hair cell function is intact, suggesting the problem may be central auditory processing or a primary social communication disorder rather than peripheral hearing loss
[D] Present OAEs indicate severe bilateral sensorineural hearing loss is the cause of the language delay

Question 4: Which immediate nursing action best aligns with safe, NGN-style priorities for this child?

[A] Start pharmacologic therapy to improve social interaction while waiting for evaluations
[B] Advise the parents to eliminate all screen exposure and return in 3 months if no change
[C] Tell the parents that because growth and motor skills are normal, no further action is needed now
[D] Document specific concerning behaviors (e.g., "no two-word phrases," "does not point," "limited eye contact"), inform the provider, and help arrange early intervention and audiology referrals

Question 5: The mother asks, "If you think this might be autism, do we have to start evaluations now, or can we wait until he's older?" Which response best reflects ethical, evidence-based nursing practice?

[A] Explain that early screening and timely referral to early intervention improves outcomes and offer to start referrals now while addressing parental questions
[B] Respectfully honor the family's wish to wait and schedule reassessment at age 3 when diagnoses are clearer
[C] Refuse to proceed without a definitive diagnosis from a specialist before making any referrals
[D] Assure the parent that a definitive diagnosis is certain today and insist on immediate long-term therapies without parental input

ANSWERS

1. Correct Answer: B

Rationale: The child's combination of limited single-word vocabulary at 24 months (<50 words/two-word phrases), lack of pointing, poor eye contact, limited social interest, and a positive M-CHAT are classic red flags for autism spectrum disorder (social communication deficits). A: Present OAEs make peripheral bilateral sensorineural hearing loss less likely as the primary cause, and hearing loss would usually impair detection on screening—though comprehensive audiology is still needed. C: Global developmental delay implies broader deficits across multiple domains including motor and growth; here motor and growth are age-appropriate. D: Selective mutism is rare in toddlers and is characterized by speaking in some settings but not others; this vignette shows pervasive social communication deficits and limited gestures.

2. Correct Answer: D

Rationale: Best practice per the chapter is to avoid "watchful waiting" when red flags for ASD or hearing concerns appear: the nurse should document specific behaviors, inform the provider, arrange comprehensive audiology testing (OAEs do not replace full audiology), and initiate early intervention/developmental referrals promptly. A: Reassurance and long delay risks missed critical early intervention window. B: Starting speech therapy alone ignores need for multidisciplinary assessment and audiology. C: Brain MRI is not the immediate next step without focal neurologic signs; prioritize screening, audiology, and developmental services first.

3. Correct Answer: C

Rationale: Present OAEs indicate functioning of cochlear outer hair cells (peripheral hearing likely intact), which suggests that the expressive/receptive concerns may stem from central auditory processing or primary social communication disorder (e.g., ASD). A: OAEs do not completely rule out all central auditory or higher-level processing disorders—further audiology evaluation (behavioral audiometry) is indicated. B: OAEs present would not indicate middle ear effusion; middle ear problems often reduce OAE amplitude or cause failure. D: Present OAEs are inconsistent with severe bilateral sensorineural hearing loss.

4. Correct Answer: D

Rationale: NGN-ready nursing priorities emphasize documenting objective behaviors, notifying the provider, and arranging appropriate referrals (early intervention, audiology, developmental assessment) to protect the child's developmental trajectory and safety. A: Pharmacologic therapy is not first-line for core ASD social communication concerns and is inappropriate without specialist input. B: Limiting screen time is reasonable counseling but insufficient as the sole action given clear red flags. C: Normal growth/motor does not rule out significant developmental or social communication disorders—further evaluation is warranted.

5. Correct Answer: A

Rationale: Ethically and evidence-based, nurses should educate caregivers that earlier screening and enrollment in early intervention when concerns are present improves developmental outcomes, and they should support informed decision-making and begin referrals with parental consent. B: Waiting risks missed critical early intervention windows. C: Refusing to refer until definitive specialist diagnosis delays needed services; referrals can be initiated while awaiting specialist evaluation. D: Forcing interventions or asserting certainty without evidence violates informed consent and family-centered care.

Clinical Vignette 2

A 24-month-old boy is brought to clinic for concerns about limited speech. He uses about 8 single words, no two-word phrases, and rarely points or waves; at daycare he plays alongside but not interactively with peers. He was born full term, passed the newborn hearing screen, has no chronic medical conditions, takes no medications, and has no drug allergies; family history is negative for developmental disorders. Over the past year he has had multiple URIs and otitis media episodes treated with two antibiotic courses. Exam: afebrile, growth at the 50th percentile, normal gross motor skills (walking, running, climbing). Otoscopy shows a dull, amber tympanic membrane with decreased mobility; tympanogram is flat (Type B). He attends to visual cues and follows simple commands but has limited spoken output; neurologic exam is nonfocal. Parents ask whether this represents autism, hearing loss, or late talking, and what next steps are needed.

Question 1: Based on the vignette, which is the most likely explanation for this child's speech delay?

[A] Autism spectrum disorder presenting with social communication deficits
[B] Conductive hearing impairment from middle ear effusion causing delayed expressive language
[C] Global developmental delay affecting multiple domains equally
[D] Selective mutism related to stranger anxiety

Question 2: What is the RN's best next action when addressing the parents' immediate concern?

[A] Arrange formal audiology testing and refer to early intervention/speech-language services while educating the family on communication strategies
[B] Reassure the parents that many children are late talkers and schedule routine follow-up in 6 months
[C] Start a 10-day course of high-dose oral amoxicillin today to clear middle ear fluid
[D] Begin speech therapy immediately without further auditory assessment

Question 3: Which pathophysiologic mechanism best explains how the clinic findings produce the child's language delay?

[A] Primary deficit in social reciprocity causing reduced language exposure and practice
[B] Central auditory processing disorder from cortical dysfunction despite normal peripheral hearing
[C] Impaired air conduction of sound through a fluid-filled middle ear reducing auditory input for speech learning
[D] Sensorineural cochlear hair-cell loss reducing perception across all frequencies

Question 4: Which pharmacologic recommendation aligns best with current first-line management for otitis media with effusion (OME) in this scenario?

[A] Initiate high-dose amoxicillin immediately to resolve the effusion and restore hearing
[B] Start an oral fluoroquinolone because of prior antibiotic exposures and recurrent infectionsC. Prescribe oral corticosteroids to hasten resolution of middle ear fluid and improve language outcomes
[C] Do not prescribe antibiotics for asymptomatic OME; use watchful waiting, analgesia as needed, and consider ENT referral if effusion persists >3 months or hearing loss is confirmed

Question 5: Which statement best reflects appropriate counseling and ethical action by the RN for this family now?

[A] Explain that immediate audiologic evaluation and early intervention referral are important because timely identification and treatment of hearing loss or persistent OME improve language outcomes, and that you will notify the provider to coordinate testing and services
[B] Advise waiting until age 3 because many toddlers spontaneously develop two-word phrases by then and early testing is usually unnecessary
[C] Recommend reducing verbal stimulation to decrease the child's frustration and encourage nonverbal communication only
[D] Tell the parents that because the newborn screen was normal, hearing problems are unlikely and no further testing is warranted

ANSWERS

1. Correct Answer: B

Rationale: The 24-month-old has <10 words, no two-word phrases, and a flat tympanogram with a dull TM—consistent with middle ear effusion causing conductive hearing loss and delayed speech. A (autism) is less likely since the child makes eye contact and follows commands. C (global delay) would involve multiple domains, not just speech. D (selective mutism) is unlikely given word use at home and no social anxiety features.

2. Correct Answer: A

Rationale: The RN's priority is referral for audiology and early intervention while teaching family strategies, since prompt action improves outcomes. B (reassurance) delays care, C (antibiotics) isn't first-line for asymptomatic OME, and D (speech therapy without hearing test) ignores the need to confirm hearing loss first.

3. Correct Answer: C

Rationale: A flat tympanogram indicates middle ear fluid causing impaired air conduction; reduced auditory input during a critical period impairs language learning (conductive hearing loss mechanism). A (primary social deficit) does not account for the audiologic findings; B (central auditory processing) implies normal peripheral hearing and cortical dysfunction, which is inconsistent with tympanometry; D (sensorineural loss) would reflect cochlear damage and usually produces different audiometric patterns, not a Type B tympanogram.

4. Correct Answer: D

Rationale: Current recommendations for otitis media with effusion without acute infection favor observation/watchful waiting (because many effusions resolve spontaneously), symptomatic care, and ENT referral if effusion or hearing loss persists beyond ~3 months or if developmental concerns continue. A (immediate high-dose amoxicillin) is indicated for acute otitis media but not for asymptomatic persistent effusion; C (oral steroids) are not routinely recommended for OME; B (fluoroquinolones) are inappropriate due to safety concerns and are not first-line for OME.

5. Correct Answer: A

Rationale: Ethically and clinically, the RN should communicate the need for timely audiology testing and early intervention because early identification/treatment of hearing loss or persistent OME improves language outcomes, and should coordinate with the provider to arrange services—this respects beneficence, promotes best outcomes, and supports informed parental decision-making. B (waiting until age 3) risks harm by delaying intervention; C (reducing verbal stimulation) is counterproductive—maximizing language exposure is recommended; D (no further testing because newborn screen was normal) is incorrect because middle ear disease can develop after the newborn period and newborn screens do not exclude later conductive losses.

Clinical Vignette 3

An 82-year-old woman is brought to the emergency department after a neighbor found her confused on the floor next to her collapsed walker; the daughter reports she lives alone and this mental change is new over the past 24 hours. Past medical history includes hypertension, osteoarthritis, and atrial fibrillation treated with warfarin; current medications are lisinopril, furosemide, and nightly over-the-counter diphenhydramine for sleep (no known drug allergies). She reports a brief episode of lightheadedness before the fall but no loss of consciousness. Vital signs: T 36.4°C, supine BP 128/72 mm Hg, standing BP 102/54 mm Hg, HR 82 irregularly irregular, RR 18, SpO2 92% on room air, fingerstick glucose 98 mg/dL. On exam she is alert but inattentive and disoriented to date, repeatedly attempts to get out of bed, and demonstrates dry mucous membranes; a gentle suprapubic fullness is palpated. A bladder scan shows approximately 450 mL retained urine. There is a small occipital scalp hematoma without focal neurologic deficit; daughter notes baseline use of a walker and that the patient did not have hearing aids in place. Urinalysis and labs are pending; a noncontrast head CT has been ordered because of warfarin use and the fall. Nursing has implemented fall precautions, a low bed, and frequent reorientation while evaluation continues.

Question 1: Based on the vignette, which is the most likely explanation for the patient's acute mental status change?

[A] Progression of Alzheimer dementia causing increasing disorientation
[B] Ischemic stroke causing acute focal neurologic deficit with global confusion
[C] Acute delirium precipitated by urinary retention and anticholinergic medication effects
[D] Spontaneous intracranial hemorrhage from warfarin anticoagulation

Question 2: Which is the most appropriate immediate nursing action to address the likely reversible cause identified in the vignette?

[A] Administer oxygen via nasal cannula to raise SpO2 before further assessment
[B] Give intramuscular haloperidol to control agitation and ensure safety
[C] Apply physical restraints to prevent further falls
[D] Perform sterile urinary catheterization per protocol to relieve retention

Question 3: Which mechanism best explains how diphenhydramine likely contributed to the patient's cognitive changes?

[A] Excess central dopamine activity causing hallucinations and agitation
[B] Enhanced GABAergic inhibition leading to somnolence and confusion
[C] Central antimuscarinic blockade reducing acetylcholine-mediated attention and cognition
[D] Increased serotonin activity producing acute confusion and autonomic instability

Question 4: Given the patient's warfarin therapy and recent fall with a scalp hematoma, what is the best immediate nursing priority related to her anticoagulation?

[A] Obtain a stat INR and initiate frequent neurological checks while awaiting imaging and provider orders
[B] Administer intravenous vitamin K empirically to reverse anticoagulation immediately
[C] Prepare protamine sulfate in case of bleeding complications from warfarin
[D] Discharge home with instructions to follow up with primary provider in 48 hours

Question 5: Ethically and practically, which action should the nurse take next regarding this patient's living situation and safety after acute issues are addressed?

[A] Arrange discharge home with a written handout on fall prevention and encourage daughter to visit daily
[B] Conduct a capacity assessment, notify social work, and arrange a home safety evaluation and support services as indicated
[C] Immediately report the daughter to Adult Protective Services for possible neglect without further assessment
[D] Allow the patient to refuse further evaluation because she is alert and oriented to person

ANSWERS

1. Correct Answer: C

Rationale: The vignette shows acute, fluctuating inattention and disorientation over 24 hours with identified reversible contributors: significant urinary retention (bladder scan ~450 mL) and recent use of diphenhydramine (an anticholinergic). These features fit delirium precipitated by medication effects and a painful/visceral trigger. A is less likely because dementia is chronic and progressive rather than an acute change. B is unlikely because exam shows no focal neurologic deficit typical of stroke. D is possible given warfarin and fall, but the absence of focal deficits and the presence of clear reversible precipitants make intracranial hemorrhage less likely as the primary cause; imaging was appropriately ordered.

2. Correct Answer: D

Rationale: Relieving urinary retention with sterile catheterization is a low-risk, corrective action that can reverse or improve delirium when retention is causative; the bladder scan supports this intervention. A (oxygen) may be appropriate if hypoxia is suspected, but SpO2 is 92% and bladder retention is a clearer reversible cause requiring prompt action. B (haloperidol) is not first-line for delirium and treats symptoms rather than addressing causes; it also carries risk in the elderly. C (physical restraints) increases risk of injury and should be avoided as a first-line safety measure.

3. Correct Answer: C

Rationale: Diphenhydramine has strong anticholinergic effects that cross the blood–brain barrier and block central muscarinic receptors, reducing acetylcholine neurotransmission important for attention and cognition, producing delirium. A (dopamine excess), B (GABAergic inhibition), and D (serotonin increase) do not accurately describe diphenhydramine's primary central mechanism related to acute anticholinergic delirium.

4. Correct Answer: A

Rationale: With warfarin use and a head injury, obtaining a stat INR and starting frequent neurological checks are appropriate priorities to assess bleeding risk and detect neurologic deterioration while awaiting the ordered head CT and provider guidance. B (empiric vitamin K) and C (protamine sulfate) are inappropriate without confirmed need—vitamin K may be indicated after lab/imaging or on provider order; protamine reverses heparin, not warfarin. D (discharge) is unsafe given the fall, anticoagulation, and acute confusion.

5. Correct Answer: B

Rationale: The patient lives alone, has acute delirium possibly related to medication use and retention, and had a recent fall; assessing decision-making capacity and involving social work for a home safety evaluation and support services is ethical, practical, and aligns with preventing future harm. A (simple discharge with handout) is insufficient given safety concerns. C (immediate report to APS) may be necessary if abuse/neglect is confirmed or strongly suspected, but the next step is a structured assessment and involvement of interdisciplinary resources per policy. D (accepting refusal without assessment) ignores possible impaired capacity during an acute episode.

Clinical Vignette 4

A 28-year-old G1P0 at 28 weeks presents for routine prenatal care before flu season. She works as a pediatric nurse, recalls childhood egg-related urticaria but no vaccine anaphylaxis, and is unsure of MMR status. Six weeks ago she received a PRBC transfusion for postpartum hemorrhage during unrelated surgery. Medications: prenatal vitamins only; no tobacco or drugs. She lives with her partner. Exam: afebrile, HR 82, BP 118/72, fundal height appropriate, lungs clear, fetal heart tones normal. She asks about receiving the intranasal "flu spray" and whether to get MMR now or wait until postpartum, expressing concern about vaccine reactions.

Question 1: Based on the vignette, which immunization approach is most appropriate to administer today?

[A] Subcutaneous MMR vaccine now, because the patient is unsure of childhood immunity.
[B] Intranasal live-attenuated influenza vaccine (LAIV), because it is effective and avoids injection pain.
[C] Defer all vaccines today because of the reported egg allergy; discuss at a later visit.
[D] Give intramuscular inactivated influenza vaccine and administer Tdap during this 27–36 week window.

Question 2: Which statement best reflects counseling you should provide the patient about her childhood egg-associated urticaria and influenza vaccination?

[A] "Because you had an allergic reaction to eggs, you should receive only the intranasal live vaccine under observation."
[B] "A history of hives with egg exposure is not a contraindication to inactivated influenza vaccine; proceed with vaccination and routine 15-minute observation."
[C] "You must be observed for 30 minutes after any vaccine because of possible egg reactions."
[D] "Egg allergy is an absolute contraindication to any influenza vaccine, so you should not be vaccinated."

Question 3: If the patient were to develop an acute anaphylactic reaction after vaccination, which statement best describes how intramuscular epinephrine treats anaphylaxis?

[A] Epinephrine stimulates alpha-1 vasoconstriction and beta-2 bronchodilation, increasing perfusion and reversing airway edema and bronchospasm.
[B] Epinephrine acts primarily as an H1 receptor antagonist to block histamine effects.
[C] Epinephrine inhibits IgE production and prevents future allergic sensitization.
[D] Epinephrine stabilizes mast cells to prevent degranulation over the next several hours.

Question 4: The patient reports a packed red blood cell transfusion six weeks ago and says she is nonimmune to rubella per uncertain records. If she remains nonimmune postpartum, what is the best plan regarding MMR vaccination after delivery?

[A] Give MMR before discharge as soon as it's confirmed she is nonimmune, because live vaccines are safe postpartum.
[B] Administer MMR two weeks after delivery to allow maternal antibody changes to stabilize.
[C] Delay live vaccines (MMR/varicella) for several months after the transfusion to allow passive antibodies to wane.
[D] Give MMR immediately and plan to repeat the dose in six months if titers remain low.

Question 5: After counseling, the patient declines the influenza vaccine today but accepts Tdap. What is the nurse's most appropriate action regarding the influenza vaccine refusal?

[A] Document the patient's informed refusal, reinforce risks/benefits, and offer to revisit vaccination at future visits.
[B] Refuse further prenatal care until she consents to all recommended vaccines.
[C] Attempt to coerce her by indicating hospital policy requires vaccination for healthcare workers.
[D] Administer the influenza vaccine without explicit consent because she works in a healthcare setting.

ANSWERS

1. Correct Answer: D

Rationale: The vignette places the patient at 28 weeks' gestation (within the 27–36 week optimal window for Tdap) and during influenza season; inactivated (IM) influenza vaccine is recommended in any trimester and is appropriate for healthcare workers. Giving both Tdap and inactivated influenza today is consistent with co-administration rules (different sites, same day allowed). A is incorrect because live MMR is contraindicated during pregnancy. B is incorrect because intranasal LAIV is a live vaccine and contraindicated in pregnancy. C is incorrect because an egg-associated urticaria is not a reason to defer inactivated influenza; mild allergy alone does not preclude vaccination.

2. Correct Answer: B

Rationale: Chapter guidance states that egg allergy limited to hives is not a contraindication to inactivated influenza vaccine; the patient can receive the IM vaccine with routine precautions and 15-minute observation. A is incorrect because intranasal LAIV is live and contraindicated in pregnancy regardless of egg allergy. C is incorrect because 30-minute observation is reserved for those with a history of anaphylaxis to vaccines or severe allergic reactions, not routine egg hives. D is incorrect because egg allergy is not an absolute contraindication to influenza vaccination with the inactivated vaccine.

3. Correct Answer: A

Rationale: Epinephrine is the first-line treatment for anaphylaxis because alpha-1 effects cause peripheral vasoconstriction (raising BP and reducing mucosal edema) and beta-2 effects cause bronchodilation, reversing bronchospasm—this addresses the life-threatening physiology of anaphylaxis. B is incorrect because H1 antagonists (antihistamines) are adjunctive and do not treat airway compromise or shock. C is incorrect; epinephrine does not directly inhibit IgE production acutely. D is incorrect because mast cell stabilization is not the primary acute mechanism; epinephrine reverses physiologic collapse.

4. Correct Answer: C

Rationale: The vignette notes a blood transfusion six weeks prior; antibody-containing blood products can neutralize live vaccines, so MMR/varicella should be delayed for several months after passive antibody exposure. Chapter guidance emphasizes delaying live vaccines after immune globulin/blood products until passive antibodies wane. A is incorrect because while postpartum is a time to give MMR if nonimmune, recent transfusion requires a delay. B is incorrect because two weeks is insufficient time for transfused antibodies to clear and is not the recommended interval. D is incorrect because giving MMR immediately risks neutralization by passive antibodies and does not follow the "delay" principle; repeating later is not routine practice.

5. Correct Answer: A

Rationale: The chapter advises documenting vaccine refusal, providing respectful evidence-based counseling, and revisiting decisions later; patient autonomy must be respected while documenting informed refusal. B is incorrect and unethical; refusing care for vaccine refusal is not appropriate. C is incorrect because coercion is unethical and ineffective; education and respectful dialogue are recommended. D is incorrect because administering a vaccine without consent is assault and violates legal and ethical standards.

Clinical Vignette 5

A 15-year-old female presents to the school sports physical clinic with her mother requesting required vaccinations before the season starts; she reports mild nasal congestion and a temperature of 100.1°F today. She was born full term with no neonatal complications and received routine childhood vaccines through age 5 but missed well-child visits after starting middle school. She received one dose of HPV vaccine at age 13; she has never received Tdap or MenACWY. She takes combined oral contraceptives, is sexually active with inconsistent condom use, and has a childhood history of hives with eggs but no history of anaphylaxis to vaccines or vaccine components. There is no history of immunodeficiency, chemotherapy, recent blood products, or pregnancy; her mother is present and willing to provide consent. On exam she is alert, cooperative, with clear lungs, mild nasal mucosal erythema, and no respiratory distress; vital signs otherwise within normal limits. No laboratory tests or imaging have been performed and none are immediately indicated. The mother asks whether vaccines should be given today given the mild cold and whether HPV can be completed now.

Question 1: Based on the vignette, which immunizations are most appropriate for the nurse to administer today?

[A] MMR and Varicella only
[B] Tdap, HPV dose 2, and MenACWY
[C] Influenza vaccine only until fully evaluated by provider
[D] Defer all vaccines until the patient is afebrile for 48 hours

Question 2: The patient has mild nasal congestion and a temperature of 100.1°F. What is the nurse's best action regarding vaccination today?

[A] Defer all vaccines until the patient is completely symptom-free for several days.
[B] Administer only inactivated vaccines today and defer any live vaccines.
[C] Proceed with administering indicated vaccines today because mild illness and low-grade fever are not contraindications.
[D] Obtain a chest x-ray and CBC before giving any vaccines.

Question 3: Which statement best describes the immunologic mechanism by which the HPV vaccine protects against cervical cancer?

[A] It uses live-attenuated HPV to produce intracellular replication and T-cell immunity.
[B] It contains inactivated whole virus that primarily stimulates cell-mediated immunity.
[C] It is a DNA vaccine that integrates into host genome to produce long-term antigen expression.
[D] It contains virus-like particles that induce neutralizing antibodies preventing viral entry into epithelial cells.

Question 4: For intramuscular administration of Tdap and MenACWY in this 15-year-old, what is the preferred route and site?

[A] A. Intramuscular injection into the deltoid muscle.
[B] B. Subcutaneous injection into the anterolateral thigh.
[C] C. Intramuscular injection into the vastus lateralis (anterolateral thigh).
[D] D. Subcutaneous injection into the deltoid region.

Question 5: The patient received her first HPV dose at age 13 and missed the scheduled second dose; she is now 15. What is the appropriate HPV catch-up plan?

[A] Restart the HPV series with a new 3-dose schedule beginning today.
[B] Wait until the patient turns 16 and then give a single booster dose.
[C] Administer the second HPV dose today and complete a 2-dose series because the series was started before the 15th birthday.
[D] No further HPV doses are needed because one dose provides adequate protection.

ANSWERS

1. Correct Answer: B

Rationale: The vignette documents that the patient received only one HPV dose at 13 and missed Tdap and MenACWY at 11–12 years; at 15 she is due for Tdap and MenACWY and is eligible to complete HPV (second dose) now. Option A is incorrect because MMR and Varicella were routinely given by age 4–6 and are not indicated here. Option C is less correct because influenza alone is incomplete—other indicated vaccines should be given if due; influenza may be added if in season but is not the only appropriate vaccine. Option D is incorrect because mild illness and a low-grade fever are not contraindications to vaccinating (per routine/catch-up principles).

2. Correct Answer: C

Rationale: The chapter emphasizes that mild illness or low-grade fever is a precaution that does not warrant delaying routine immunizations; therefore the nurse should proceed with indicated vaccines. Option A is incorrect because deferring for several days is unnecessary for mild illness and could delay protection. Option B is too restrictive—unless a true contraindication exists, inactivated and live vaccines may be given when illness is mild; also the vaccines due here are inactivated/recombinant, not live. Option D is inappropriate and not indicated for a mild upper respiratory symptom; unnecessary testing would delay needed immunization.

3. Correct Answer: D

Rationale: HPV vaccines are virus-like particle (VLP) recombinant vaccines that induce neutralizing antibodies to prevent viral attachment/entry into epithelial cells, reducing infection and subsequent cancer risk. Option A is incorrect—HPV vaccines are not live-attenuated. Option B is misleading because they are not inactivated whole-virus vaccines and the primary protective mechanism is antibody-mediated rather than solely cell-mediated. Option D is incorrect—current HPV vaccines are not DNA vaccines integrating into the host genome.

4. Correct Answer: A

Rationale: For adolescents with adequate deltoid muscle mass, intramuscular injection into the deltoid is the preferred route and site for Tdap and MenACWY. Option B is incorrect—subcutaneous thigh is not the recommended site for these IM vaccines. Option C is more appropriate for infants (vastus lateralis) rather than a 15-year-old with adequate deltoid muscle. Option D is incorrect because these vaccines should be given intramuscularly, not subcutaneously.

5. Correct Answer: C

Rationale: Because the patient began the HPV series before her 15th birthday (first dose at 13), she qualifies for a 2-dose schedule; the second dose can be given now to complete the series per catch-up rules. Option A is incorrect—the series is not restarted (never restart a vaccine series). Option B is incorrect—waiting is unnecessary and delays protection. Option D is incorrect—one dose does not provide adequate routine protection; a second dose is required when started before age 15.

Clinical Vignette 6

A 52-year-old man presents for an annual physical requesting routine screening and asking specifically whether he should have a PSA test. He reports a 30 pack-year smoking history and quit 8 years ago, drinks alcohol socially, and works as an accountant; he takes no regular medications and has no medication allergies. Family history is notable for a father who had colorectal cancer at age 68 and a brother with hyperlipidemia. Vital signs show BP 152/94 mm Hg, pulse 82, BMI 32 kg/m2. Exam is otherwise unremarkable with clear lungs and no abdominal masses. He completed a home fecal immunochemical test last week that returned positive and brings the result today. Recent labs in the clinic show A1c 6.2% and fasting lipid panel with LDL 150 mg/dL. He asks about lung cancer screening given his prior smoking and whether to start a statin or get PSA screening now.

Question 1: Referencing the vignette, what is the nurse's most appropriate next action regarding the positive fecal immunochemical test?

[A] Arrange a diagnostic colonoscopy promptly.
[B] Repeat the FIT to confirm before further evaluation.
[C] Order a guaiac fecal occult blood test to compare results.
[D] Advise watchful waiting and repeat stool testing in 6 months.

Question 2: Based on the vignette, which screening is indicated now because of the patient's smoking history?

[A] Obtain a chest x-ray as an initial screening.
[B] Offer annual low-dose CT scan of the chest.
[C] Perform sputum cytology annually.
[D] No lung cancer screening is indicated because he quit smoking.

Question 3: The patient's A1c is 6.2% and BMI is 32 kg/m2. Which physiologic process best explains his current glucose elevation?

[A] Peripheral insulin resistance associated with adiposity leading to higher fasting glucose.
[B] Autoimmune destruction of pancreatic beta cells causing insulin deficiency.
[C] Pancreatic exocrine insufficiency decreasing insulin secretion.
[D] Increased insulin clearance by the liver reducing circulating insulin levels.

Question 4: Considering the vignette's age and LDL of 150 mg/dL, what is the most appropriate next nursing action regarding primary prevention with statin therapy?

[A] Initiate high-intensity statin therapy immediately without further assessment.
[B] Defer lipid management until LDL exceeds 190 mg/dL.
[C] Calculate the 10-year ASCVD risk and discuss statin therapy based on risk and shared decision-making.
[D] Start ezetimibe monotherapy instead of a statin for primary prevention.

Question 5: The patient asks the nurse whether he should have a PSA test today. What is the best response consistent with screening guidance and ethical nursing practice?

[A] "Yes—men over 50 should have an annual PSA as routine."
[B] "No—PSA testing is never recommended because harms always outweigh benefits."
[C] "Only if you have urinary symptoms; otherwise PSA is unnecessary."
[D] "Explain that PSA screening is preference-sensitive and generally offered with shared decision-making for men aged 55–69; discuss risks and benefits and document his preferences."

ANSWERS

1. Correct Answer: A

Rationale: A positive FIT is a stool-based screening positive result that requires prompt diagnostic colonoscopy rather than repeating stool tests; the vignette's positive FIT and family history of colorectal cancer support immediate colonoscopic evaluation. B is incorrect because repeating FIT after a positive result is inappropriate—positive stool tests should lead to colonoscopy. C is less correct because guaiac tests are not needed and are less specific; they do not replace diagnostic colonoscopy. D is incorrect because watchful waiting delays necessary diagnostic evaluation and risks missed lesions.

2. Correct Answer: B

Rationale: Current guidelines recommend annual low-dose CT for adults aged 50–80 with at least a 20 pack-year history who currently smoke or quit within the last 15 years; this patient is 52 with a 30 pack-year history and quit 8 years ago, making annual LDCT indicated. A is incorrect because chest x-ray is not an effective screening tool for lung cancer. C is incorrect because sputum cytology is not recommended as routine screening. D is incorrect because quitting within 15 years still qualifies the patient for screening.

3. Correct Answer: A

Rationale: Elevated A1c in the setting of obesity (BMI 32) is most consistent with peripheral insulin resistance related to adiposity, which raises fasting and overall glucose and is typical of type 2 diabetes pathophysiology. B is incorrect because autoimmune beta-cell destruction describes type 1 diabetes and is less likely in an obese 52-year-old with gradual hyperglycemia. C is incorrect as exocrine insufficiency does not commonly cause this pattern of A1c elevation. D is incorrect because increased hepatic insulin clearance is not the primary mechanism in obesity-related glucose intolerance.

4. Correct Answer: C

Rationale: For adults 40–75 with LDL <190, clinical guidelines recommend calculating the 10-year ASCVD risk to guide statin initiation and engage in shared decision-making; the vignette's age and LDL 150 mg/dL warrant risk calculation before starting therapy. A is incorrect because immediate high-intensity statin without risk assessment is not standard for primary prevention in average-risk patients. B is incorrect because waiting until LDL >190 ignores risk-based indications for earlier therapy. D is incorrect because ezetimibe is not first-line monotherapy for primary prevention in this scenario.

5. Correct Answer: D

Rationale: PSA screening is preference-sensitive and generally discussed with shared decision-making for men aged 55–69; the nurse should explain risks/benefits, support informed choices, and document preferences—this aligns with ethical practice and chapter guidance. A is incorrect because routine annual PSA for all men over 50 is not recommended. B is incorrect because PSA is not universally contraindicated; it can be appropriate after shared decision-making in the 55–69 age group. C is incorrect because PSA may be considered for asymptomatic men within the recommended age range after discussion; limiting to only symptomatic men is not consistent with guidance.

CHAPTER 4

Client Needs III — Psychosocial Integrity

4.1 Therapeutic Communication (Best vs. Worst Answers List)

On the NCLEX, communication items are high-yield because they test how you protect psychosocial integrity while using clinical judgment. You are expected to default to client-centered, empathetic, nonjudgmental, and trauma-informed language. The reliable rule: feelings first, facts second; safety always. Think "assess emotion and risk → invite expression → maintain reality and boundaries → teach and plan last." Avoid advice, reassurance, and "why" questions. When safety signals appear—suicidal/homicidal ideation, abuse, psychosis—move immediately to clear, direct assessment.

A quick CJMM mini-approach helps you choose the best response:

1. Recognize cues: What emotion or state is present (fear, grief, anger, panic, hopelessness)? Any immediate safety risk (suicide/homicide, abuse, command hallucinations, severe agitation)?
2. Analyze cues: What does the client need now—ventilate feelings, feel understood, clarify events, or be kept safe?
3. Generate and prioritize options: Prefer responses that invite expression, validate feelings, and assess risk. Avoid those that judge, fix, or minimize.
4. Take action and evaluate: Pick the least restrictive, boundaries-preserving, reality-based answer that de-escalates and protects safety. Teaching and problem-solving come after assessment and validation.

Below are patterns the exam repeatedly rewards and penalizes. Use them to scan choices quickly.

Therapeutic Communication: Patterns That Help or Harm

On the NCLEX, communication items consistently reward certain therapeutic patterns and penalize others. The goal is to recognize which approaches foster safety, trust, and expression, and which ones shut clients down or create risk.

Helpful approaches include open-ended invitations that allow clients to lead, such as "Tell me more about what's worrying you right now" or "Help me understand what the nights are like for you." Reflection and validation are also rewarded, for example: "You sound overwhelmed with everything happening" or "It's understandable to feel scared before surgery." Restating and clarifying ensures shared understanding: "So you're saying the pain gets worse when you stand, and that worries you?"

Therapeutic presence—silence, attentive posture, and moving from broad exploration to specific follow-up—encourages deeper sharing. Safety must always be assessed directly if risk is suspected: "Are you thinking about harming yourself? Do you have a plan?" For psychotic symptoms, presenting reality without arguing is key: "I believe you're hearing voices; I don't hear them. You are safe here." When anxiety or mania runs high, simple and calm statements such as "You're safe. Breathe with me. In through the nose, out through the mouth" are more effective than complex explanations. Communication should also remain culturally responsive, using professional interpreters when needed and addressing the client directly. Above all, the nurse supports autonomy and boundaries: "These are your options. What feels right to you?"

Unhelpful approaches are just as important to recognize. These include "why" questions, moralizing, offering advice or personal opinions, giving false reassurance, or minimizing concerns. Arguing, challenging, or testing the client undermines trust, as does teaching or problem-solving before feelings and safety have been addressed. Other red flags include premature self-disclosure, promises of secrecy, use of jargon, or speaking to family instead of the client.

Situational adaptations are worth remembering. With suicidal or homicidal ideation, ask directly about thoughts, plan, and means, and never leave the client alone. With hallucinations or delusions, acknowledge feelings but do not validate false content. With anger or agitation, allow venting, remain calm, and set clear limits while prioritizing safety. During panic or acute anxiety, use short statements, grounding, and guided breathing. Grief calls for silence, presence, and invitations to share, while children may need drawings or play and adolescents privacy. For older adults, avoid elderspeak, allow more time, and adapt to sensory deficits.

On test items, apply these rules systematically. Select options that validate feelings, assess safety, invite exploration, present reality without arguing, and set boundaries respectfully. Discard those that judge, probe "why," offer false reassurance, or jump prematurely into teaching. When arranging steps, think in order: identify emotion → assess safety → invite expression → maintain reality and limits → teach or plan last.

Mini-scenarios illustrate this principle:

- A suicidal client saying, "I don't see a reason to go on" should be met with "Those are serious feelings. Are you thinking about harming yourself? Do you have a plan?" rather than "Don't say that—your family needs you."
- A client with schizophrenia stating, "The TV is sending me messages" calls for "That sounds unsettling. I don't receive messages from the TV, and you're safe here" rather than confrontation.
- An anxious client before MRI benefits from "The machine can feel confining. Let's practice slow breathing together" instead of "There's nothing to worry about."

4.2 Safety, Coping, Grief, and Abuse

Think "safety first, least restrictive, and legally clean." Use the clinical judgment sequence: recognize cues, analyze risk level, prioritize immediate safety, act with the least-restrictive effective measures, and evaluate whether risk has dropped and supports are in place.

Start every psychosocial assessment with a brief, behavior-focused safety screen. Ask directly about suicide, homicide, and recent agitation. Use simple, clear language, and document verbatim responses.

Immediate safety screening always centers on whether the patient is an imminent danger to self or others. For suicide, high-yield cues include a specific plan, access to means, immediacy or recent preparation behaviors, a history of past attempts, a sudden brightening in mood after severe depression, giving away belongings, increased isolation, and access to firearms or lethal medications. If imminent risk is present, move to 1:1 observation, remove ligature and lethal means, provide a safe environment, notify the provider, and prepare for possible involuntary hold if criteria are met. Do not rely on "contracts for safety." When the acute risk subsides and discharge is appropriate, a written safety plan includes lethal means restriction, crisis numbers, and rapid follow-up appointments within a short interval.

Homicide and violence risk go up with command hallucinations telling the person to harm others, identification of a specific target, access to weapons, escalating agitation, and substance intoxication. The duty to protect or warn activates when there is a credible, imminent threat to an identifiable third party. Involve security per policy and law enforcement if required by your facility's protocol. Share only the minimum necessary information to protect life and follow chain-of-command.

Crisis and agitation follow observable phases—trigger, escalation, crisis, and recovery. Effective de-escalation uses a calm tone, short one-step directions, generous personal space, nonthreatening posture, and environmental control (reduce noise, remove audience). Offer choices that preserve autonomy, and consider oral PRN medication before any injectable. Seclusion and restraints are last-resort interventions for violent or self-destructive behavior when lesser measures fail and there is imminent danger. They require time-limited orders, ongoing assessment, continuous monitoring, meticulous documentation of behaviors and alternatives tried, and strict protection of patient rights. For violent/self-destructive restraints, an order cannot be PRN, must be time-limited (adults typically up to 4 hours; 9–17 years up to 2 hours; under 9 years up to 1 hour), requires continuous monitoring and a timely face-to-face evaluation by a qualified practitioner. Once behavior is controlled, remove restraints promptly—always least restrictive, minimum duration.

A quick "Do/Avoid" for acute safety clarifies priorities:

- Do: ask directly about suicide/homicide; institute 1:1 for imminent risk; remove means; notify provider; involve security per policy; use de-escalation; document cues, actions, and responses; plan lethal means restriction at discharge.
- Avoid: minimizing threats; relying on no-harm contracts; leaving the patient alone when risk is high; using restraints without exhausting less-restrictive measures and required monitoring; threatening or confrontational communication.

Coping and adaptation are best handled by recognizing what reduces versus increases risk. Adaptive coping includes problem-solving, paced breathing, grounding techniques (for example, identify five things you can see, four you can touch, three you can hear), structured routines for sleep and meals, activity scheduling, and appropriate use of social support. These skills are brief, teachable, and safe to recommend at the bedside. Maladaptive patterns include substance use or escalation of use, self-injury, binge–purge behaviors, compulsive gambling or spending, and violent acting out. Identify and redirect these toward safer skills; if substance use or self-harm is present, the safety plan must escalate. Defense mechanisms are testable mainly when they increase risk or derail care: denial commonly appears in substance use disorders and mandates firm but empathetic feedback linked to safety (e.g., "drinking despite withdrawals is dangerous; let's consider detox supports"), and splitting in borderline traits requires consistent limit-setting and team communication to prevent staff-splitting. Label mechanisms only to inform your response; don't pathologize normal stress reactions.

Grief and loss show wide normal variability. Expect waves of sadness, guilt, sleep/appetite changes, and intermittent functioning. Red flags for complicated grief include persistent, intense impairment, inability to function in basic roles for a prolonged period, preoccupation with death of the loved one that doesn't soften, and any suicidal ideation. Nurses support by being present, validating the loss, avoiding clichés or "fixing," encouraging rituals and cultural practices meaningful to the patient, and connecting to supports (family, spiritual care, bereavement groups). In perinatal loss, offer options without pressure: seeing or holding the baby if desired, memory items (photos, footprints, lock of hair), naming opportunities, and time for farewell. Document the family's choices and provide resources. During pediatric death, communicate honestly using developmentally appropriate language, invite questions, involve child life when available, and support parents' presence and participation in care to the extent they wish. In any bereavement with noticeable hopelessness, substance escalation, or talk of "not wanting to go on," perform a suicide risk assessment and escalate as needed.

Abuse assessment is trauma-informed: safety first, privacy, choice, and nonjudgment. Intimate partner violence often presents with injuries inconsistent with the story, frequent ED visits for vague complaints, a controlling partner who refuses to leave the room, and hypervigilance or fearfulness. Approach privately and ask normalized, direct questions. Child abuse or neglect cues include bruises on protected areas (torso, ears, neck), patterned injuries (loop marks), immersion burns, spiral fractures, delay in seeking care, and STIs; always consider whether the child's developmental abilities match the reported mechanism. Elder or vulnerable adult abuse may show as dehydration, pressure injuries, poor hygiene, over- or under-medication, unexplained fractures or bruises, sudden financial changes, or exhausted caregivers. With any suspected abuse, stabilize medical needs, ensure immediate safety, interview the patient alone, use a validated screening tool if available, and avoid pressuring a victim to leave; empower them with options.

Safety planning is concrete and should be offered whenever IPV is suspected or disclosed: discuss a code word with trusted contacts, identify safe exits, gather a go-bag (IDs, cash, meds, keys), and provide hotlines, shelter contacts, and information on protective orders and legal resources. Respect the patient's readiness; your role is to keep the door open and provide resources. Use certified medical interpreters; do not use family members.

Sexual assault care prioritizes consent and control. Explain each step, obtain consent for exam and evidence collection, and avoid retraumatizing language or touch. Preserve evidence by advising against bathing, changing clothes, eating, or brushing teeth if possible; if the patient has already done so, proceed—assistance is still appropriate. Arrange a timely forensic exam by a trained clinician (SANE where available), maintain chain of custody for evidence, and administer prophylaxis per orders (STIs, emergency contraception, HIV post-exposure prophylaxis when indicated). Offer crisis resources and follow-up. Document objectively, including the patient's words.

Mandatory reporting and legal/ethical essentials guide what must be disclosed. Nurses are mandated reporters for suspected child abuse/neglect and elder/vulnerable adult abuse; suspicion is enough—you do not need proof. Follow facility policy and state law for reporting while providing ongoing care and safety. Document objectively using body maps and photos per policy, include verbatim quotes, and note who you notified and when. Duty to warn or protect applies when there is a credible, imminent threat to an identifiable person; notify the provider and appropriate authorities according to policy, and take steps to protect potential victims. Involuntary commitment criteria generally include danger to self, danger to others, or grave disability (unable to provide for basic needs due to mental illness). Even under an involuntary hold, maintain the least-restrictive environment, protect rights to informed consent, and remember that medication may be refused unless an emergency exists or a court order is obtained. Confidentiality has limits in these scenarios—suicidal or homicidal risk, mandated reporting, or court orders. Always use certified interpreters for consent and screening.

Write notes as if they will be scrutinized in court. Strong documentation is objective, factual, and time-stamped. Record the patient's exact words in quotes, describe injuries with size, location, shape, and color, include diagrams or photos if policy allows, list all safety measures taken and the patient's response, and note notifications (provider, security, social work, protective services, law enforcement) with times. If restraints or seclusion were used, document the behaviors that led to use, less-restrictive measures attempted, monitoring data, care provided (fluids, toileting, ROM), and criteria for release.

To integrate clinical judgment quickly in NGN scenarios, use compact if–then maps that guide first actions and legal steps:

- If suicidal ideation includes a specific plan and means now, then do not leave the patient alone, initiate 1:1 observation, remove means, notify the provider, obtain a time-limited order for any required emergency measures, consider involuntary hold criteria, and begin a collaborative safety plan for ongoing care. Evaluate by confirming reduced access to means, stable observation, and arranged rapid follow-up.
- If child abuse is suspected (injury inconsistent with developmental ability or story), then stabilize medical needs, separate child and caregiver for history, document objectively with quotes and body maps, notify the provider, and file a mandated report to child protective services per policy—do not confront the alleged abuser or promise confidentiality beyond legal limits. Evaluate by confirming the report was submitted and that the child's immediate safety plan is in place.
- If agitation is escalating with threats or weapon access, then clear the area, call for help/security, use calm one-step directions and space, offer oral PRN medication, and move toward seclusion/restraints only if imminent harm persists after lesser measures. Obtain a time-limited order, initiate continuous monitoring, and protect rights. Evaluate by ensuring behavior has de-escalated and restraints are removed as soon as safely possible.
- If IPV is disclosed, then ensure a private setting, provide validation and options without pressure, conduct safety planning (code word, exits, go-bag), offer resources (hotline, shelters, legal), document objectively, and assess for co-occurring suicide risk. Evaluate by confirming the patient leaves with a plan and resources and understands options.

Throughout, prioritize using ABCs alongside imminent violence or self-harm cues. Choose the least-restrictive effective action first and escalate only as needed. Always finish by asking, "Is risk lower now? What follow-up or protections are in place?" That question anchors both bedside care and test answers to safe, legal, and compassionate nursing practice.

4.3 Knowledge Check

Clinical Vignette 1

A 34-year-old woman presents to the ED tearful, stating "I don't see a reason to go on" after a fight with her partner. She has major depressive disorder previously treated with sertraline 50 mg daily, stopped 2 weeks ago due to cost. For the past month she reports poor sleep, appetite loss, and low energy. She discloses her partner "hit me last night" but is vague about injuries; two children (ages 6 and 8) live at home. Exam: thin, tearful, slow speech, depressed affect; vitals stable, pregnancy test negative. She endorses passive suicidal thoughts ("maybe it would be better if I weren't here") and occasional voices calling her "worthless," but no commands or homicidal intent. No acute medical findings; labs are normal. She has no drug allergies and no nearby family support.

Question 1: Based on the vignette, which is the most likely clinical diagnosis for this patient?

[A] Major depressive episode with suicidal ideation
[B] Adjustment disorder with depressed mood
[C] Posttraumatic stress disorder (PTSD)
[D] Schizoaffective disorder

Question 2: Referencing the vignette, what is the nurse's next best immediate action at the bedside?

[A] Reassure the patient that "everything will be okay" and offer to call her partner to come to the ED.
[B] Ask, "Why would you think that?" and explore triggers in detail.
[C] Tell the patient she should leave her partner right away and make a safety plan later.
[D] Validate her feelings and directly assess suicide risk: "I hear you saying you don't see a reason to go on; are you thinking about ending your life? Do you have a plan or access to means?"

Question 3: The patient stopped taking sertraline 2 weeks ago. Which statement best describes sertraline's primary mechanism of action relevant to her depressive symptoms?

[A] It inhibits monoamine oxidase, increasing availability of multiple monoamines.
[B] It blocks presynaptic serotonin reuptake, increasing serotonin in the synaptic cleft.
[C] It antagonizes postsynaptic serotonin (5-HT2) receptors, reducing anxiety.
[D] It increases norepinephrine release from presynaptic terminals.

Question 4: Which of the following nurse responses best follows therapeutic-communication principles from the chapter when the patient says, "I don't see a reason to go on"?

[A] "Don't talk like that—your children need you."
[B] "You should leave him; staying is unsafe."
[C] "Why are you feeling so hopeless?"
[D] "I can see you're feeling hopeless and scared. I'm glad you told me. Are you thinking about hurting yourself now?"

Question 5: The patient discloses that her partner hit her last night and that the children were present. Which action is ethically and legally appropriate for the nurse to take first?

[A] Ensure immediate safety for the patient and children, explain limits of confidentiality, provide resources and a safety plan, and notify appropriate protective services if children are at risk.
[B] Honor the patient's request for confidentiality and do not notify anyone unless she asks you to call the police.
[C] Contact the partner to inform him the patient is in the ED and request he come to the hospital for a family meeting.
[D] Promise not to tell anyone and place the patient on home safety precautions with outpatient follow-up only.

ANSWERS

1. Correct Answer: A

Rationale: The patient has a history of major depressive disorder, stopped sertraline 2 weeks ago, and now reports anhedonia, sleep/appetite disturbance, low energy, passive suicidal ideation, and depressed affect—features most consistent with a major depressive episode with suicidal ideation. B (Adjustment disorder) is less likely because symptoms are more pervasive and meet criteria for a major depressive episode rather than a short-term stress reaction. C (PTSD) would require re-experiencing, avoidance, and hyperarousal tied to a traumatic event; the vignette centers on depressive symptoms and suicidality. D (Schizoaffective disorder) requires prominent mood and persistent psychotic symptoms outside mood episodes; she reports occasional non-command auditory perceptions but not persistent psychosis independent of mood.

2. Correct Answer: D

Rationale: The chapter emphasizes "assess emotion and risk → invite expression," and safety always: validate feelings and ask directly about suicidal thoughts, plan, and means. Asking directly (D) assesses immediate risk and guides next steps. A is false reassurance and inappropriately involves the partner; B is a "why" question and can be judgmental; C gives premature advice and skips immediate safety assessment.

3. Correct Answer: B

Rationale: Sertraline is a selective serotonin reuptake inhibitor (SSRI) that blocks presynaptic serotonin reuptake, increasing serotonin availability in the synaptic cleft—this underlies its antidepressant effect. A describes MAOI activity (incorrect). C refers to 5-HT2 antagonism (not sertraline's primary action). D is more consistent with drugs that increase norepinephrine (e.g., SNRIs or stimulants), not SSRIs.

4. Correct Answer: D

Rationale: Option D follows the chapter's "feelings first, facts second" rule: it validates emotion, expresses presence, and directly assesses safety—an empathic, trauma-informed approach. A is judgmental/minimizing and may shame the patient; B gives advice and bypasses assessment; C uses a "why" question, which is probing and can increase defensiveness.

5. Correct Answer: A

Rationale: The nurse must prioritize immediate safety for patient and children, disclose limits of confidentiality (safety reporting), provide resources and a safety plan, and notify protective services if children are at risk—this aligns with ethical duty to protect vulnerable individuals. B wrongly promises confidentiality despite potential child risk. C would breach safety by contacting the alleged perpetrator. D inappropriately promises secrecy and delays addressing imminent safety needs.

Clinical Vignette 2

A 28-year-old woman presents to the emergency department with the chief complaint, "I don't want to live anymore." She has a history of major depressive disorder and started sertraline 6 days ago; allergies: NKDA. She reports heavy drinking most evenings and had several drinks last night. Her partner accompanied her and initially refused to leave the room; when asked privately, she becomes tearful, says, "He has a gun at home," and reports giving away her wedding ring "a few days ago." On exam she is tearful, hypervigilant, and avoids eye contact; there are multiple bruises of varying ages on the left forearm and right lateral ribs; she says she "fell down the stairs" but is vague about timing. Vital signs are T 37.1°C, HR 98, BP 126/78, RR 18, SpO2 99% on room air. A urine pregnancy test is negative; a breath alcohol screen is positive at 0.06%. She denies current hallucinations or wanting to harm anyone else, but when asked directly about suicide she says, "I plan to go soon" without providing timeline. The ED nurse documents the patient's exact words and requests a private interview when the partner is asked to step into the waiting area.

Question 1: Based on the vignette, which initial nursing action is the highest priority for safety?

- [A] Ask directly about a specific suicide plan and access to lethal means and institute constant observation if imminent risk is confirmed.
- [B] Arrange a forensic sexual assault exam and collect evidence.
- [C] Discharge the patient with a safety contract and outpatient psychiatry follow-up.
- [D] Allow the partner to remain in the room to provide emotional support while the nurse completes documentation.

Question 2: In the private interview the patient adds, "He hits our 3-year-old when I'm not looking." Referencing the vignette, which action should the nurse take next?

- [A] Confront the partner and demand an explanation before reporting.
- [B] Promise the mother confidentiality and do not report to avoid breaking trust.
- [C] Advise the mother to take the child home and monitor for further injuries.
- [D] Stabilize immediate medical needs if present, interview child and caregiver separately as appropriate, document objectively, and file a mandated report to child protective services per facility/state policy.

Question 3: Which element of the vignette most significantly increases this patient's acute risk for suicide?

- [A] Recent initiation of sertraline 6 days ago without follow-up.
- [B] Positive breath alcohol screen (0.06%) on arrival.
- [C] Patient report of access to a firearm at home in the context of a stated plan.
- [D] Presence of multiple bruises on exam and an inconsistent history.

Question 4: The patient states, "I plan to go soon," and appears increasingly agitated when the partner re-enters the room. Which immediate intervention aligns best with least-restrictive, legally clean practice?

- [A] Place the patient in wrist and ankle restraints to prevent self-harm.
- [B] Administer an intramuscular sedative without attempting oral medication first.
- [C] Leave the patient alone with the partner to calm down while waiting for the provider.
- [D] Do not leave the patient alone, remove access to lethal means (ask about firearm location and secure), initiate 1:1 observation, notify the provider, and document verbatim statements.

Question 5: Which documentation practice best follows the chapter guidance for legal defensibility and supports continuity of care for this vignette?

- [A] Write a subjective summary that "patient denies intent" and list observed bruising as "old injuries."
- [B] Record paraphrased statements about the firearm and omit exact times to protect privacy.
- [C] Time-stamp and record the patient's exact quoted statements, describe bruises with size/location/appearance or body map, note who was notified and when, and list safety measures implemented.
- [D] Enter only the provider's assessment and plan in the chart and keep nursing notes brief to avoid redundancy.

ANSWERS

1. Correct Answer: A

Rationale: The vignette includes an explicit suicidal statement ("I don't want to live anymore," "I plan to go soon") plus access to a firearm; asking directly about a specific plan and means and initiating observation when imminent risk is present is the priority per safety-first rules. B is incorrect because a forensic sexual assault exam is not indicated by this vignette. C is incorrect—safety contracts are unreliable and discharging a patient with active plan and means would be unsafe. D is incorrect because leaving the partner in the room risks coercion and interferes with private assessment; the partner should be asked to step out for safety screening.

2. Correct Answer: D

Rationale: Disclosure of child abuse mandates reporting; the correct legal/ethical sequence is to address immediate medical needs, separate interviews as appropriate, document objectively (quotes, body maps), and file a mandated report to child protective services per policy. A is inappropriate and may escalate risk; B is incorrect because suspicion is sufficient to report—confidentiality has limits. C is unsafe—advising the child return home without reporting could leave the child at risk.

3. Correct Answer: C

Rationale: Access to firearms in the context of a stated plan is among the highest-leverage risk factors for completed suicide and requires immediate lethal-means restriction. A (recent SSRI start) can be a risk modifier but is less immediately dangerous than current access to lethal means. B (alcohol) increases risk but is less specific than firearm access. D (bruises/inconsistent history) suggests abuse and safety concerns but does not directly increase lethality of a suicide plan as much as firearm access.

4. Correct Answer: D

Rationale: The least-restrictive, legally clean immediate actions when imminent self-harm risk is present are to stay with the patient, remove or secure lethal means, initiate constant observation (1:1), notify the provider, and document—this follows de-escalation and safety-first protocols. A is incorrect because restraints are a last resort after less-restrictive measures fail and have legal/time limits. B is incorrect—injectables should be considered only after offering oral meds and when necessary; also no medication orders are documented yet. C is unsafe—leaving the patient with the partner may increase coercion and risk.

5. Correct Answer: C

Rationale: Legally defensible documentation includes time-stamped verbatim quotes, objective descriptions of injuries (size, location, color, body map/photo per policy), record of notifications (who/when), and actions taken for safety—matching chapter guidance. A is incorrect because vague or inaccurate descriptions can be challenged in court. B is incorrect—paraphrasing and omitting times weakens the record; exact quotes and times are required. D is incorrect—nursing documentation must include the nursing assessment and interventions, not only the provider's notes.

CHAPTER 5

Client Needs IV — Physiological Integrity

5.1 Basic Care & Comfort (Positioning, Diets, Enteral Feeding, Ostomy)

Basic Care and Comfort questions reward nurses who prevent problems before they happen. Use clinical judgment to recognize cues that signal airway/aspiration risk, skin breakdown, malnutrition, or dehydration; prioritize the safest first action; perform it; then evaluate if risk has decreased. Stable cues allow teaching and routine care. Unstable cues (respiratory changes, new bleeding/ischemia, sudden neurological change, high-output losses) demand immediate safety moves and reassessment.

Start with positioning and mobility because safe position often is the first, fastest risk reducer. High-Fowler's is the default for dyspnea and aspiration risk: it maximizes lung expansion and helps protect the airway during meals, tube feeds, or emesis. If the patient has decreased level of consciousness or is vomiting, side-lying reduces aspiration by allowing secretions to drain. For increased intracranial pressure, keep the head midline with the head of bed about 30 degrees to promote venous drainage and avoid jugular compression. In hypotension, supine with legs elevated improves venous return; avoid Trendelenburg, which is not recommended and can worsen respiratory status. If you suspect a venous air embolism (for example, after central line removal with sudden dyspnea), first position the patient in left lateral Trendelenburg to trap air in the right ventricle and call for help.

Post-procedure positioning often shows up as "what is the first action?" After a liver biopsy, position on the right side to tamponade the site. After a lumbar puncture, keep the patient flat to reduce CSF leak and headache as ordered. Following a thyroidectomy, use semi-Fowler's with the neck neutral to reduce strain on the incision and maintain airway access. For epistaxis, lean forward and apply pressure—never tilt back. For total hip arthroplasty, prevent dislocation with an abduction pillow, avoid hip flexion beyond 90 degrees, no adduction or internal rotation, and use raised seats. After mastectomy, elevate the affected arm to promote lymphatic drainage and reduce edema.

Preventing pressure injuries combines schedule and support. Reposition at least every two hours in bed and every hour in a chair, float the heels, pad bony prominences, and keep the skin clean and dry with moisture barriers. Adequate protein and hydration support skin integrity; cue malnutrition (weight loss, poor intake, muscle wasting) should prompt a nutrition referral and a higher-protein meal plan if not contraindicated.

Ambulation safety is another frequent test angle. A cane is held on the strong side; the sequence is cane, weak leg, then strong leg. With a walker, move the walker first, then the weak leg, then the strong leg while keeping the back of the chair behind the knees when standing up. On stairs, remember "up with the good, down with the bad": the stronger leg leads when going up; the weaker leg and device lead when going down. Teach the sequence and stand slightly behind and on the weaker side with a gait belt.

Diet orders protect against aspiration and metabolic complications. Know the progression: NPO, then clear liquids, full liquids, pureed/mechanically altered/soft, and regular as tolerated. Cardiac diets restrict sodium and saturated fat. Renal diets commonly restrict potassium, phosphorus, and sodium with fluids individualized to labs and output. Diabetic diets maintain consistent carbohydrates. Celiac disease requires strict gluten avoidance (no wheat, barley, or rye). Neutropenic precautions mean no raw or undercooked meats, unwashed produce, or unpasteurized products.

Dysphagia is an airway issue until proven otherwise. Screen for swallow safety; during meals, keep the patient fully upright at 90 degrees and remain upright for 30–60 minutes afterward. Provide small bites and sips without rushing. Use a chin-tuck if prescribed and the consistency recommended by speech therapy (nectar/honey-thick liquids, pureed textures). Avoid straws unless specifically allowed. Stop immediately if you see coughing, a wet or gurgly voice, pocketing food, or a drop in oxygen saturation, and reassess the plan with SLP/HCP. For patients with high metabolic demand or poor appetite, small, frequent, high-calorie, high-protein options help; manage nausea with cool, bland foods and antiemetics as ordered.

Enteral feeding requires verification and vigilance. Confirm tube placement by x-ray before the first feed—never use an air "whoosh." For ongoing checks, assess aspirate pH if appropriate, confirm external length, and ensure securement has not changed. Prevent aspiration by keeping the head of bed at 30–45 degrees during feeds and for 30–60 minutes afterward, verifying tube position, assessing bowel sounds and abdominal distention, and avoiding oversedation. Follow facility policy for gastric residuals; large residuals (for example, over 500 mL) or symptoms such as nausea and distention warrant holding the feed, reassessment, and notifying the provider. Use continuous feeding for high aspiration risk rather than large boluses.

Medication administration via tubes is testable detail: flush 15–30 mL of water before, between, and after each medication to maintain patency and prevent interactions; give meds separately; do not crush enteric-coated or sustained-release forms; and consider known drug–feed interactions—phenytoin often requires holding feeds around dosing and monitoring levels. Common complications include aspiration, for which the first action is to stop the feed, sit the patient up, suction as needed, assess breath sounds and oxygen saturation, and notify the provider. For a clogged tube, use warm water flushes with gentle back-and-forth; never force. Diarrhea often stems from rapid rates, formula osmolarity, or medications; evaluate these factors and adjust. Hyperglycemia requires monitoring and formula/rate review. In malnourished patients, start slowly and monitor phosphorus, potassium, and magnesium for refeeding syndrome. If the tube is for decompression, a Salem sump is attached to low intermittent suction; keep the blue air vent above stomach level and do not clamp it.

Ostomy care centers on protecting the stoma and skin, managing output, and teaching self-care. A healthy stoma is beefy red and moist; pallor, cyanosis, or black discoloration suggests ischemia and requires urgent provider notification. Mild oozing early post-op is expected, but brisk bleeding is not. Cut the wafer about 1/8 inch (3 mm) larger than the stoma for a snug fit, use barrier products, empty the pouch when it is one-third to one-half full, and change the system every three to five days or with any leak. Expect liquid, higher-volume output from an ileostomy with an associated risk of dehydration and electrolyte loss; a colostomy becomes more formed the more distal it is; a urostomy has continuous urine with mucus strands. Teach ileostomy patients to increase fluids and salt unless contraindicated, avoid very high-fiber or gassy foods early (like nuts, popcorn, celery), add foods gradually, and identify odor or gas producers. High-output losses should be treated with oral rehydration solutions and reported if persistent. Signs of blockage—no output with cramping—call for fluids, knee-chest positioning to relieve pressure, and contacting the provider. Irrigation is only appropriate for a sigmoid or descending colostomy; never irrigate an ileostomy. Address clothing options, body image, activity resumption, and clear thresholds for seeking care: persistent peristomal skin breakdown, no output, severe cramps, or signs of dehydration.

Use a CJMM mindset for fast, safe decisions. If a patient coughs and desaturates during a tube feeding, recognize aspiration risk, prioritize airway protection, act by stopping the feed and elevating the head, suction and assess, then evaluate oxygenation and breath sounds before notifying the provider. If a new stoma looks dusky, recognize ischemia, assess vital signs and perfusion, and escalate promptly. If dysphagia signs appear during a meal, stop feeding, keep the patient upright, and re-engage the swallow plan. When an immobile, undernourished patient arrives with moisture-associated skin damage, schedule repositioning, apply protectants, and optimize nutrition and hydration immediately—then reassess the skin for improvement.

Test-ready do/don't reminders:

- Do confirm enteral tube placement by x-ray before the first feed, maintain head-of-bed elevation for feeding and aspiration risks, give enteral meds separately with flushes, protect peristomal skin with a well-fitted wafer, and teach practical self-care sequences for devices and diets.
- Don't use air boluses to verify tube placement, flatten hypotensive patients in Trendelenburg, crush enteric-coated or sustained-release meds for tube delivery, irrigate an ileostomy, or ignore new signs of aspiration or stoma ischemia.

Basic care done early and correctly prevents emergencies. On test day, let the cues tell you whose airway or skin is at risk, take the simplest position or diet action that reduces that risk first, and then check that your action worked.

5.2 Pharmacological & Parenteral Therapies (Safety First)

Every medication in the NCLEX world runs through the same safety filter: use the Clinical Judgment Measurement Model to recognize, analyze, prioritize, implement, and evaluate. Before you touch a medication, recognize the cues: is the order complete and appropriate; do the client's diagnosis and indication match; any allergies or prior adverse reactions documented; what are the vital signs, pain score, mental status, urine output, and focused assessment; what do labs show (renal/hepatic function, coagulation, drug levels, electrolytes); are there pregnancy or lactation considerations; what access do you have (IV type and patency); and what other medications or infusions are running that could interact or be incompatible. As you analyze, ask "Is it safe to give now?" This includes dosing and frequency for age and organ function, interaction checks (pharmacodynamic synergists like CNS depressants together; pharmacokinetic issues like CYP inhibitors; food-drug effects like grapefruit), and for IV medications, line compatibility and the right route. Prioritize threats next: life-threatening risks (airway compromise, bleeding, arrhythmia, severe hypotension, hypoglycemia) always come before symptom control. The implement step is mechanical and non-negotiable: perform the 10 rights and three checks using two identifiers, use aseptic technique, barcode scanning, smart pump guardrails, and independent double-checks for high-alert medications. Finally, evaluate: did the expected therapeutic effect occur, did any adverse effects appear, and what are your next actions—continue, slow/hold, stop and treat, notify, or escalate care.

Core safety pillars are testable and must be automatic. Use two identifiers (name and DOB or medical record number, never a room number). The 10 rights include right client, right medication, right dose, right route, right time, right indication, right assessment, right education, right evaluation, and right documentation. Complete three checks against the MAR: when you pull the medication, when you prepare it, and at the bedside before you give it (barcode scanning supports but never replaces your checks). Clarify allergy versus side effect: an allergy implies immune-mediated symptoms such as rash, hives, bronchospasm, angioedema, or anaphylaxis; nausea or constipation alone is a side effect. Reconcile the MAR to the provider order if anything is inconsistent; use read-back for any telephone or verbal orders; avoid do-not-use abbreviations (U for unit, IU, QD/QOD, trailing zeros like 1.0, or missing a leading zero like .5, and ambiguous drug abbreviations such as MS, MSO4, MgSO4). Treat alert overrides with respect, especially for dose, route, allergy, and duplication. Know look-alike/sound-alike risks (for example, hydrALAzine vs hydrOXYzine; buPROPion vs busPIRone) and rely on Tall Man lettering cues.

Your pre-administration "green light" check is where many NCLEX items live. Confirm that the medication has a valid indication in this client and that baseline assessments are done and acceptable: check blood pressure and heart rate for antihypertensives or beta-blockers; check pain score and sedation for opioids; check respiratory status before opioids or benzodiazepines; check blood glucose before insulin; check aPTT/INR/platelets for anticoagulants; check potassium and renal function for ACE inhibitors, ARBs, potassium supplements, or spironolactone; check digoxin level and apical pulse before digoxin; check magnesium level and deep tendon reflexes in clients on magnesium sulfate; check liver enzymes for hepatotoxic medications. Review hold parameters that may be explicitly ordered or implied by standard of care: for example, hold a beta-blocker for bradycardia or hypotension, hold opioids for respiratory depression or excessive sedation, hold heparin/warfarin if active bleeding or dangerously elevated coagulation tests, hold potassium if serum potassium is high or if the client is oliguric. Screen for high-risk interactions such as multiple CNS depressants, anticholinergic stacking in older adults, duplicative anticoagulants or antiplatelets, and QT-prolonging combinations. Confirm route appropriateness and line access: is the IV patent, do you have a central line if the medication requires one, and are other medications in the line compatible. Keep time-critical medications on schedule: antibiotics, insulin, anticoagulants, antiepileptics, and immunosuppressants should not be delayed; these affect safety and therapeutic levels.

Parenteral routes require attention to site selection, volumes, technique, and labeling. Intradermal injections go into the dermis for small volumes (often 0.1 mL), bevel up at a shallow angle, producing a wheal; they are used for tests rather than therapy. Subcutaneous injections go into fatty tissue for small volumes (generally up to 1 mL in adults); rotate sites; do not aspirate for vaccines, insulin, or heparin; and do not massage after heparin to prevent bleeding and bruising. Intramuscular injections accept larger volumes depending on the site (deltoid typically up to 1 mL; vastus lateralis and ventrogluteal up to 2–3 mL in most adults), use the Z-track method for irritating solutions to reduce leakage into subcutaneous tissue, and rotate sites. Intravenous administration demands patency, correct dilution, and correct rate; IV push medications require confirmation that IV push is safe for that drug, adherence to dilution and rate recommendations, flushing the line appropriately, and giving via the closest port to the client unless contraindicated by the line type; IV piggyback medications hang higher than the primary solution and require compatibility checks with the primary solution. Label all syringes and lines with the medication name and concentration, date and time, and your initials. Maintain aseptic technique throughout preparation and administration.

Smart pump and infusion safety prevent many errors. Use guardrails by selecting the correct drug library entry and concentration; input the correct dose and rate; and avoid bypassing limits unless verified. Independent double-checks are expected for high-alert infusions and titrations (insulin, heparin, some vasopressors, patient-controlled analgesia, chemotherapy, and often total parenteral nutrition) and must include verifying the medication, concentration, pump programming, and patient against the MAR. Label tubing and ports; trace the line from the bag to the patient before connecting anything; and minimize free-flow risk by using clamps and back-check valves correctly.

High-alert medication groups require clear first actions and stop/hold rules. Insulin always gets a two-RN check for type, dose, timing, and route. Do not mix long-acting analogs (glargine, detemir, degludec) with other insulins. Check blood glucose and ensure meal availability for prandial doses; use facility hypoglycemia protocols to treat low blood glucose quickly, choosing oral carbohydrate if the patient is awake and IV dextrose or IM glucagon if not. Monitor for hypokalemia and hypoglycemia after insulin infusions. With anticoagulants, always verify bleeding risk, labs, and indications. For heparin infusions, check aPTT and platelets; hold and notify for active bleeding, severely elevated aPTT, or suspected heparin-induced thrombocytopenia (sudden platelet drop or thrombosis). For warfarin, review INR and assess for bleeding or drug-diet interactions; consistent intake of vitamin K foods is key, but active bleeding with high INR requires provider notification and reversal per protocol. Direct oral anticoagulants depend on renal function and have fewer labs; hold for active bleeding and before invasive procedures as ordered. Opioids and sedatives demand a focus on sedation and respirations; assess pain, sedation, respiratory rate, and oxygenation before giving; hold for excessive sedation or low respiratory rate; have naloxone immediately available; and after reversal, monitor closely for renarcotization once naloxone wears off. Concentrated electrolytes such as potassium chloride, magnesium sulfate, and hypertonic saline are never given IV push. Use a pump, follow concentration and rate limits per policy, monitor ECG and serum levels, and stop the infusion and evaluate if the client develops arrhythmias, hypotension, flushing, or worsening symptoms. Recognize magnesium toxicity by depressed reflexes, respiratory depression, and oliguria; the first steps are to stop the infusion, support airway, and prepare to give calcium gluconate per protocol. TPN and lipids require a dedicated line, frequent glucose and electrolyte monitoring, no piggyback medications into the TPN line, and a backup plan to prevent abrupt discontinuation—D10 infusion may be used if TPN is interrupted per policy. Chemotherapy administration requires certification, appropriate personal protective equipment, closed-system transfer devices when available, and readiness for spills and extravasation; verify orders using two qualified staff and oncology protocols, and keep extravasation antidotes and kits available.

Know how to separate expected effects, side effects, allergies, and anaphylaxis. Mild nausea, diarrhea, or headache are common adverse effects depending on the drug class. Urticaria, angioedema, bronchospasm, or hypotension suggest allergic reaction; if severe and multisystem, treat as anaphylaxis. The first actions for anaphylaxis are to stop the medication, maintain airway and breathing with high-flow oxygen, call for help (notify provider and activate the rapid response team), give intramuscular epinephrine per protocol, maintain IV access and begin fluids for hypotension, and prepare adjuncts such as antihistamines and corticosteroids. Document the reaction as a true allergy and educate the patient afterward.

Infusion and injection sites offer cues you must act on immediately. Infiltration presents as cool, pale swelling with discomfort and slowed or stopped infusion; stop the infusion, elevate the limb, and restart at a different site. Extravasation involves a vesicant drug and can cause tissue damage; stop the infusion, leave the catheter in place, aspirate any drug if possible, and initiate the antidote and heat/cold per protocol before removing the catheter; notify the provider and document. Phlebitis presents with redness, warmth, and a tender cord; stop the infusion, remove the catheter, apply warm compresses, and monitor; consider a new site. Signs of local infection include purulent drainage, warmth, and fever; remove the catheter, notify the provider, possibly send the tip for culture, and monitor. In central lines, maintain sterile technique for access, scrub the hub, change dressings per policy, and watch closely for signs of CLABSI.

Certain populations require modified dosing and monitoring. Pediatric dosing is based on weight in mg/kg or body surface area; calculate carefully and use the correct formulation and equipment (oral syringes with mL markings, small-volume syringes and low-dead-space needles). Double-check doses with another RN for high-alert medications. Older adults require "start low, go slow" dosing given reduced renal and hepatic clearance, altered body composition, and high sensitivity to sedatives, anticholinergics, and hypotensives; assess for orthostatic hypotension and falls; simplify regimens and watch for polypharmacy. Clients with renal or hepatic impairment need dose or interval adjustments and sometimes drug selection changes; monitor drug levels when applicable (vancomycin, aminoglycosides, anticonvulsants) and stop or hold if toxicity signs appear. In pregnancy and lactation, avoid teratogens, use the lowest effective dose, and time doses around feeds to minimize infant exposure when safe; consult reliable lactation resources if the scenario provides them.

Effective patient education prevents harm. Always teach the purpose of the medication, how and when to take it, what to do if a dose is missed, and which adverse effects are common versus which are red flags requiring immediate help (for example, bleeding with anticoagulants; chest tightness or swelling with antibiotics; severe rash; suicidal ideation with some psychotropics; profound dizziness or syncope with antihypertensives). Reinforce adherence strategies such as pill organizers, alarms, and synchronized refills. Show safe storage, including childproof containers, refrigeration if needed, and sharps disposal for injections. Confirm understanding using teach-back and correct misunderstandings before discharge.

Preventing and responding to errors is part of safe RN practice. Foster a just culture by reporting near-misses and hazards. Never document a medication as administered until it is given. If an error or adverse event occurs, stabilize the client first, notify the provider and leadership per policy, complete an incident report factually and objectively, disclose to the client/family according to policy, and never conceal or alter records.

To sharpen your CJMM, tie cues to actions. If you see a potassium level of 5.8 mEq/L in a client taking an ACE inhibitor or spironolactone, hold any potassium supplements and potassium-sparing agents and notify the provider. If you see an INR of 4.5 on warfarin without bleeding, hold the dose and notify; if bleeding is present, stop the drug and prepare for reversal and supportive care. If respiratory rate is 8/min with pinpoint pupils after an opioid, stop opioid administration, support breathing, give naloxone per protocol, and monitor for recurrence. If a client on insulin is diaphoretic and confused with a blood glucose of 52 mg/dL, give quick-acting carbohydrate if able to swallow or initiate IV dextrose if not, recheck glucose, and reassess. If a client on magnesium sulfate develops absent deep tendon reflexes and respirations slow to 10/min, stop the infusion, support the airway, and prepare calcium gluconate.

Finally, document promptly, completely, and objectively. Include the medication, dose, route, time, site (for injections), pre- and post-administration assessments (vital signs, pain/sedation scores, pertinent labs or ECG strips), patient response (therapeutic effect and any adverse reactions), interventions taken, and education provided with the patient's teach-back. Good documentation communicates clinical judgment and protects the client.

A few additional parenteral specifics are frequently tested. Never piggyback anything into a TPN line; it is dedicated. For potassium chloride, use a pump with appropriate concentration; typical adult peripheral rates do not exceed 10 mEq per hour, and central lines may allow higher rates per protocol; ECG monitoring is prudent for significant replacement. For vancomycin and other vesicants or irritants, infuse slowly, monitor for red-man syndrome, and assess the IV site; checking trough levels ensures therapeutic range and limits nephrotoxicity. For benzodiazepines and opioids together, anticipate compounded sedation and respiratory depression; prefer non-opioid adjuncts when appropriate and monitor closely if combined. For immunosuppressants like tacrolimus or cyclosporine, keep dosing regular and avoid missed doses; monitor trough levels and kidney function. For antiepileptics such as phenytoin, avoid rapid IV push due to hypotension and arrhythmias; ensure compatible solutions (phenytoin is incompatible with dextrose solutions) and monitor for CNS toxicity.

Tie back to basics and do not let the exam bait you into skipping steps. Two identifiers, 10 rights, three checks, and an allergy check happen every single time. Look for the one cue that makes the dose unsafe right now and act conservatively: hold, assess, and notify rather than blindly administering. Use the pump guardrails and independent double-checks. Stop infusions when you suspect harm, and treat the immediate threat. Educate every time you can, and document what you saw, did, and taught. This safety-first pattern is exactly what NCLEX wants you to demonstrate.

5.2.1 Medication Math & High-Alert Medications

The NCLEX expects you to prevent dosing errors and mitigate harm—especially with high-alert medications. Approach every calculation and high-risk drug the same way you approach a clinical judgment item: recognize the key cues in the order, analyze the units and the patient factors, prioritize safety steps, act with clean math and clean technique, and evaluate by monitoring the right outcomes. Dimensional analysis is your default tool; an estimate before you calculate is your safety net for catching 10× errors.

Start by reading the order like a nurse, not a calculator. Pull out the essential cues: the drug, strength and concentration on hand, the prescribed dose and time unit, the patient's weight and organ function, the route, and whether the medication is a known high-alert. Estimate what seems reasonable before you compute. For example, if a 70-kg patient is ordered heparin at 18 units/kg/hr, your rough mental math says around 1,200 units/hr. If your final pump rate translates to 12,000 units/hr, you know you've made a unit or decimal slip. This estimate-before-calc habit is a simple but powerful layer of risk reduction.

Dimensional analysis keeps the units honest. Line up what you're given and cancel the units until you're left with what the question asks for. The core relationships you'll use repeatedly are straightforward: Dose = (Desired/Have) × Volume; mL/hr = total mL ÷ hours; gtt/min = (mL × drop factor) ÷ minutes. When weight is involved, attend to dose versus day: mg/kg/dose multiplied by the number of doses per day is not the same as mg/kg/day. Always check the computed dose against the safe range for that patient before you decide to administer.

Keep your conversions tight and consistent. For weight, 1 kg = 2.2 lb, and you should convert to kilograms and round the weight to the nearest tenth kg unless otherwise specified. For mass, 1 g = 1,000 mg and 1 mg = 1,000 mcg. For volume, 1 L = 1,000 mL; household measures convert as 1 tsp = 5 mL, 1 tbsp = 15 mL, and 1 oz = 30 mL. For gravity infusions, know your drop factors: macrodrip sets are commonly 10, 15, or 20 gtt/mL; microdrip is 60 gtt/mL. When you're asked for gtt/min, you round to a whole number because you can't count fractions of drops. Pump rates are typically rounded to the tenth as needed. And keep your entries safe: never use trailing zeros (2 not 2.0) and always lead with a zero for decimals (0.5 not .5).

Weight-based dosing is a frequent NCLEX testing ground because pediatric prescriptions and organ impairment are error-prone. Convert weight to kilograms, compute mg/kg/dose or mg/kg/day as ordered, and compare to the safe range for that age and condition. If the prescribed amount exceeds the safe range or the patient has cues for reduced clearance (older adult, renal impairment, hepatic dysfunction), you hold and clarify. For pediatric patients, the trap is dose versus day: an order may be written per dose while your reference states a daily range, or vice versa. Normalize them to the same time base before judging safety, and do not give until you are certain the dose falls within the safe range.

Many vasoactive and endocrine infusions use mcg/min or mcg/kg/min dosing. You must be comfortable converting those to mL/hr using the bag concentration. Here's a clean example with dimensional analysis: A patient is ordered dopamine 5 mcg/kg/min. The patient weighs 70 kg. The bag is 400 mg in 250 mL. First, compute the drug requirement in mcg/min: 5 mcg/kg/min × 70 kg = 350 mcg/min. Convert the bag concentration: 400 mg = 400,000 mcg; 400,000 mcg ÷ 250 mL = 1,600 mcg/mL. Now, mL/min = 350 mcg/min ÷ 1,600 mcg/mL = 0.21875 mL/min. Convert to an hourly pump rate: 0.21875 mL/min × 60 = 13.125 mL/hr. Round sensibly to 13.1 mL/hr if your pump allows tenths. Before you press start, you recognize this as a high-alert vasopressor, prioritize an independent double-check and correct line selection (central line preferred), then act by programming the smart pump guardrails, and evaluate by monitoring BP, HR, and perfusion while watching the IV site for extravasation.

Safe dose decision-making is not only math—it is clinical judgment. After you compute the dose, compare it with the safe range for that patient. If it is out of range, do not administer. Hold the medication and clarify the order with read-back. Document the rationale: "Prescribed dose exceeds pediatric mg/kg/day maximum," or "Dosing not adjusted for eGFR; increased risk of accumulation and toxicity." Look for cues that increase risk even when the dose is technically within range: for example, an older adult with decreased renal function ordered enoxaparin at the full weight-based dose, or a patient with rising aPTT on a heparin drip. The right action on NCLEX is to recognize those cues, prioritize holding and clarifying, and facilitate a safer plan (dose reduction, baseline labs, pharmacy verification).

Preventing error begins with the order itself. The do-not-use abbreviations U (units), IU (international units), QD/QOD, and trailing zeros are constant traps. Look-alike/sound-alike risks include insulin types (Humalog vs Humulin), heparin concentrations (1,000 vs 10,000 units/mL), and U-500 concentrated insulin. If an order reads "10 U regular insulin now" or ".5 mg hydromorphone," you clarify and require a read-back. On test day, choose the answers that specify contacting the prescriber for ambiguous orders, using the complete drug name, dose, route, and time with read-back, and employing pharmacy-prepared admixtures when appropriate.

High-alert medications are drugs that bear a heightened risk of causing significant patient harm when used in error. The list most likely to appear on NCLEX includes insulins (IV and subQ), anticoagulants (heparin, warfarin, enoxaparin), opioids and sedatives, neuromuscular blockers, concentrated electrolytes (potassium chloride, magnesium sulfate, hypertonic saline), vasopressors, chemotherapy agents, and parenteral nutrition. These drugs demand standardized, safety-forward handling. The actions the exam favors are consistent: perform an independent double-check before initiation and with titration that confirms the correct drug, concentration, dose, pump rate, and patient. Use smart pump guardrails and standardized concentrations; prefer pharmacy-prepared infusions. Never administer potassium chloride IV push. Keep concentrated electrolytes off the unit floor unless required for codes and secure them distinctly. Label all prepared syringes and IV lines at both ends; titration orders must include parameters such as target range, titration increments, and maximum rate. Bar-code scanning is a support, not a substitute; you still verify allergies, indications, labs, and the five rights.

Monitoring must be aligned to the drug class risk and your first actions must mitigate harm. With insulin, you watch for hypoglycemia—diaphoresis, tremor, confusion, seizures, and decreased level of consciousness—and you verify meal timing for prandial doses. IV insulin for DKA is typically 0.1 units/kg/hr using a standardized 1 unit/mL infusion; you monitor blood glucose hourly, potassium levels frequently, and add dextrose when glucose falls to around 200–250 mg/dL per protocol. For heparin and other anticoagulants, observe for bleeding (gums, urine, stool, bruising, drop in hemoglobin), and adjust the infusion based on aPTT or anti-Xa per protocol; if labs are supratherapeutic or bleeding is suspected, you hold and notify. Warfarin requires INR monitoring and consistent dietary vitamin K instruction; low-molecular-weight heparins like enoxaparin are weight-based and require careful dosing in renal impairment. Opioids and sedatives require ongoing assessment of respiratory rate and level of consciousness with dose holds for respiratory depression and immediate naloxone access for severe depression. Concentrated electrolytes demand cardiac monitoring for potassium and magnesium; do not exceed safe IV rates (for potassium: typically ≤10 mEq/hr via peripheral line, up to 20 mEq/hr via central line with continuous monitoring) and reassess serum levels. Vasopressors require vigilant BP, HR, and perfusion checks; use a central line when possible and treat extravasation per protocol. Chemotherapy and TPN require handling precautions, intact dedicated lines, and infection and metabolic monitoring (glucose, electrolytes, liver function, triglycerides). For magnesium sulfate, especially in obstetric patients, watch for loss of deep tendon reflexes and respiratory depression; have calcium gluconate available for toxicity.

Know the antidotes by name for quick decision-making: naloxone for opioids, protamine for heparin, vitamin K for warfarin, calcium gluconate for magnesium toxicity, and dextrose or glucagon for insulin-induced hypoglycemia. On NCLEX, if a prompt mentions worsening respiratory depression after IV morphine, selecting naloxone readiness or administration is often the safest first action after assessing airway and breathing.

When you see a calculation item, apply a repeatable NGN tactic. Extract the cues first: the drug name, order units (mg vs mcg; per dose vs per day), concentration on hand, time base (per minute vs per hour), route, weight in kilograms, and whether the infusion is gravity or pump. Convert your units up front. Make a quick estimate to anchor your answer. Perform the calculation with dimensional analysis and round only at the end, using whole numbers for gtt/min and tenths for pump rates if requested. Immediately compare the result to the safe range. Then decide: administer, hold and clarify, or adjust per protocol. Your final action should reflect risk prevention as much as arithmetic.

Common traps are almost always unit mismatches. Don't mix mg and mcg; reconcile hour and minute bases; convert pounds to kilograms before computing a weight-based dose; distinguish dose versus day and divide or multiply by the dosing frequency accordingly. With reconstitution, compute the final concentration after adding diluent, not the powder amount. When calculating drops per minute, confirm your tubing's drop factor and whether it is microdrip or macrodrip. And for insulin, don't confuse U-100 and U-500 products: the same "units" have very different volumes and risks.

A few short cases illustrate how the math drives the decision:

A pediatric antibiotic order arrives for ceftriaxone 1.5 g IV once daily for a child weighing 18 kg. The common pediatric safe range for ceftriaxone is approximately 50–75 mg/kg/day. Compute the safe daily range: 50 mg/kg × 18 kg = 900 mg/day to 75 mg/kg × 18 kg = 1,350 mg/day. The ordered dose is 1,500 mg/day, which exceeds the upper limit. What do you do first? You hold and clarify with the prescriber, citing the weight-based safe range; you do not administer.

A heparin infusion order prescribes 18 units/kg/hr for a 70-kg adult. The IV bag is 25,000 units in 250 mL (100 units/mL). Compute the hourly units: 18 × 70 = 1,260 units/hr. Convert to mL/hr: 1,260 units/hr ÷ 100 units/mL = 12.6 mL/hr. This is a high-alert anticoagulant. What do you do first? You perform an independent double-check of drug, concentration, rate, and patient, ensure baseline labs (aPTT or anti-Xa, CBC, platelets) are in place, and then program the smart pump guardrails.

A patient with DKA weighing 90 kg is ordered an insulin infusion at 0.1 units/kg/hr. The standard bag is 100 units regular insulin in 100 mL NS (1 unit/mL). Compute: 0.1 × 90 = 9 units/hr. Convert to mL/hr: 9 units/hr ÷ 1 unit/mL = 9 mL/hr. What do you do first? You verify the standardized concentration and pump setup, confirm potassium is ≥3.3 mEq/L and blood glucose monitoring is ordered hourly, and begin the infusion with hypoglycemia management supplies ready; if hypoglycemia develops, you follow protocol to administer dextrose and adjust the rate.

An order requests adding 30 mEq KCl to 500 mL NS to infuse over 3 hours. Vials are 10 mEq/5 mL. Compute the volume of KCl to add: 30 mEq × (5 mL/10 mEq) = 15 mL. The infusion rate will be 500 mL ÷ 3 hr ≈ 167 mL/hr, delivering 10 mEq/hr. What do you do first? You confirm the route and rate are appropriate (never IV push KCl), ensure a pump and cardiac monitoring are used as indicated, and verify adequate renal function and urine output before administration.

To round out your calculation skill set, practice a gravity example: infuse 500 mL over 4 hours using 15 gtt/mL tubing. gtt/min = (500 mL × 15 gtt/mL) ÷ (240 min) = 31.25 gtt/min. You set 31 gtt/min because drops are whole numbers. If a pump rate is requested, you would answer 125 mL/hr instead, matching the unit asked for.

Tie your process to a short, memorable checklist you can use for any calculation or high-alert medication: check–calc–check–act–label–monitor. First, check the order and the patient, pulling out all dosing, time, and risk cues and estimating what makes sense. Then calculate using dimensional analysis. Check again by comparing your result to the safe range and the patient's risk profile. Act by implementing high-alert safety practices—independent double-checks, smart pump guardrails, standardized concentrations, and correct line selection. Label every prepared syringe and line at both ends with drug, concentration, and rate. Finally, monitor the class-specific outcomes and adverse effects, and be ready with antidotes or protocol-driven responses. This six-step rhythm embodies clinical judgment: you are not just getting the math right—you are preventing harm.

5.2.2 System Drug Classes (Test-Frequent Only)

How to read this section: For each class, know the prototype/suffix and why it's given; what to assess before/after; when to hold or notify the provider; the high-risk adverse effects and toxicity cues; key labs and interactions; the first safe action if something goes wrong; and one must-teach point. Safety first, recognize deterioration, and know the antidotes.

Cardiovascular medicines are frequent and safety-critical. ACE inhibitors (ending -pril, prototype lisinopril) and ARBs (ending -sartan, prototype losartan) treat hypertension, heart failure, and kidney protection in diabetes. Red flags are cough and life-threatening angioedema (especially with ACEi), first-dose hypotension, and hyperkalemia; creatinine can rise slightly but a notable bump warrants evaluation. They are contraindicated in pregnancy and used cautiously in renal artery stenosis. Hold for facial/lip swelling, a potassium above normal, or symptomatic hypotension; assess airway if swelling occurs. Avoid potassium supplements/salt substitutes; teach to rise slowly and report swelling immediately.

Beta-blockers (ending -lol; metoprolol, atenolol, nonselective propranolol) are used for rate control, hypertension, and post-MI. Watch for bradycardia, AV block, hypotension, and bronchospasm with nonselective agents; they can mask hypoglycemia symptoms. Hold if HR <60 or SBP <90, or for new wheezing in asthma patients. Do not stop abruptly due to rebound ischemia; teach to check pulse and to call for dizziness, fainting, or worsening shortness of breath.

Calcium channel blockers include **dihydropyridines** (amlodipine, nifedipine) and **non-DHPs** (diltiazem, verapamil). They treat hypertension and angina; non-DHPs also control rate. Red flags are hypotension, peripheral edema, constipation (verapamil), and brady/heart block with non-DHPs. Hold for symptomatic hypotension or bradycardia. Avoid grapefruit with diltiazem/verapamil; teach orthostatic precautions and to report swelling.

Diuretics are test favorites. Loop diuretics (furosemide) can cause hypokalemia, dehydration, hypotension, and ototoxicity at high/rapid doses; thiazides (hydrochlorothiazide) cause hyponatremia, hypokalemia, and photosensitivity; potassium-sparing (spironolactone) risks hyperkalemia and gynecomastia. Monitor BP, daily weights, I&Os, and electrolytes (especially K+). Hold spironolactone for K+ ≥5 or with ACEi/ARBs if hyperkalemia is present; hold loops/thiazides if severe hypovolemia or K+ is low and patient symptomatic. Teach high-K diet with loops/thiazides and to avoid salt substitutes with spironolactone.

Nitrates (nitroglycerin) relieve angina via vasodilation. Expect headache and flushing; red flags are profound hypotension and syncope. They absolutely interact with phosphodiesterase-5 inhibitors (sildenafil, tadalafil) within the prior 24–48 hours—do not give. For hypotension or dizziness, have the patient lie down, hold the next dose, and reassess BP. Teach a daily patch-free interval (10–12 hours) to prevent tolerance.

Digoxin improves symptoms in heart failure and controls ventricular rate in atrial fibrillation. Hold if apical HR <60. Toxicity cues include anorexia, nausea, vomiting, visual halos, confusion, and arrhythmias; risk increases with hypokalemia and renal impairment. Monitor levels (therapeutic 0.5–2 ng/mL), K+, and renal function. First action for toxicity cues is to hold and obtain a level and ECG; digoxin immune Fab is the antidote in severe toxicity. Teach patients to take a daily pulse and to avoid taking extra doses.

Anticoagulants and **antiplatelets** demand precision. Heparin (unfractionated) is titrated to aPTT 1.5–2.5 times control; watch for bleeding and heparin-induced thrombocytopenia (a >50% platelet drop or platelets <150,000). Protamine sulfate reverses heparin. Warfarin targets INR 2–3 for most indications (2.5–3.5 for mechanical valves); vitamin K is the antidote. Warfarin is teratogenic; maintain consistent dietary vitamin K and beware interactions (e.g., **TMP-SMX** increases INR). Direct oral anticoagulants (apixaban, rivaroxaban, dabigatran) have bleeding risk;

dabigatran is reversed with idarucizumab; apixaban/rivaroxaban with andexanet alfa (or PCC if not available). Avoid NSAIDs and many herbals that increase bleeding. First action for serious bleeding: hold drug, apply pressure, assess hemodynamics, and prepare reversal as appropriate.

Amiodarone treats arrhythmias but brings multisystem toxicity. Red flags include new cough/dyspnea (pulmonary), thyroid dysfunction (hypo/hyper), liver injury, photosensitivity, and corneal deposits; QT prolongation is possible. It has a long half-life and many interactions (warfarin, digoxin). Obtain baseline and periodic tests (CXR/PFTs, LFTs, TSH) and ECGs. First action for new respiratory symptoms is to hold and notify the provider.

Respiratory drugs are about quick relief versus control. Short-acting beta-agonists such as albuterol are rescue inhalers; tremor and tachycardia are common. If using more than two times per week (not counting before-exercise), asthma control is inadequate—assess and escalate. Use SABA before inhaled corticosteroids so airways are open.

Inhaled corticosteroids (fluticasone, budesonide) are controllers, not for acute relief. They increase thrush risk; have patients rinse and spit after use. Monitor for hoarseness; systemic effects are limited but hyperglycemia can occur at higher doses. Teach daily adherence and proper device technique.

Anticholinergic bronchodilators (ipratropium, tiotropium) can cause dry mouth and caution is needed in angle-closure glaucoma and BPH due to urinary retention. Avoid spraying in eyes; ensure the patient can achieve a full inhalation. In acute bronchospasm, use SABA first; ipratropium may be added.

Leukotriene modifiers (montelukast) are maintenance agents. Watch for neuropsychiatric changes (agitation, depression, suicidal thoughts); if present, stop and notify. Take nightly; not for acute attacks.

Endocrine medications require timing and vigilance. Insulins differ by onset and peak: rapid-acting (lispro/aspart) onset ~15 minutes, peak ~1 hour; regular onset 30–60 minutes, peak 2–4 hours; NPH peaks 4–12 hours; glargine has no pronounced peak. Hypoglycemia cues are sweating, tremor, confusion, and palpitations; the first action is to check blood glucose and give rapid-acting carbs if the patient is awake (glucagon if not). Glargine is never mixed and is not given IV. Rotate sites and teach recognition and treatment of hypoglycemia.

Metformin reduces hepatic glucose output. Red flags are lactic acidosis (malaise, myalgias, respiratory distress) and renal impairment. Hold before and 48 hours after iodinated contrast until renal function is confirmed; avoid if eGFR <30. GI upset is common; vitamin B12 deficiency can occur with long-term use. Teach to take with meals and to report unexplained fatigue or shortness of breath.

Sulfonylureas (glipizide, glyburide) cause hypoglycemia and weight gain; glyburide is discouraged in older adults. Alcohol may provoke a disulfiram-like reaction. Take with breakfast and monitor for low blood sugars. The first action for symptomatic hypoglycemia is to treat immediately.

SGLT2 inhibitors (canagliflozin, empagliflozin) increase urinary glucose excretion. Risks include mycotic GU infections, volume depletion, and euglycemic DKA (nausea, abdominal pain, tachypnea with normal glucose). Hold during acute illness or surgery; check renal function. Teach hydration and to report genital symptoms or signs of DKA.

Thyroid agents require precision. Levothyroxine is taken on an empty stomach in the morning, 30–60 minutes before food or other meds; separate from calcium/iron by 4 hours. Over-replacement causes palpitations, weight loss, and insomnia; dose is titrated with TSH. Antithyroid drugs (methimazole, PTU) risk agranulocytosis (fever, sore throat) and PTU is hepatotoxic. The first action for fever or sore throat while on these drugs is to hold and get a CBC; for jaundice or dark urine on PTU, hold and obtain LFTs.

Neuro/psych drugs often cross safety domains. Antiepileptics: phenytoin has a therapeutic range of 10–20 mcg/mL; toxicity presents with nystagmus, ataxia, confusion, and can cause rash (SJS) and gingival hyperplasia. It interacts with tube feeds—separate by 1–2 hours. Valproate carries hepatic and pancreatic toxicity and thrombocytopenia; monitor LFTs and platelets. Levetiracetam can cause mood changes and somnolence with few interactions. For rash, severe CNS depression, or rising LFTs/bleeding, hold and notify.

SSRIs/SNRIs (sertraline, fluoxetine; duloxetine, venlafaxine) risk serotonin syndrome (agitation, hyperreflexia, fever, diarrhea, diaphoresis). They cause sexual dysfunction and take 4–6 weeks for full effect. Maintain a 2-week washout for MAOIs (5 weeks for fluoxetine). First action for suspected serotonin syndrome is to stop the serotonergic agent and support airway/breathing/circulation.

TCAs (amitriptyline) cause anticholinergic effects and orthostasis; overdose is lethal due to arrhythmias and widened QRS. Baseline ECG is wise in at-risk patients. In overdose, prioritize cardiac monitoring and sodium bicarbonate if indicated per provider order.

MAOIs (phenelzine, tranylcypromine) require strict dietary avoidance of tyramine (aged cheeses, cured meats) to prevent hypertensive crisis (severe headache, hypertension). Avoid many drugs (decongestants, other antidepressants); keep a 2-week washout window. Teach the diet and to seek immediate help for severe headache.

Antipsychotics: typicals (haloperidol) cause EPS (dystonia, akathisia, parkinsonism) and rarely NMS (fever, rigidity, AMS, autonomic instability). First action in NMS is to stop the drug, support ABCs, cool, and expect dantrolene/bromocriptine per orders. Atypicals (olanzapine, risperidone) cause metabolic syndrome and can prolong QT. Clozapine requires ANC monitoring due to agranulocytosis; hold for ANC below the safe threshold and for any fever/sore throat.

Benzodiazepines (lorazepam) depress CNS; co-use with opioids/alcohol can cause respiratory depression. Flumazenil can precipitate seizures in chronic users—use cautiously. First action for oversedation is to support airway and breathing and hold further doses; taper with chronic use to prevent withdrawal.

Pain and anti-inflammatory agents carry bleeding and breathing risks. Opioids (morphine, hydromorphone) require respiratory rate and sedation assessment; hold if RR <12 or the patient is difficult to arouse. Naloxone is the antidote for life-threatening respiratory depression. Start bowel prophylaxis to prevent constipation; teach not to mix with alcohol or drive while sedated.

NSAIDs (ibuprofen, naproxen) increase GI bleeding risk, impair renal perfusion, and can raise BP and worsen heart failure; avoid in CKD, peptic ulcer disease, late pregnancy, and after CABG. Aspirin is unique for platelet inhibition; avoid in children with viral illness due to Reye's syndrome. Avoid combining with anticoagulants unless directed; teach to take with food and to report black stools.

Acetaminophen is hepatotoxic in overdose; keep total daily dose ≤4 g (≤3 g in older adults or liver disease). N-acetylcysteine is the antidote and works best early. Check hidden acetaminophen in combination products; avoid alcohol overuse.

Infectious disease drugs are about allergies, kinetics, and organ toxicity. Penicillins and cephalosporins can cause allergic reactions; serious penicillin anaphylaxis is a caution for cephalosporins (greatest with first-generation). Observe for rash, hives, wheezing, or angioedema; stop and treat anaphylaxis if present. Complete the full course and consider backup contraception.

Macrolides (azithromycin, erythromycin) can prolong QT and interact via CYP3A4 (raising warfarin and other drug levels); monitor for palpitations and avoid with other QT-prolonging agents when possible. GI upset is common; take as directed.

Aminoglycosides (gentamicin) are nephrotoxic and ototoxic; rising creatinine or new tinnitus/vertigo are red flags—hold and notify. Trough and peak monitoring guide dosing. Avoid combining with other nephro/ototoxins when possible.

Fluoroquinolones (ciprofloxacin, levofloxacin) carry risks of tendonitis/rupture (higher with steroids), QT prolongation, peripheral neuropathy, photosensitivity, and rare aortic aneurysm issues in high-risk patients. At first tendon pain or swelling, stop the drug. Separate from mineral supplements/antacids. Avoid in children and pregnancy.

Tetracyclines (doxycycline) cause photosensitivity and tooth/bone effects; avoid in pregnancy and in children under 8. Take with water, stay upright for 30 minutes, and separate from dairy/iron/antacids. Reduce sun exposure.

Sulfonamides (TMP-SMX) can cause severe rash (SJS/TEN), hyperkalemia, and crystalluria; hydrate and stop immediately for rash. It increases INR with warfarin—monitor closely. Avoid late in pregnancy; check for sulfa allergies.

Vancomycin can cause red man syndrome if infused too quickly (flushing, pruritus)—stop/slow infusion and premedicate if needed; distinguish from anaphylaxis (wheezing, hypotension, angioedema). Monitor trough levels and renal function; watch for ototoxicity.

TB drugs: isoniazid is hepatotoxic and can cause peripheral neuropathy; give pyridoxine (B6) to prevent neuropathy and avoid alcohol. Rifampin turns body fluids orange, induces metabolism (reducing efficacy of OCPs and other drugs), and is hepatotoxic. Teach adherence to multidrug therapy and to report jaundice.

GI medications balance symptom control and risk. PPIs (omeprazole) increase risks of C. difficile, fractures, and hypomagnesemia; use the lowest effective dose and duration. Monitor magnesium if long-term and report persistent diarrhea.

H2 blockers (famotidine preferred) reduce acid; cimetidine has numerous interactions and CNS effects in older adults. Dose adjust in renal impairment. Teach to avoid simultaneous antacids around dosing.

Antiemetics: ondansetron can prolong QT; monitor ECG in patients with electrolyte abnormalities or long QT syndrome. Metoclopramide risks EPS and tardive dyskinesia; hold for facial spasms or rigidity and treat acute dystonia with diphenhydramine or benztropine per orders. Contraindicated in suspected bowel obstruction/bleed.

Laxatives differ by type. Bulk-forming (psyllium) require adequate fluids; osmotics (PEG) can disturb electrolytes; stimulants (senna, bisacodyl) can cause cramping and dependence. Do not give if there is severe undiagnosed abdominal pain or suspected obstruction; first action is to hold and assess.

OB and newborn pharmacology emphasizes maternal-fetal safety. Tocolytics: terbutaline (beta-agonist) can cause maternal tachycardia, hyperglycemia, and hypokalemia; hold if maternal HR >120, chest pain, or arrhythmia. Nifedipine can cause hypotension and headache; monitor maternal BP and fetal status.

Uterotonics: oxytocin can cause uterine tachysystole and fetal distress; continuous FHR and contraction monitoring is required. First action for tachysystole or nonreassuring FHR is to stop the infusion, reposition, give IV fluids/oxygen as ordered, and notify the provider. Methylergonovine is contraindicated in hypertension or preeclampsia; carboprost is contraindicated in asthma; misoprostol is used for cervical ripening and postpartum hemorrhage—avoid for induction in patients with a prior uterine scar without provider oversight due to rupture risk.

Magnesium sulfate prevents eclamptic seizures. Toxicity presents with loss of deep tendon reflexes, respiratory depression (<12/min), hypotension, and decreased urine output. Stop the infusion immediately, call the provider, support airway, and give calcium gluconate as the antidote. Always assess DTRs, RR, and urine output before each dose escalation.

Other high-yield agents round out the essentials. **Systemic corticosteroids** (prednisone) increase infection risk and blood glucose and can cause mood changes and osteoporosis. Taper to avoid adrenal crisis; take with food; avoid live vaccines on high-dose therapy. Teach to report signs of infection and to wear a medical alert if chronic therapy.

Immunosuppressants such as **cyclosporine** and **tacrolimus** are nephrotoxic and increase infection and malignancy risk. Monitor trough levels and creatinine, and avoid grapefruit. Cyclosporine can cause gingival hyperplasia; emphasize oral hygiene. Fever or signs of infection warrant prompt evaluation.

Bisphosphonates (alendronate) reduce fracture risk but can cause esophagitis. Take first thing in the morning with a full glass of water, on an empty stomach, and remain upright for at least 30 minutes; avoid if esophageal stricture or severe renal impairment. Dental evaluation is prudent due to rare osteonecrosis of the jaw.

Gout drugs include allopurinol for urate lowering and colchicine for flares. Allopurinol hypersensitivity (rash that can evolve to SJS) is a stop-now emergency; maintain hydration and dose-adjust in CKD. Colchicine toxicity begins with GI diarrhea and can progress to myelosuppression; reduce dose with renal impairment and avoid chronic high-dose use.

NGN/CJMM tie-ins occur everywhere: a client on an ACE inhibitor with new lip swelling—stop the drug, assess the airway, prepare for emergent management, and notify the provider. A patient on magnesium sulfate with RR 8 and absent patellar reflexes—stop the infusion, call the provider, and administer calcium gluconate. A patient on gentamicin whose creatinine rises from 0.9 to 1.6 with new tinnitus—hold the dose and notify. Someone on warfarin with INR 5.2 and gum bleeding—hold warfarin and notify the provider; anticipate vitamin K administration if significantly elevated or if bleeding is present. A patient using albuterol rescue inhaler six times a day—recognize poor control, assess adherence/technique and triggers, and anticipate adding or optimizing controller therapy. Always prioritize "stop the offending agent," assess stability (ABCs, vital signs), obtain focused labs/ECG as indicated, and escalate care early.

5.3 Reduction of Risk Potential

Reduction of Risk Potential is the RN's proactive playbook: anticipate complications, prevent them when possible, detect early when not, and act before harm escalates. On the NCLEX, this shows up as questions that ask who is highest risk, what to do first, whether to assess or intervene, and which option is the least invasive and most safety-protective. Apply clinical judgment at the bedside: recognize cues, analyze trends and risk multipliers, choose preventive actions, intervene for deterioration, and re-evaluate for effect. Think: safety first, simple before complex, noninvasive before invasive, and verify new changes from baseline before irreversible actions—unless ABCs are threatened.

Begin by scanning for rapid risk stratifiers. Certain client factors multiply risk and therefore raise priority for surveillance and prevention: extremes of age (infant/older adult), recent surgery or trauma, immobility, the presence of invasive lines or tubes, cardiopulmonary or renal/hepatic compromise, pregnancy and the postpartum period, anticoagulation or bleeding disorders, immunosuppression, altered level of consciousness or impaired swallow, and known or suspected electrolyte or acid–base imbalance. On test day and in practice, a new change from baseline and trends over time carry more weight than a single value. An isolated abnormal finding in a stable, asymptomatic client often yields to monitoring; an abnormal with symptoms or a downward trend deserves earlier action.

Preventive bundles are your backbone. Master the principles so you can apply them to any setting or device.

Bleeding precautions center on minimizing trauma and detecting hidden bleeding early. Avoid intramuscular injections and limit venipunctures; use a soft toothbrush and an electric razor; apply prolonged, firm pressure after any needle sticks or line removal; avoid rectal temperatures and suppositories; and screen for occult bleeding by monitoring stool and urine color, gingival bleeding, easy bruising, or new, severe headache. If a client on antiplatelets or anticoagulants shows bleeding cues, hold the next dose and notify the provider. Before invasive procedures, verify if anticoagulants should be paused and for how long. Teach clients to report melena, hematuria, coffee-ground emesis, or dizziness/syncope promptly.

Thrombosis prophylaxis is about blood flow. Get clients moving early if not contraindicated, encourage frequent leg and ankle pumps when in bed, ensure sequential compression devices are on and functioning, and maintain adequate hydration. Never massage a painful or swollen calf; unilateral warmth, tenderness, or swelling are red flags for deep vein thrombosis. If you see sudden dyspnea, tachycardia, pleuritic chest pain, or hemoptysis in a high-risk client, escalate immediately—this may be pulmonary embolism. In all cases, avoid constrictive devices and ensure proper fitting and continuous use of prophylactic measures as ordered.

Aspiration precautions protect the airway during eating and feeding. Screen swallow function after stroke, head/neck surgery, or sedation, and only advance diet when safe. Keep the client fully upright for all oral intake and at least semi-Fowler's for tube feeds; offer slow, small bites and sips with appropriate texture and thickening as indicated. Keep suction and oxygen at the bedside for high-risk clients. Stop feeding and notify if coughing, a wet/gurgly voice, drooling, pocketing food, or decreased level of consciousness occurs—resume only after reassessment. For nasogastric or gastrostomy feeds, verify tube placement per facility policy before each feeding and hold feeds for high gastric residuals if paired with regurgitation, aspiration signs, or decreasing mental status.

Seizure precautions aim to prevent injury and maintain airway. Set up the room: padded side rails, suction and oxygen at the bedside, and bed in the lowest position. If a seizure occurs, turn the client to the side, protect the head, note the onset and duration, and avoid restraining limbs or placing anything in the mouth. After the event, ensure airway patency, check vital signs, reorient, and assess for triggers or injury. Know the location of rescue medications if ordered and recognize postictal somnolence as expected; persistent confusion, focal deficits, or recurrent seizures require prompt escalation.

Neutropenic and immunocompromised clients need infection prevention tailored to their vulnerability. Place in a private room when possible, enforce strict hand hygiene for everyone who enters, and avoid raw or unwashed foods, unpasteurized products, live plants and flowers, and sick visitors. Perform daily skin and oral assessments and encourage gentle oral care. Fever in these clients is an emergency—report promptly and obtain cultures after orders; do not delay notifying the provider.

Delirium prevention in older adults focuses on orientation, mobility, and minimizing iatrogenic harm. Promote daytime alertness and nighttime sleep (lights by day, quiet at night), use glasses and hearing aids, and reorient with clocks, calendars, and family photos. Mobilize early and often, minimize unnecessary lines and tethers, treat pain, constipation, and urinary retention, maintain hydration and nutrition, and avoid or limit sedatives and anticholinergics. Reserve restraints for last resort; they often worsen agitation and risk.

Sedation and opioid safety requires vigilant monitoring for hypoventilation and oversedation. Assess sedation level and respiratory status at regular intervals and after any dose change; have naloxone immediately available and know the dosing protocol. If a client is difficult to arouse, has shallow respirations, or develops a falling oxygen saturation or rising carbon dioxide, stimulate, support the airway, apply oxygen, consider bag-valve-mask ventilation if needed, and call for help. Hold the next dose and notify the provider. For procedural sedation, ensure continuous pulse oximetry and appropriate capnography if available, maintain IV access, and keep emergency equipment at the bedside.

Surveillance and timely escalation tie prevention to outcomes. Watch the ABCs first, followed by mental status changes and signs of perfusion. Restlessness, anxiety, or a subtle increase in work of breathing often precede overt hypoxia; a thready pulse, cool clammy skin, delayed capillary refill, or a downward trend in urine output can signal shock before blood pressure falls. New, severe, or disproportionate pain suggests compartment syndrome, ischemia, or uncontrolled bleeding and should not be dismissed. Monitor drainage and device outputs for sudden increases, bright red color, stoppage of expected output, or dislodgement—all require assessment and often a call.

Deciding whether to reassess or intervene hinges on stability. If there is acute compromise of airway, breathing, or circulation, stabilize first—open the airway, provide oxygen, control bleeding, elevate the head of bed for respiratory distress, and call for a rapid response. If the client is stable but a complication is possible, verify with assessment before acting—check breath sounds before calling for diuretics, reassess pain patterns before escalating opioids, or recheck a suspicious monitor reading manually. If a therapy or infusion is suspected as the source of a complication, stop the source first while maintaining ABCs, then notify the provider for further orders.

Communication should be precise and ready with data. Structure your call using SBAR: succinctly state the situation, give relevant background, present current assessment findings, and recommend or request what you need. Before calling, gather recent vital signs and oxygen saturation, mental status, intake and output trends, pertinent device settings and outputs (such as infusion rates, drains, or oxygen delivery), time course of changes, last medication doses including anticoagulants or sedatives, allergies, and code status. Anticipate what might be ordered and prepare likely supplies, such as IV fluids, blood tubes for labs, or supplemental oxygen.

Certain "never do" cautions reliably protect clients and save points on the NCLEX. Do not take blood pressure or perform venipuncture on the side of a mastectomy, an arteriovenous fistula, or established lymphedema. Avoid rectal temperatures in neutropenic or thrombocytopenic clients, those post–rectal surgery, or with severe diarrhea. Avoid nasopharyngeal airways or blind nasal tube insertions with suspected basilar skull fracture; do not place nasogastric tubes with severe midface trauma until cleared. Do not clamp a chest tube for a suspected air leak and do not strip chest tubes; both can precipitate tension physiology—maintain the system below the chest and intact, and call for help when problems arise. Avoid straining and Valsalva maneuvers with increased intracranial pressure or after eye or cranial surgery; stool softeners and gentle bowel regimens are safer. Do not reposition, advance, or remove newly placed surgical drains or central lines; secure them, monitor output and site, and call if malposition, bleeding, or dislodgement is suspected.

Test-taking cues that align with clinical judgment will steer you to the safest answer. Prefer preventive, least invasive, and highest-safety options first—positioning, oxygen, and stopping a problematic infusion often precede medications or invasive steps. Prioritize new or worsening cues and unstable clients over chronic and stable conditions. Choose trending abnormalities with symptoms over isolated abnormal numbers without symptoms. If a therapy appears to be causing harm, stop the source first, maintain ABCs, and then notify for further orders. When unsure, ask: does this action validate the problem safely, prevent harm while I confirm, or buy time for definitive care?

To cement the mindset, consider a few micro-scenarios that require recognizing risk and acting early:

- A client with thrombocytopenia is scheduled to receive an intramuscular vaccine. Cue: bleeding risk and invasive route. Action: hold the IM injection and notify the provider for an alternative route or timing. Expected outcome: prevent hematoma or bleeding.
- A post-stroke client takes a sip of water and develops a wet, gurgly voice with light coughing. Cue: aspiration risk and sign of impaired swallow. Action: stop oral intake, keep the client upright, perform oral suction if needed, and notify for a formal swallow evaluation. Expected outcome: prevent aspiration pneumonia.
- A postoperative client with an indwelling urinary catheter has had steadily declining urine output for 3 hours and now has cool, clammy skin and new restlessness. Cue: perfusion risk and early shock signs. Action: assess ABCs, verify catheter patency quickly, elevate legs if appropriate, obtain current vitals, and activate rapid response while preparing for orders. Expected outcome: early resuscitation and prevention of decompensation.
- A client on a patient-controlled analgesia pump is difficult to arouse, with slow, shallow breathing and oxygen saturation trending down. Cue: opioid-induced respiratory depression. Action: stimulate, support the airway, apply oxygen, stop or pause the opioid infusion, call for help, and prepare naloxone per protocol. Expected outcome: reversal of oversedation and safe ventilation.
- A client on bed rest after trauma complains of new unilateral calf pain and warmth. Cue: DVT risk with classic signs. Action: stop any walking orders, keep the client at rest, do not massage the area, notify the provider, and anticipate diagnostic confirmation and anticoagulation if not contraindicated. Expected outcome: prevent embolization.

Reduction of Risk Potential questions reward a consistent, prevention-first approach: scan for multipliers, protect the airway and circulation, position and mobilize, limit invasive trauma and infection exposure, monitor for early deterioration, stop harmful sources, and communicate clearly. When you pair cue recognition and risk trend analysis with the least invasive, highest-yield action, you will choose the safest answer—and safer care follows.

5.3.1 Labs & Diagnostics: Normals and Actions

Use labs to recognize risk early, link cues to likely causes, act on the highest threat first, and then reassess to confirm improvement. Ranges vary slightly by lab; know typical adult values and anchor your actions to the patient's symptoms and trends.

CBC: Hemoglobin, hematocrit, white blood cells, platelets, and ANC are frequent decision-makers. Typical hemoglobin is about 12–16 g/dL in females and 13.5–17.5 g/dL in males; hematocrit roughly 36–46% in females and 41–53% in males. A falling hemoglobin/hematocrit with tachycardia, hypotension, or overt bleeding signals acute blood loss or hemolysis; when symptomatic or very low (for many institutions, hemoglobin around 7 g/dL), anticipate PRBC transfusion, apply oxygen for hypoxemia, obtain large-bore IV access, and assess for the bleeding source. White blood cells normally range 4,000–11,000/mm³; elevations suggest infection, inflammation, or stress, while severe leukopenia raises infection risk. Platelets are typically 150,000–400,000/mm³; thrombocytopenia under 50,000/mm³ markedly increases bleeding risk. The absolute neutrophil count (ANC) is critical for infection risk: ANC below 1,000/mm³ indicates neutropenia, and below 500/mm³ is severe. In severe neutropenia, institute neutropenic precautions immediately—private room if available, meticulous hand hygiene, avoid sick visitors and raw fruits/vegetables/flowers, and wear a mask when leaving the room. Fever is an emergency: obtain cultures and anticipate rapid antibiotics. In thrombocytopenia, initiate bleeding precautions: avoid IM injections and unnecessary venipunctures, hold anticoagulants when appropriate, use a soft toothbrush and electric razor, apply pressure longer after any sticks, and avoid rectal temperatures/suppositories. Notify the provider or rapid response for ANC below 500 with fever, platelets below 50,000 with bleeding, or rapidly falling hemoglobin/hematocrit with instability.

Coagulation: Link the number to the drug and the bleeding risk. PT/INR guides warfarin; a normal INR is around 0.8–1.1 off therapy. Most warfarin goals are INR 2.0–3.0; mechanical mitral valves often need 2.5–3.5. aPTT is used for unfractionated heparin; a typical normal is 25–35 seconds, with a therapeutic range about 1.5–2.5 times control (often 46–70 seconds; follow protocol). Fibrinogen usually ranges 200–400 mg/dL and can fall in DIC; D-dimer rises when significant clot breakdown occurs and prompts evaluation for VTE/PE or DIC in the right clinical context. Safety rules are straightforward: if the client on warfarin shows bleeding or an INR well above goal, hold warfarin, check for interactions, and prepare to administer vitamin K for significant elevations and FFP if actively bleeding per orders. If aPTT is markedly high on heparin with bleeding, stop heparin and anticipate protamine sulfate. For clinically significant bleeding from any cause, prepare blood products (PRBCs, FFP, platelets, or cryoprecipitate) as ordered and monitor for DIC if there is diffuse bleeding, low platelets, low fibrinogen, and elevated D-dimer. Notify promptly for supratherapeutic anticoagulation with any bleeding, sudden neuro changes suggesting intracranial hemorrhage, or signs of DIC.

Electrolytes: The sodium range is 135–145 mEq/L. Severe hyponatremia, especially below 120 or any level with acute neuro changes (headache, confusion, seizures), is dangerous; implement seizure precautions, restrict free water, and anticipate hypertonic saline (3%) per protocol, correcting slowly to avoid osmotic demyelination. Hypernatremia often reflects dehydration; treat with oral or IV free water replacement depending on volume status. Potassium ranges 3.5–5.0 mEq/L. Hyperkalemia above 5.5, and especially any level with ECG changes (peaked T waves, widening QRS), demands immediate cardiac monitoring, IV calcium to stabilize membranes, and measures to shift potassium intracellularly (IV insulin with dextrose, plus possible nebulized albuterol and sodium bicarbonate if acidotic). Remove potassium with loop diuretics, sodium polystyrene sulfonate, or dialysis in refractory cases. Hypokalemia raises arrhythmia risk; replace potassium carefully—never IV push—and follow safe rates (generally ≤10 mEq/hr peripheral; up to 20 mEq/hr via central line with cardiac monitoring), rechecking levels and magnesium as needed. Total calcium is 8.6–10.2 mg/dL; symptomatic hypocalcemia (tetany, stridor, seizures, prolonged QT) calls for IV calcium, while hypercalcemia often warrants fluids and evaluation for malignancy or hyperparathyroidism. Magnesium is 1.5–2.5 mEq/L; hypermagnesemia presents with loss of deep tendon reflexes, bradycardia, hypotension, and respiratory depression—stop magnesium and give IV calcium gluconate while supporting airway and ventilation. Hypomagnesemia predisposes to torsades de pointes; treat with magnesium replacement. Phosphate is 2.5–4.5 mg/dL; severe hypophosphatemia can cause respiratory muscle weakness, especially in refeeding—replace cautiously. Call for help rapidly for potassium ≥6.0 with ECG changes, sodium <120 with seizures, or magnesium toxicity with respiratory depression.

Renal: Use creatinine and eGFR together; creatinine typically ranges 0.6–1.3 mg/dL, BUN 7–20 mg/dL, and eGFR should be above 60 mL/min/1.73 m². A rise in creatinine of ≥0.3 mg/dL in 48 hours suggests acute kidney injury. When creatinine is rising and eGFR is falling, hold nephrotoxins (NSAIDs, aminoglycosides, IV contrast) and adjust medication doses. Before contrast studies, check renal function, optimize hydration, and follow metformin protocols to reduce lactic acidosis risk. Urine output is a frontline cue: less than 0.5 mL/kg/hr or under 30 mL/hr for two consecutive hours needs prompt evaluation for hypovolemia, obstruction, or AKI. Notify for abruptly worsening kidney labs, oliguria, or uremic signs (pericarditis, altered mental status).

ABGs: Think oxygenation and ventilation first. Normal pH is 7.35–7.45; PaCO2 35–45 mm Hg; HCO3 22–26 mEq/L; PaO2 80–100 mm Hg; SaO2 95–100%. Hypoxemia (PaO2 <80 or low pulse oximetry) calls for supplemental oxygen and evaluation of airway, breathing, and circulation. Hypercapnia with somnolence and rising PaCO2 suggests ventilatory failure—elevate the head of bed, apply oxygen, and prepare to support ventilation (consider BiPAP if appropriate; call rapid response if deteriorating). Metabolic acidosis (low pH, low HCO3) often stems from DKA, sepsis, or renal failure; treat the cause (fluids and insulin for DKA; sepsis bundle; dialysis when indicated). Reassess with repeat ABG or oximetry after interventions.

Cardiac markers: Troponin I/T is normally undetectable or very low; any rise above the lab's reference with ischemic cues (chest pain, dyspnea, diaphoresis, ECG changes) is concerning. Act quickly: obtain a 12-lead ECG, place the client on a cardiac monitor, start oxygen only if hypoxemic, establish IV access, keep NPO for possible catheterization, and notify the provider. Anticipate aspirin if not contraindicated and follow facility reperfusion pathways for ST-elevation. BNP under 100 pg/mL is expected; markedly elevated values support heart failure. With high BNP and symptoms of fluid overload, position upright, give oxygen as needed, and anticipate diuretics and afterload reduction per orders. Monitor I/O, daily weights, and electrolyte trends.

Endocrine/glucose: Fasting glucose should be about 70–110 mg/dL; A1c under 7% reflects good control for many adults. TSH is commonly 0.4–4.0 mIU/L with free T4 around 0.8–1.8 ng/dL. Hypoglycemia below 70 mg/dL requires immediate correction: if the patient is awake and can swallow, give 15 g of fast-acting carbohydrates and recheck in 15 minutes; if altered, administer IV dextrose (e.g., 25 g of D50) or IM glucagon and secure the airway. Hyperglycemia with positive ketones or high anion gap suggests DKA; begin isotonic fluids first, then regular insulin infusion, monitor potassium closely (replace if needed before insulin), and add dextrose to fluids when glucose approaches 200 mg/dL to continue clearing ketones. Notify urgently for severe hypoglycemia, DKA, or suspected hyperosmolar hyperglycemic state.

Hepatic/pancreas: AST/ALT are usually about 10–40 U/L; total bilirubin 0.2–1.2 mg/dL. Ammonia is roughly 15–45 µmol/L (lab-dependent). Elevated ammonia with confusion or asterixis indicates hepatic encephalopathy; administer lactulose and titrate to two to three soft stools per day, consider rifaximin, check neuro status frequently, and avoid sedatives that mask decline. Watch for coagulopathy and low fibrinogen in advanced liver disease. Lipase (0–160 U/L) is the preferred marker for pancreatitis; when elevated with severe epigastric pain, keep the patient NPO, initiate aggressive IV fluids (often lactated Ringer's), provide pain control, and monitor for complications like hypocalcemia, ARDS, or sepsis.

Infection/sepsis markers: Lactate above 2 mmol/L is concerning and ≥4 indicates severe tissue hypoperfusion until proven otherwise. Procalcitonin rises with bacterial infection; WBC may be high or paradoxically low in sepsis. Start the sepsis bundle rapidly: draw blood cultures before antibiotics, give broad-spectrum antibiotics promptly, administer 30 mL/kg of isotonic crystalloid for hypotension or lactate ≥4, and escalate to vasopressors to maintain MAP ≥65 mm Hg if shock persists. Apply oxygen, monitor urine output, trend lactate, and reassess vitals frequently. Call rapid response for hypotension unresponsive to fluids, rising lactate, or worsening mental status.

Urinalysis: A quick, rich source of cues. Specific gravity should be 1.005–1.030; high values suggest dehydration while very low values point to diabetes insipidus or overhydration. Nitrites and leukocyte esterase suggest bacterial UTI; protein should be negative—persistent proteinuria raises concern for kidney disease. Ketones should be negative; ketonuria indicates fat breakdown and warrants evaluation for DKA in diabetics. Obtain a clean-catch specimen and send promptly; collect urine culture before starting antibiotics to avoid false negatives. In older adults, new confusion plus positive UA could be UTI; still assess for other causes of delirium and avoid anchoring.

Therapeutic drug levels: Many NCLEX decisions hinge on recognizing toxicity and acting. Digoxin's therapeutic range is about 0.8–2 ng/mL; toxicity presents with anorexia, nausea/vomiting, visual halos, and arrhythmias, and risk increases with hypokalemia and hypomagnesemia. Hold the dose, obtain a level, correct electrolytes, place on a monitor, and anticipate digoxin-specific antibody fragments for severe toxicity. Lithium should be 0.6–1.2 mEq/L; toxicity (tremor, GI upset, confusion, ataxia, seizures) generally appears above 1.5 mEq/L, and severe toxicity above 2.0 is an emergency. Maintain consistent sodium and hydration, avoid NSAIDs when possible, hold the dose, check a level, and prepare for supportive care or dialysis in severe cases. Phenytoin's range is 10–20 mcg/mL; toxicity causes nystagmus, ataxia, confusion; ensure tube feeds are held 1–2 hours before and after dosing to improve absorption. Vancomycin troughs usually target 10–20 mcg/mL depending on infection; draw trough just before the next dose, monitor creatinine, and recognize that red man syndrome is an infusion reaction managed by slowing the rate and giving antihistamines rather than being a "level" problem. Theophylline 10–20 mcg/mL has a narrow window, with arrhythmias and seizures in toxicity; avoid caffeine and many drug interactions. Aminoglycosides require low troughs (often <2 mcg/mL) to reduce nephro- and ototoxicity; verify correct timing of peak/trough draws, monitor renal function, and report tinnitus or vertigo.

High-yield diagnostics: Read the cue and act for safety. An ECG that shows peaked T waves points to hyperkalemia—put the patient on a cardiac monitor, repeat potassium to confirm if discordant with the clinical picture, and begin stabilization and shifting measures. ST-segment elevation in a regional pattern is an emergency: activate the reperfusion pathway, obtain the first troponin and 12-lead promptly, keep NPO, and prepare for PCI if indicated. On a chest X-ray, a visible pleural line with absent lung markings suggests pneumothorax; apply high-flow oxygen, assess for tension physiology (tracheal deviation, hypotension), and prepare for chest tube or emergent decompression per orders. CT with IV contrast requires checking creatinine/eGFR, screening for prior contrast reactions, verifying consent, ensuring IV access, and promoting hydration before and after. Follow metformin protocols (often holding on the day of contrast and for 48 hours if kidney function may be impaired). Ultrasound prep depends on the study: NPO is common for gallbladder evaluation to enhance visualization; a full bladder may be required for pelvic imaging—confirm orders and teach accordingly. A lumbar puncture demands platelet/coagulation assessment and a brief neuro check beforehand; position the client lateral and flexed, maintain sterile technique, and after the procedure lay the client flat as ordered, increase fluids, and monitor for post-LP headache, CSF leak, or neuro changes. For cultures, draw blood cultures before antibiotics, use two sets from separate sites with meticulous asepsis, and label/time specimens accurately to preserve diagnostic value.

Specimen and timing pearls: Some tests require fasting—follow orders carefully for fasting glucose and many lipid panels. Hormones have diurnal patterns; morning cortisol and ACTH are typically drawn early (around 8 a.m.). Hemolysis can falsely elevate potassium; if the number is unexpectedly high without clinical correlation or ECG changes, request a redraw. Therapeutic trough levels are drawn immediately before the next dose; peak times are drug-specific and must match the protocol. Communicate abnormal or critical values promptly using SBAR, document actions, and always reassess after an intervention to ensure the physiologic change matches your expectation. Trend lines are stronger than single dots—worsening patterns deserve urgent attention even if values are "still within normal."

Micro-checklist: Recognize the critical value and connect it to the patient's cues; verify the patient and specimen details; recheck any implausible result or one that doesn't match the clinical picture; act with safety first (protect airway and breathing, place on a monitor, stop the offending agent, start reversal or corrective therapy, prepare needed products); communicate clearly and promptly; reassess to confirm improvement and continue monitoring trends.

Once you've mastered prevention at the bedside, your next layer of safety comes from reading data early—labs, diagnostics, and vital trends that reveal risk before symptoms explode.

5.3.2 Pre/Post-Op Risks

Use the same fast, safety-first logic from clinical judgment: recognize the unstable cue, decide if it threatens airway/breathing/circulation right now, and take the first safe nursing actions while you alert the provider and anticipate orders. Think in a short cycle: recognize key data, analyze what it means (time-sensitive or not), prioritize the next safe step, act, and evaluate the response. Test-wise, if a finding delays surgery, your best "first" is to notify the surgeon/anesthesia and hold until clarified; if a finding kills fast post-op, first protect the ABCs before calling. Evaluate by measurable targets (SpO2, MAP, urine output, drain trends) to know the action worked.

Start with the pre-op screen. The RN's job is to catch red flags before a patient ever gets to the OR, because anything that increases anesthesia risk, bleeding risk, aspiration risk, or hemodynamic instability may delay or cancel the case. Recognize the "don't proceed" cues and document accurately so the team can act.

Pre-op risk screen starts with infection prevention and instability. Fever above 38°C, a new productive cough, purulent urine, chest pain, dyspnea, uncontrolled hypertension, or a new arrhythmia are not "routine" findings; they increase peri-anesthesia risk. First action: stop the line toward the OR, place a call to the surgeon and anesthesia, and be prepared to collect ordered specimens (urine, sputum) or an ECG. Analyze quickly: is the patient unstable (chest pain, dyspnea, arrhythmia)? If yes, treat as an acute problem: obtain vital signs, apply oxygen if hypoxic, place on a monitor, and escalate. Evaluate by resolution of symptoms, stable vital signs, and a clear plan. For low-grade symptoms, anticipate postponement, targeted treatment, and repeat labs before rescheduling.

Abnormal labs are another stop sign. Potassium less than 3.0 or greater than 5.5 mEq/L, sodium less than 130 or greater than 150 mEq/L, glucose above 180 mg/dL, hemoglobin less than 8 g/dL, hematocrit less than 24%, platelets less than 100,000, INR above 1.5 in a non-anticoagulated patient, aPTT above 40 sec, an upward-creeping creatinine, and a positive pregnancy test all trigger a pause. First action: hold progression, highlight the value to the surgical and anesthesia team, and verify whether the patient was supposed to be anticoagulated. Anticipate specific orders: electrolyte repletion (e.g., IV potassium if low), insulin to keep glucose between 80–180 mg/dL, vitamin K or reversal planning if INR is elevated, repeat labs after correction, and a clarified anticoagulation strategy. Evaluate by corrected values on repeat tests and a documented green light to proceed.

Medications and substances can amplify surgical risk. Recognize recent intake of anticoagulants or antiplatelets, long-acting insulin or oral hypoglycemics, MAOIs, herbal supplements that increase bleeding (e.g., ginkgo, garlic, ginseng), heavy alcohol use or withdrawal risk, and any history of obstructive sleep apnea with benzodiazepines or opioids on board. First action: verify last doses and hold parameters; confirm patient-specific instructions were followed. Notify anesthesia for glucose and insulin plans and for withdrawal prophylaxis if needed. Evaluate by a clear medication reconciliation and an individualized anesthetic plan, not by guessing that "it's probably fine."

Aspiration risk is fundamentally about gastric contents and airway protection. If the patient had solids within 6–8 hours or clear liquids within 2 hours of anesthesia start, or if they have gastroparesis, symptomatic GERD, or pregnancy, maintain NPO status and alert anesthesia. Anticipate aspiration prophylaxis (e.g., H2 blocker, prokinetic) and possible delay. Evaluate by revised timing or protective strategies being implemented.

Allergies and reactivity also matter. Latex, chlorhexidine or povidone-iodine sensitivity, and any prior anesthesia complication (malignant hyperthermia in the patient or family, severe nausea, difficult intubation) must be surfaced. First action: apply allergy bands, ensure non-latex supplies are planned, and relay the history. Anticipate premedication orders if appropriate and a documented MH precaution if indicated. Evaluate by the OR team acknowledging and preparing for the risk.

Baseline status informs everything post-op. Document airway and neck mobility, dentures or loose teeth, known OSA, mobility aids needed, and skin integrity. These baselines become your comparison points later; a mismatched assumption post-op can cost you time.

Once the patient arrives from the OR to PACU or the unit, shift to the top life threats. Airway and breathing come first. Recognize obstruction and hypoventilation early: snoring or gurgling, stridor, SpO2 below 92% (or below patient baseline if they live lower), shallow respirations, agitation, or cyanosis. Act immediately: position the patient lateral or with the head of bed up 30–45°, perform a jaw thrust (avoid head tilt if cervical spine precautions are in place), insert an oral or nasal airway if trained and indicated, suction secretions, and apply oxygen. If obstruction persists or you hear stridor, call anesthesia promptly; this is not a watch-and-wait moment. As the patient awakens, coach incentive spirometry and deep breathing. Evaluate with objective targets: SpO2 at or above 92% (or baseline), respiratory rate 12–20, clear or improving breath sounds, and the patient maintaining the airway independently.

Next, circulation and bleeding. Recognize shock by tachycardia, narrow pulse pressure, hypotension, cool clammy skin, decreasing level of consciousness, increasing drain output or rapidly saturating dressings, and oliguria defined as less than 0.5 mL/kg/hr. Act fast: expose and assess the surgical site and all drains, trace tubes and connections, and apply direct pressure to an accessible bleeding site without disturbing the operative field. Trend vital signs every 5–15 minutes, ensure a large-bore IV is patent or place a second site if ordered/within scope, and initiate an isotonic fluid bolus per protocol while you notify the surgeon. Draw labs if ordered and prepare a type and screen. Evaluate by achieving MAP of at least 65 mmHg, stabilizing heart rate, urine output returning to at least 0.5 mL/kg/hr, and drain output that is stable and not rapidly rising.

Malignant hyperthermia requires rapid recognition and protocolized response. Early cues are rising end-tidal CO2 if being monitored, generalized or masseter muscle rigidity, and tachycardia; hyperthermia is a late sign. If suspected, call the MH emergency, stop triggering anesthetics, deliver 100% oxygen, administer dantrolene per protocol, begin active cooling, and treat the metabolic derangements (hyperkalemia, acidosis) per orders. Evaluate by falling ETCO2, improving rigidity and vital signs, and stabilization of labs.

Pain and sedation safety are a balancing act. Recognize over-sedation by a decreasing respiratory rate and level of consciousness, and uncontrolled pain by tachycardia, hypertension, and splinting. Titrate opioids cautiously, especially in obstructive sleep apnea; use multimodal analgesia if ordered. If the patient is oversedated with compromised respirations, administer naloxone per protocol and support the airway. Reassess frequently—pain and sedation are dynamic—and evaluate by adequate analgesia without respiratory depression.

As you move into the first hours to the second post-op day, look for preventable complications. Atelectasis and pneumonia show up as tachypnea, low-grade fever on day 1–2, and crackles or diminished breath sounds. The best actions are preventive: scheduled incentive spirometry every 1–2 hours while awake, coached cough with abdominal splinting for comfort, early and frequent ambulation, and adequate pain control to permit deep breathing, with oxygen as needed. Evaluate by improving breath sounds, better oxygenation, and resolution of fever trends.

Deep vein thrombosis and pulmonary embolism require vigilance. Unilateral leg swelling, warmth, and pain suggest DVT; sudden dyspnea, pleuritic chest pain, tachycardia, and hypoxemia suggest PE. Do not massage a suspected DVT. Keep the patient on bedrest, elevate the head of bed, apply oxygen, and notify the provider emergently. Anticipate orders for imaging and anticoagulation. Preventively, apply sequential compression devices if not contraindicated and mobilize early. Evaluate by stabilized oxygenation, relief of dyspnea, and a definitive plan underway.

Nausea, vomiting, and aspiration risk are common as anesthesia wears off. Recognize a depressed gag reflex or active emesis. First action: place the patient side-lying to protect the airway and suction promptly. Administer antiemetics as ordered and slow or space opioids if they are contributing. Keep NPO until a safe swallow is demonstrated. Evaluate by cessation of vomiting, protected airway, and return of protective reflexes.

Urinary retention can emerge within 6–8 hours post-op, often visible as suprapubic fullness and discomfort. Scan the bladder, assist to void with privacy and normal cues (upright position, running water), and perform straight catheterization if the volume exceeds protocol thresholds and noninvasive measures fail. Evaluate by comfortable bladder emptying and avoidance of overdistention.

Ileus presents with absent or hypoactive bowel sounds, abdominal distention, and nausea. Keep the patient NPO, anticipate an NG tube for decompression if vomiting or significant distention occurs, encourage ambulation, provide IV fluids and electrolyte management, and minimize opioids when possible. Evaluate by passage of flatus, return of bowel sounds, decreasing distention, and comfort.

Wound complications require quick differentiation. Dehiscence or evisceration can be heralded by a sudden "pop" sensation and increased serosanguineous drainage. Place the patient in low Fowler's with the knees slightly flexed to reduce tension, cover exposed viscera with sterile normal saline–moistened gauze, keep the patient NPO, and notify the surgeon immediately. Evaluate by protection of the viscera and rapid surgical response. Infection typically appears after 48–72 hours with redness, warmth, purulent drainage, and fever. Notify the provider, obtain cultures if ordered, and perform wound care per orders. Evaluate by decreasing local signs and systemically improving temperature.

Positioning matters across procedures. Initially recover in a lateral position to protect the airway and transition to head-of-bed elevation after extubation. Avoid prone positioning in anyone with airway risk. Know the specific cautions: never hyperextend the neck after thyroid surgery because of airway edema risk; teach abdominal splinting for coughing after abdominal surgery; and use a logroll with spinal precautions when indicated. These are first-line safety measures that appear frequently on exams.

Tailor vigilance to high-risk populations. Older adults are vulnerable to delirium (waxing/waning level of consciousness), dehydration, and hypothermia. Reorient frequently, ensure glasses and hearing aids are available, mobilize early, and use warm blankets. Patients with OSA or obesity are prone to airway collapse and opioid sensitivity; minimize sedatives, maintain continuous oximetry, and apply CPAP if ordered. Those with diabetes face hyper- or hypoglycemia and infection risk; maintain glucose between 80–180 mg/dL with protocols and monitor the wound closely. Renal or cardiac disease creates a narrow window between fluid overload and hypovolemia; measure intake and output meticulously, weigh daily, assess for edema and crackles, and titrate fluids as ordered. Your evaluation targets are objective: stable oxygenation, steady hemodynamics, appropriate urine output, and no new pulmonary congestion.

Monitoring must be intentional. Follow postoperative vital sign frequency (typically every 5–15 minutes in PACU, then spacing on the unit), assess pain and neurological status, watch urine output for at least 0.5 mL/kg/hr, keep SpO2 at or above 92% or the patient's baseline, track temperature between 36.0–38.0°C, and trend bleeding and drain output rather than relying on single numbers. Readiness for discharge from PACU centers on a stable airway with adequate oxygenation and ventilation, hemodynamic stability without escalating support, controlled pain and nausea, and intact protective reflexes; many institutions use Aldrete-type scoring systems to standardize this decision.

To internalize the "what to do first" steps, rehearse a few mini-algorithms. When you suspect hemorrhage: assess the surgical site immediately for bleeding, apply direct pressure if the site is accessible, obtain rapid vital signs and recognize the shock pattern, call the surgeon, and initiate IV fluids while preparing a type and screen. When an airway obstruction develops: reposition to lateral or elevate the head of bed, perform a jaw thrust, insert an oral airway and suction if indicated, apply oxygen, and call anesthesia if there is no rapid improvement. For a possible PE: apply oxygen, elevate the head of bed, stay with the patient, notify the provider urgently, and anticipate anticoagulation workup and therapy. With evisceration: place in low Fowler's with knees flexed, cover with sterile normal saline–moistened dressings, keep NPO, and notify the surgeon immediately.

What ties all of this together is disciplined cue recognition and tight first actions. On the exam, unstable cues (airway noises, SpO2 below target, MAP dropping, rising drain outputs, altered LOC, rigidity with hypercarbia) demand immediate ABC-focused interventions you can do now as the RN, not passive observation or delayed calls. Stabilize first, then notify, and always know how you will evaluate success: a number you can measure, a breath you can hear, a drain that has slowed, a patient who is awake enough to protect their own airway.

5.3.3 Recognizing Deterioration (Electrolytes, ABGs, OB Red Flags)

Use a rapid, action-first approach that mirrors the Clinical Judgment Measurement Model. When something is "off," move through these steps without delay:

1. Recognize cues. Look for trends (getting worse), big or out-of-range numbers, and any new neuro or respiratory change. Verify accuracy: recheck vital signs, assess the patient yourself, and consider lab error (e.g., hemolyzed sample causing false hyperkalemia).
2. Analyze. Apply ABCs and identify unstable features: airway/stridor, RR <12 or >30, SpO2 falling on oxygen, new arrhythmia, hypotension, acute confusion, seizure, heavy bleeding, severe pain out of proportion. Consider likely causes (electrolyte, bleed, drug effect).
3. Prioritize actions. Secure airway/oxygen first, stop offending agents (meds/infusions), ensure safety (seizure precautions, fall risk), then give the targeted fix (e.g., antidote, electrolyte replacement).
4. Evaluate. Reassess vital signs, tele, mental status, urine output; repeat key labs/ABGs after interventions; and escalate with SBAR to the provider. Document response and trends.

Electrolytes are classic deterioration triggers. Know normal ranges, dangerous cutoffs, hallmark cues, and first-line actions. Treat abnormal numbers only when clinically appropriate, but respond immediately when red flags are present.

Potassium (3.5–5.0 mEq/L). Hyperkalemia becomes dangerous at >6.0 or with ECG changes such as peaked T waves and widened QRS. Expect muscle weakness and paresthesias; the true danger is lethal arrhythmias. First actions are to place the client on a cardiac monitor and stop potassium sources (supplements, ACE inhibitors, ARBs, spironolactone). Stabilize the myocardium with IV calcium gluconate, shift potassium intracellularly with IV insulin and dextrose and consider nebulized albuterol, then remove potassium with a loop diuretic, cation-exchange resin, or dialysis if renal failure. Hypokalemia <3.0 may show U waves, PVCs, weakness, ileus, and increases digoxin toxicity risk. Place on telemetry, replace potassium—never IV push—and use a pump: no more than 10 mEq/hour peripherally, up to 20 mEq/hour via central line with continuous monitoring. Evaluate and correct magnesium, which impairs potassium repletion if low.

Sodium (135–145 mEq/L). Hyponatremia becomes a cerebral edema emergency when <120 or when seizures or pronounced LOC changes occur. Initiate seizure precautions, maintain airway, restrict free water, and for severe symptomatic cases anticipate hypertonic saline (3%) with careful monitoring; correction must be slow to prevent osmotic demyelination. Hypernatremia >160 causes neuro irritability, thirst, dry mucosa, and can lead to hemorrhage in the brain if corrected too rapidly. Restore volume first with isotonic fluids if hypovolemic, then gradually lower sodium with hypotonic solutions and treat the cause (e.g., diabetes insipidus, dehydration). Monitor neuro status closely.

Calcium (8.6–10.2 mg/dL). Hypocalcemia presents with tetany, perioral numbness, stridor/laryngospasm, Chvostek and Trousseau signs, and QT prolongation. Airway is priority—prepare suction and oxygen, and give IV calcium gluconate; check and correct magnesium; implement seizure precautions. Hypercalcemia causes weakness, constipation, polyuria, stones, shortened QT, and confusion. Treat with IV isotonic fluids to promote calciuresis, add a loop diuretic (not thiazides), and anticipate bisphosphonates for malignancy-associated cases. Encourage mobility if appropriate.

Magnesium (1.5–2.5 mg/dL). Hypermagnesemia, often iatrogenic in obstetrics, is signaled by absent or decreasing deep tendon reflexes, bradypnea (RR <12), hypotension, flushing, and lethargy progressing to respiratory arrest. Immediately stop magnesium, support airway and ventilation as needed, and administer IV calcium gluconate as the antidote. Hypomagnesemia produces hyperreflexia, tremors, ventricular ectopy, and torsades de pointes. Begin IV magnesium sulfate with continuous telemetry and frequent reflex and respiratory checks.

Phosphate (2.5–4.5 mg/dL). Severe hypophosphatemia causes respiratory muscle weakness and failure, often in refeeding. Replete phosphate cautiously while monitoring calcium, which inversely changes; watch for tetany if calcium drops. Improving respiratory effort is a key evaluation point.

Arterial blood gases and oxygenation require a quick, structured read to catch impending failure. Scan the pH first to identify acidemia or alkalemia, then decide whether CO_2 (respiratory) or HCO_3 (metabolic) is the primary driver. Consider compensation next, and then judge oxygenation using PaO_2 and SpO_2. Red flags include pH <7.25, $PaCO_2$ >50 with a low pH indicating acute ventilatory failure, PaO_2 <60 or SpO_2 <90% despite supplemental oxygen, and rising CO_2 with decreasing LOC. Immediate actions are to position the airway (head-tilt/chin-lift or jaw thrust if trauma suspected), administer oxygen and titrate to effect—target 88–92% in COPD exacerbations to avoid CO_2 retention—and suction secretions if needed. Treat the cause: give naloxone for suspected opioid overdose, bronchodilators and steroids for bronchospasm, diuretics for pulmonary edema, antibiotics for pneumonia as ordered. Prepare for noninvasive ventilation or intubation if there is worsening work of breathing, refractory hypoxemia, or altered mental status. Reassess with repeat ABG after interventions to confirm improvement.

Obstetric deterioration carries two patients at once. Rapid recognition and intrauterine resuscitation while calling for help can be lifesaving. In hypertensive disorders of pregnancy, severe features include BP ≥160/110, severe headache, vision changes, right upper quadrant or epigastric pain, hyperreflexia with clonus, proteinuria, and thrombocytopenia. Implement seizure precautions, place the client in the left lateral position, begin IV antihypertensives per order, administer magnesium sulfate for seizure prophylaxis, maintain strict I&O to watch for oliguria, and ensure continuous fetal heart rate monitoring. Be prepared for delivery if maternal or fetal status is unstable. If magnesium toxicity develops—diminishing or absent DTRs, respiratory rate <12, or urine output <30 mL/hr—stop magnesium and give IV calcium gluconate while supporting airway and ventilation.

Hemorrhage before or after birth presents with heavy bleeding, a boggy fundus postpartum, tachycardia, hypotension, and pallor. Massage a boggy uterus, empty the bladder, and administer oxytocin as first line. If bleeding persists, add methylergonovine if hypertension is not present, carboprost if the client does not have asthma, or misoprostol per protocol. Start large-bore IVs, infuse isotonic fluids, quantify blood loss, type and cross, and prepare for transfusion while monitoring for shock.

Fetal distress consistent with Category III tracing—absent variability with recurrent late or variable decelerations or bradycardia—requires intrauterine resuscitation immediately: turn the client to the left lateral position, stop oxytocin, apply oxygen at 10 L via nonrebreather, give an IV fluid bolus, and consider a tocolytic if there is tachysystole. Notify the provider and be ready for operative delivery if the tracing does not recover.

Cord prolapse is a time-critical emergency marked by sudden decelerations and a palpable or visible cord. Call for help, move the client to knee-chest or steep Trendelenburg, and with a sterile-gloved hand elevate the presenting part off the cord without removing pressure until birth. Cover any exposed cord with a sterile, moist dressing, apply oxygen, and prepare for an emergent cesarean.

Shoulder dystocia shows the turtle sign (head retracts against the perineum). Perform the McRoberts maneuver and apply suprapubic pressure; never use fundal pressure. Continue communicating clearly and prepare for neonatal resuscitation.

Uterine rupture or amniotic fluid embolism presents as sudden severe pain, abnormal fetal heart rate, maternal hypotension, hypoxia, and possible DIC. Stop oxytocin, apply high-flow oxygen, establish or add large-bore IV access, initiate massive transfusion if indicated, call a code, and prepare for rapid transfer to the operating room.

Safety principles on the NCLEX are nonnegotiable. Do not delegate unstable clients, acute changes, or initial assessments. Never IV push potassium; always use a pump and double-check rates for all high-alert infusions. Stabilize life-threatening airway, breathing, and circulation problems before calling the provider, then communicate with SBAR including what you recognized, what you did, and how the patient responded. Remember that trends matter more than a single normal value; treat new confusion, arrhythmias, stridor, rapid oxygen desaturation, severe blood pressure derangements, heavy bleeding, and seizure activity as top-tier priorities. Throughout deterioration, the RN's role is immediate recognition and first-line stabilization, rapid interruption of the cause when possible, and continuous evaluation. These are the actions that save lives—and score points—because they reflect safe, timely clinical judgment.

5.4 Physiological Adaptation (Acute/Chronic High-Yield)

On NCLEX, physiological adaptation is about recognizing when a client is decompensating and implementing the safest, first-line responses. Think in Clinical Judgment terms: collect and trend cues (not single vitals in isolation), determine what you must rule in or rule out right now (threatened airway? shock? stroke?), anticipate the next complication, and act in ABCs order while prioritizing unstable over stable. Frame your first minute: reposition for airway and perfusion, titrate oxygen appropriately, secure IV access, begin indicated isotonic fluids (unless signs of overload/cardiogenic failure), stop the offending agent/bleed source, and prepare for the time-sensitive therapy (reperfusion, insulin infusion, epinephrine) while continuously reassessing.

Universal deterioration cues to trend include sudden mental status change; increased work of breathing or an SpO2 drop; respiratory rate >30/min or <12/min; new stridor or wheezes; systolic BP <90 mm Hg or MAP <65 mm Hg; heart rate >130/min or <50/min; chest pain; unilateral neurologic deficits; urine output <30 mL/hr; temperature >38.5°C with hypotension; or new, uncontrolled bleeding. Activate a rapid response team for threatened airway, hypoxia unresponsive to oxygen, RR >30 or <8, HR >140 or <40 with symptoms, SBP <90 or MAP <65 after initial measures, acute mental status change, new seizure, chest pain unrelieved by initial measures, or significant bleeding. In triage terms, ESI-1 requires immediate life-saving intervention; ESI-2 is high risk, confused/lethargic, severe pain/distress—do not delay evaluation.

Use the following compact "condition cards" to recognize patterns quickly and act safely.

Airway/breathing emergencies

Upper airway obstruction (foreign body, edema, anaphylaxis). What's happening: airflow blocked at or above the larynx; risks include surgery of head/neck, allergic exposure. Red flags: stridor, drooling, "can't speak," retractions, cyanosis. First actions: call RRT, high-flow oxygen, upright positioning with jaw thrust, suction as needed, prepare for emergent advanced airway; for choking with ineffective cough, perform abdominal thrusts. Monitor: SpO2, work of breathing, voice quality. Escalate: inability to ventilate, SpO2 <90% despite oxygen, rapidly worsening edema. Pitfalls: do not leave the client; do not attempt blind finger sweeps.

Status asthmaticus. What's happening: severe bronchospasm/mucus plugging refractory to usual therapy. Red flags: silent chest, RR >30, accessory muscle use, SpO2 falling, pulsus paradoxus. First actions: high-flow oxygen, upright position, continuous short-acting bronchodilator via nebulizer, prepare for systemic steroids; prepare for intubation if fatigue/CO2 retention. Monitor: SpO2 ≥94%, wheeze air movement improving, ability to speak phrases. Escalate: deteriorating mentation, rising CO2, persistent hypoxemia. Pitfalls: avoid sedatives that depress respirations; avoid beta-blockers.

COPD exacerbation. What's happening: acute worsening of airflow limitation and gas exchange. Red flags: increased dyspnea, wheeze, purulent sputum, drowsiness (hypercapnia). First actions: upright tripod position, titrate oxygen to 88–92% using Venturi if available, encourage pursed-lip breathing, airway clearance/nebulized bronchodilator per orders. Monitor: mentation, SpO2 88–92%, RR and accessory use. Escalate: progressive somnolence, acidosis, SpO2 <88% despite oxygen—prepare for NIV (BiPAP) or intubation. Pitfalls: avoid excessive oxygen and supine positioning.

Acute pulmonary edema (cardiogenic). What's happening: fluid floods alveoli due to left-sided failure. Red flags: pink frothy sputum, crackles, severe dyspnea, orthopnea, S3. First actions: sit upright legs dependent, high-flow oxygen (consider CPAP/NIV if available), prepare for IV diuretics and vasodilators per orders; Foley for accurate UOP. Monitor: SpO2 ≥94%, work of breathing, MAP ≥65, UOP ≥30 mL/hr. Escalate: refractory hypoxemia, hypotension—consider intubation/ICU. Pitfalls: avoid large fluid boluses and Trendelenburg.

Pulmonary embolism. What's happening: clot obstructs pulmonary circulation. Red flags: sudden pleuritic chest pain, dyspnea, tachycardia, hypoxemia, hemoptysis, anxiety. First actions: high-flow oxygen, elevate HOB, stay with the client, establish IV access, notify HCP for anticoagulation/thrombolysis, consider hemodynamic support.

Monitor: SpO2, hemodynamics, pain, respiratory status. Escalate: hypotension, syncope—RRT, prepare for thrombolysis/embolectomy. Pitfalls: do not ambulate or massage legs; avoid SCDs if DVT suspected.

ARDS. What's happening: noncardiogenic inflammatory lung injury with refractory hypoxemia. Red flags: severe dyspnea, high oxygen needs, bilateral infiltrates, decreased compliance. First actions: high-flow oxygen, prepare for intubation/low tidal volume ventilation; conserve fluids unless in shock; prone positioning per team. Monitor: SpO2, ventilator parameters, hemodynamics. Escalate: persistent hypoxemia, rising plateau pressures. Pitfalls: avoid aggressive fluid overload and high tidal volumes.

Circulation/perfusion emergencies

Shock (hypovolemic, cardiogenic, distributive). What's happening: inadequate tissue perfusion. Red flags: MAP <65, tachycardia, cool clammy skin (warm in early distributive), altered mental status, oliguria. First actions: two large-bore IVs; for hypovolemic/distributive, rapid isotonic boluses; control bleeding/stop source; supine with legs elevated; oxygen. For cardiogenic, oxygen, gentle diuresis/inotropes per orders—avoid large boluses. Monitor: MAP ≥65, lactate trend if available, UOP ≥30 mL/hr, mental status. Escalate: persistent hypotension → vasopressors, ICU. Pitfalls: do not delay fluids for labs; do not start vasopressors before volume in hypovolemia.

Acute coronary syndrome/MI. What's happening: myocardial ischemia from plaque rupture. Red flags: chest pressure radiating to arm/jaw, diaphoresis, dyspnea, nausea, ST-T changes. First actions: semi-Fowler, oxygen if SpO2 <90%, obtain 12-lead ECG, IV access, chewable aspirin unless contraindicated, prepare for reperfusion. Monitor: pain relief without hypotension, rhythm, hemodynamics. Escalate: VT/VF, shock—defibrillation; ongoing ischemia—cath lab. Pitfalls: avoid nitroglycerin if hypotensive or recent PDE5 inhibitor use; no IM injections.

Acute decompensated heart failure. What's happening: inability to maintain cardiac output; congestion. Red flags: dyspnea, crackles, JVD, weight gain, edema. First actions: upright, oxygen, prepare for diuresis, sodium/fluid restriction, Foley for strict I&Os. Monitor: daily weight, UOP, crackles, SpO2. Escalate: hypotension, escalating oxygen need—ICU. Pitfalls: avoid fluid boluses; avoid NSAIDs.

Hypertensive crisis. What's happening: severe BP elevation with target-organ injury. Red flags: HA, visual change, neuro deficits, chest pain, BP ≥180/120. First actions: verify BP with correct cuff and position HOB ~30°, quiet environment, IV access, prepare for IV antihypertensives; continuous monitoring. Monitor: gradual BP reduction, neuro status, renal function. Escalate: encephalopathy, chest pain—ICU. Pitfalls: do not lower BP too fast.

Neurologic emergencies

Stroke (suspected). What's happening: ischemia or hemorrhage. Red flags: sudden unilateral weakness, facial droop, aphasia, visual loss; time last known well. First actions: stroke alert; NPO; head midline, HOB ~30°; oxygen to keep SpO2 >94%; IV access; check glucose; prepare for CT. Monitor: neuro checks, BP (permissive hypertension often for ischemic), airway protection. Escalate: decreased LOC, vomiting—prepare suction/intubation. Pitfalls: no PO/meds until swallow screen; do not aggressively lower BP pre-CT.

Increased ICP. What's happening: volume increase in skull reduces perfusion. Red flags: declining LOC, headache, vomiting, unequal pupils, Cushing triad. First actions: HOB ~30°, head midline, avoid neck flexion; minimize stimulation; oxygenation; only brief, pre-oxygenated suction as needed. Monitor: neuro status, MAP/CPP if available. Escalate: herniation signs—RRT, prepare for hyperosmolar therapy/intubation. Pitfalls: avoid hypotonic fluids and lumbar puncture in mass effect.

Seizures/status epilepticus. What's happening: abnormal electrical activity; prolonged seizure threatens airway. Red flags: tonic–clonic activity, cyanosis, salivation, postictal confusion. First actions: protect from injury, turn to side, suction ready, oxygen; time the seizure; prepare benzodiazepines per protocol. Monitor: airway, oxygenation, neuro recovery. Escalate: >5 minutes or recurrent seizures—status; RRT. Pitfalls: no restraints; nothing in the mouth.

Autonomic dysreflexia (SCI at/above T6). What's happening: uncontrolled sympathetic discharge to noxious stimuli below lesion. Red flags: severe headache, hypertension, bradycardia, flushing/sweating above level, piloerection.

First actions: sit upright immediately; loosen clothing; check/remove triggers (kinked catheter, bladder distention, fecal impaction); monitor BP frequently; notify HCP. Monitor: BP trending down, symptom relief. Escalate: refractory hypertension—antihypertensives per orders. Pitfalls: do not lay flat; do not ignore bladder.

Endocrine/metabolic emergencies

DKA vs HHS. What's happening: insulin deficit; DKA with ketosis/acidosis, HHS with extreme hyperglycemia and dehydration. Red flags: DKA—Kussmaul respirations, abdominal pain, fruity breath; HHS—profound dehydration, neuro deficits, minimal ketones. First actions: airway, isotonic fluid resuscitation first; IV access; check K and glucose; prepare insulin infusion after initial fluids and potassium assessment; cardiac monitoring. Monitor: improving mentation, closing anion gap (trending), UOP. Escalate: shock, altered mental status—ICU. Pitfalls: do not start insulin before addressing potassium and volume.

Thyroid storm vs myxedema coma. What's happening: extremes of thyroid dysfunction. Red flags: storm—fever, tachyarrhythmias, agitation; myxedema—hypothermia, bradycardia, hypoventilation. First actions: ABCs; for storm, cooling measures and prepare beta blockade/antithyroid per orders; for myxedema, warming and ventilatory support, prepare IV thyroid hormone. Monitor: temperature, heart rhythm, mental status. Escalate: arrhythmias, respiratory failure. Pitfalls: avoid aspirin in storm; avoid sedatives in myxedema.

Adrenal crisis. What's happening: acute cortisol deficiency. Red flags: hypotension refractory to fluids, hyponatremia, hyperkalemia, abdominal pain, history of steroid use. First actions: isotonic fluids (consider dextrose), draw labs but do not delay steroids, administer stress-dose corticosteroid per orders; cardiac monitoring. Monitor: MAP ≥65, electrolytes, glucose, UOP. Escalate: persistent shock—ICU. Pitfalls: do not postpone steroids for diagnostics.

Severe hyperkalemia. What's happening: elevated serum potassium threatens cardiac conduction. Red flags: muscle weakness, peaked T waves, widened QRS. First actions: cardiac monitor; repeat lab to rule out hemolysis; stop potassium sources; prepare membrane stabilization and shift therapies per orders. Monitor: rhythm normalization, K trending down, UOP. Escalate: arrhythmias, AKI—dialysis. Pitfalls: avoid potassium-containing IV fluids.

Renal/hepatic/GI emergencies

AKI with oliguria. What's happening: abrupt kidney injury with reduced output. Red flags: UOP <0.5 mL/kg/hr, fluid overload or hypovolemia, rising creatinine. First actions: assess volume status; strict I&O; avoid nephrotoxins/contrast; isotonic bolus if hypovolemic; dose-adjust meds. Monitor: UOP ≥30 mL/hr, weights, electrolytes. Escalate: refractory hyperkalemia, uremic symptoms—dialysis. Pitfalls: avoid excess potassium/Mg.

Upper GI bleed/varices. What's happening: hemorrhage from mucosa or portal hypertension. Red flags: hematemesis, melena, hypotension, tachycardia. First actions: two large-bore IVs, oxygen, NPO, type and crossmatch, prepare for endoscopy; position on side if vomiting, consider balloon tamponade prep per team. Monitor: MAP ≥65, H/H trends, UOP. Escalate: continued bleeding, shock—massive transfusion protocol. Pitfalls: avoid NG tube in known/suspected varices without orders.

Acute pancreatitis. What's happening: autodigestion/inflammation of pancreas. Red flags: severe epigastric pain radiating to back, N/V, hypocalcemia signs. First actions: NPO, aggressive isotonic fluids if hypotensive, pain control, side-lying with knees flexed for comfort. Monitor: pain, hemodynamics, electrolytes, UOP. Escalate: hypoxia, hypotension, sepsis—ICU. Pitfalls: avoid alcohol/fatty intake education; avoid unnecessary opiates commentary—follow orders.

Hepatic encephalopathy. What's happening: neurotoxicity from ammonia and triggers. Red flags: confusion, asterixis, fetor hepaticus; precipitated by GI bleed, infection, constipation. First actions: safety precautions, lactulose as ordered to achieve 2–3 soft stools/day, correct triggers (treat bleed, avoid constipation), monitor electrolytes. Monitor: mentation improving, stool goals, potassium. Escalate: worsening LOC—airway protection. Pitfalls: avoid sedatives; avoid protein restriction unless severe.

Infectious/immune/burns/onc emergencies

Sepsis. What's happening: dysregulated infection with organ dysfunction. Red flags: fever or hypothermia, tachycardia, hypotension, altered mental status, oliguria, elevated lactate. First actions: RRT; oxygen; two sets of blood cultures then broad-spectrum antibiotics without delay; 30 mL/kg isotonic fluids; vasopressors if MAP <65 after fluids. Monitor: MAP, UOP, mentation, lactate trend. Escalate: persistent shock—ICU. Pitfalls: do not delay antibiotics; avoid hypotonic fluids.

Anaphylaxis. What's happening: IgE-mediated multisystem reaction. Red flags: urticaria, angioedema, wheeze/stridor, hypotension. First actions: stop exposure; call RRT; IM epinephrine; high-flow oxygen; airway adjuncts/suction; IV access and isotonic fluids; prepare adjunct meds per orders. Monitor: airway patency, BP, SpO2. Escalate: refractory symptoms—repeat epinephrine, advanced airway. Pitfalls: do not remove epinephrine from plan; observe for biphasic reaction.

Early burn fluid shift (24–48 h). What's happening: capillary leak causing hypovolemia; inhalation injury risk. Red flags: hoarseness, soot, singed hairs; tachycardia, hypotension; circumferential burns. First actions: secure airway early if inhalation injury suspected; two large-bore IVs; initiate fluid resuscitation per formula; elevate burned limbs; keep warm; tetanus status. Monitor: UOP (0.5–1 mL/kg/hr adults), MAP, airway edema progression. Escalate: deteriorating airway—intubate; compartment syndrome signs—escharotomy. Pitfalls: no ice; no prophylactic antibiotics.

Oncologic metabolic/compressive syndromes. Tumor lysis syndrome: after chemo—hyperkalemia, hyperphosphatemia, hypocalcemia, AKI. First actions: cardiac monitoring, aggressive hydration, manage electrolytes per orders. Pitfalls: avoid K-containing fluids. SIADH: hyponatremia with low serum osmolality, confusion, seizures. First actions: fluid restriction, seizure precautions, hypertonic saline cautiously per orders; monitor sodium correction rate. SVC syndrome: facial/upper extremity edema, dyspnea, distended neck veins. First actions: HOB up, oxygen, minimize upper extremity venipuncture, notify for emergent radiation/stenting. Spinal cord compression: new back pain, weakness, bowel/bladder changes. First actions: spine precautions, notify HCP, prepare for steroids/imaging. Pitfalls: do not delay steroids for imaging when compression strongly suspected.

Across these scenarios, your first actions are anchored to safety: position to support airway/ICP/cardiac output, titrate oxygen to the right target (≥94% for most; 88–92% in COPD), open the airway and suction as needed, obtain two large-bore IVs, give isotonic fluids when indicated (avoid boluses in cardiogenic overload), stop the trigger (offending drug, bleeding source), and prepare for time-sensitive therapies while verifying contraindications. Reassess continuously and document response.

Evaluate your interventions by looking for improving mentation, a stable airway/ventilation with appropriate SpO2, RR easing, hemodynamics with MAP ≥65, urine output ≥30 mL/hr, and pain relief without hemodynamic compromise.

Prevent chronic-to-acute spirals with focused teaching: in heart failure, daily weights and call for >2–3 lb/day or >5 lb/week gain, increased dyspnea, or edema; for COPD/asthma, correct inhaler and spacer technique, a written action plan, and early use of rescue inhaler with prompt follow-up; for diabetes, sick-day rules (never stop basal insulin, hydrate, monitor glucose/ketones, seek help for persistent vomiting or ketones), and hypoglycemia recognition; with cirrhosis, avoid constipation and GI bleeding triggers, take lactulose as prescribed, and report confusion early; across conditions, emphasize adherence, early symptom recognition, and escalation before instability.

NGN/CJMM angle—linking cues to the first safe action: Post-op day 1, HR 128, BP 86/50, cool clammy skin, UOP 15 mL/hr: this cue cluster rules in hypovolemic shock/bleeding. First action is to support circulation—lay supine with legs elevated, call RRT, obtain two large-bore IVs and start isotonic bolus while quickly assessing the surgical site/drains and applying pressure to any external bleeding; then notify the surgeon and prepare for blood products. In COPD exacerbation with increasing somnolence and SpO2 88% on 2 L, prioritize airway/ventilation: sit upright, titrate oxygen to 88–92% (consider Venturi), prepare for BiPAP, and notify the provider; avoid supine sedation.

Select-all prioritization—suspected pulmonary embolism: immediate steps include apply high-flow oxygen, elevate HOB, stay with the client, assess vitals and perfusion, establish IV access, and notify the HCP/RRT to prepare for anticoagulation and imaging. Later tasks include obtaining informed consent for CT angiography, comprehensive risk-factor teaching, and applying SCDs (contraindicated when acute DVT/PE is suspected).

5.4.1 Cardio/Resp, Neuro, Endocrine/Renal (Red Flags + First Actions)

How to use this page: See the cue, decide stability, act in ABC order, and escalate early. Rapid Response is for acute deterioration with a pulse/breathing; call a Code Blue for unresponsive/no pulse or agonal/no breathing. Anchor your decisions in clinical judgment: recognize key cues, prioritize the unstable finding, implement safe first actions, then evaluate and escalate.

Cardiovascular/Respiratory. The fastest points you earn in this system come from catching time-sensitive, high-mortality problems and doing the first right things. Start with a focused assessment: airway patency, work of breathing, circulation (skin, pulses, cap refill), level of consciousness, vital signs with SpO2. Keep the head of bed elevated unless contraindicated. Place the patient on continuous cardiac and pulse oximetry monitoring and obtain IV access.

Know the red flags you cannot miss. Acute coronary syndrome and MI show up as crushing or pressure-like chest pain, diaphoresis, nausea, and often ST elevation or new LBBB. Pulmonary embolism presents with sudden dyspnea, pleuritic chest pain, tachycardia, hypoxemia, and sometimes hemoptysis or anxiety. Tension pneumothorax produces severe respiratory distress with absent breath sounds on one side, tracheal deviation away from the affected side, hypotension, and distended neck veins. Cardiac tamponade signals with hypotension, JVD, muffled heart sounds, pulsus paradoxus, and narrowing pulse pressure. Acute pulmonary edema or flash heart failure is pink frothy sputum, severe dyspnea, orthopnea, crackles, and anxiety. Life-threatening dysrhythmias include unstable bradycardia or tachycardia (hypotension, altered LOC, chest pain, signs of shock), and pulseless VT/VF. A hypertensive emergency is severe BP elevation with end-organ symptoms such as severe headache, visual changes, chest pain, dyspnea, or neurologic deficits. Status asthmaticus is severe bronchospasm with minimal air movement—a "silent chest"—and rising CO2; in advanced COPD, CO2 narcosis shows as somnolence with elevated PaCO2.

Move immediately to the first actions. Ensure airway patency and apply oxygen; titrate to SpO2 ≥ 94% for most adults, targeting 88–92% if the patient is a known chronic CO2 retainer, but do not withhold oxygen in severe hypoxemia. Sit the patient upright to decrease work of breathing; in pulmonary edema, dangle the legs if tolerated to reduce preload. Obtain a 12-lead EKG for chest pain or dysrhythmia concerns without delay and start continuous cardiac monitoring. Establish one or two large-bore IV lines. Prepare high-yield medications per protocol: chewable aspirin for suspected ACS if no allergy or active bleeding; nitroglycerin for chest pain if systolic BP is adequate and the patient has not taken phosphodiesterase-5 inhibitors; bronchodilators and systemic corticosteroids for asthma; IV diuretics for pulmonary edema if ordered; beta-blockade and IV antihypertensives as ordered for hypertensive emergency; heparin for suspected PE per provider order. For suspected PE, maintain bedrest, apply oxygen, and do not massage the legs. In suspected tension pneumothorax, provide high-flow oxygen, prepare for immediate needle decompression by a provider, and do not delay for imaging if the patient is crashing. In suspected cardiac tamponade, provide oxygen, maintain hemodynamic monitoring, and prepare for pericardiocentesis; avoid large fluid boluses unless specifically ordered as a bridge. Call the Rapid Response Team early for any unstable pattern, and if you encounter pulseless VT/VF or asystole/PEA, activate a Code and start high-quality CPR; defibrillate VT/VF as soon as the defibrillator arrives.

Keep the pitfalls in mind. Do not delay oxygen or a bedside EKG in a patient with chest pain. Do not ambulate a suspected PE; keep on bedrest. Be cautious with nitrates in right-sided MI and with hypotension. For tension pneumothorax or tamponade, recognize that definitive treatment is decompression or pericardiocentesis; prepare equipment and the patient while maintaining oxygenation and hemodynamics.

Neurologic. Life-threatening neuro events announce themselves with time-critical cues; your job is to protect the brain and buy time for definitive therapy. Stroke recognition starts with FAST: facial droop, arm weakness, speech difficulty, time last known well. Add any unilateral weakness or numbness, aphasia, visual field cuts, severe sudden headache, or acute confusion to your mental list. Increased intracranial pressure appears as Cushing's triad—bradycardia, widening pulse pressure, and irregular respirations—along with worsening headache, vomiting, and decreased LOC. Status epilepticus is a seizure lasting more than five minutes or recurrent seizures without recovery. Meningitis often brings fever, severe headache, nuchal rigidity, photophobia, and in meningococcal disease, a petechial rash with rapid deterioration. In high spinal cord injury with neurogenic shock, anticipate hypotension, bradycardia, warm dry skin, and loss of sympathetic tone.

Begin with airway protection. Position a seizing patient on the side, pad the bed, and clear the area to prevent injury; time the seizure and apply oxygen. Have suction ready for secretions and be prepared to administer a benzodiazepine per order, establishing IV access quickly. For suspected stroke, check blood glucose immediately and correct hypoglycemia; keep the patient NPO, perform a rapid neuro check, place the head of bed around 30 degrees, administer oxygen only if hypoxic, establish IV access, and prepare for immediate noncontrast CT. Note the exact last known well time and obtain vital signs; avoid administering anticoagulants or antiplatelets until intracranial hemorrhage is ruled out. For increased ICP, elevate the head of bed to about 30 degrees, keep the neck midline to promote venous drainage, minimize suctioning and stimulation, control pain and agitation, and notify the provider urgently; anticipate orders for hyperosmolar therapy and avoid hypotonic fluids. When meningitis is suspected, initiate droplet precautions immediately, obtain cultures if feasible without delay, then administer antibiotics promptly—do not hold antibiotics if the patient is unstable. With possible spinal cord injury or neurogenic shock, maintain spinal immobilization, support the airway, provide oxygen, initiate IV fluids per order to support perfusion, and monitor mean arterial pressure to maintain spinal cord perfusion.

Avoid common missteps. Do not give anything by mouth to a patient with acute neurologic change. Do not aggressively hyperventilate a patient with suspected elevated ICP unless there are signs of impending herniation and it's specifically ordered as a short-term bridge. Avoid hypotonic fluids in increased ICP. Do not delay antibiotics in suspected bacterial meningitis when the patient is unstable.

Endocrine. Critically ill endocrine patients deteriorate because of hypoglycemia, acidosis/dehydration, hormone excess, or deficiency. DKA and HHS share profound dehydration, polyuria, polydipsia, tachycardia, hypotension, and altered mental status; DKA typically adds Kussmaul respirations and ketone breath. Severe hypoglycemia presents with diaphoresis, tremor, palpitations, confusion, slurred speech, seizures, or coma. Thyroid storm is hypermetabolic—high fever, agitation/delirium, tachyarrhythmias, and heart failure signs. Myxedema coma is the opposite—hypothermia, bradycardia, hypotension, hypoventilation, and obtundation. Adrenal crisis features refractory hypotension, abdominal pain, hyponatremia, hyperkalemia, and possible hypoglycemia. Diabetes insipidus shows massive polyuria with hypernatremia and dehydration; SIADH shows dilutional hyponatremia with confusion, headache, and possibly seizures.

Act quickly and target the cause. Any altered mental status gets a bedside glucose first; treat hypoglycemia immediately: if the patient is awake and can swallow, give 15 grams of rapid-acting carbohydrate and recheck in 15 minutes; if unable to swallow or unconscious, protect the airway and give glucagon IM or D50 IV per protocol, then follow with complex carbs once alert and swallowing. For DKA/HHS, stabilize the airway and breathing, begin isotonic fluid resuscitation first, place the patient on a cardiac monitor, and draw labs including electrolytes and ketones. Begin insulin therapy per protocol after the initial fluid bolus, but monitor potassium closely; if potassium is critically low, replace potassium before starting insulin to prevent life-threatening arrhythmias. Treat precipitating factors such as infection. In thyroid storm, secure ABCs, apply cooling measures (tepid cooling, antipyretics—avoid aspirin), place on a cardiac monitor, and anticipate beta-blockers and antithyroid medications followed by iodine; corticosteroids may be ordered. In myxedema coma, support the airway and ventilation—these patients hypoventilate—apply passive warming measures, avoid external heating pads on the skin, and anticipate IV levothyroxine and stress-dose steroids. For adrenal crisis, give rapid isotonic fluids, correct hypoglycemia, place on a cardiac monitor, and prepare to administer hydrocortisone; monitor electrolytes and treat hyperkalemia as needed. For DI, replace free water and anticipate desmopressin; for SIADH, implement fluid restriction, perform frequent neurologic checks, place the patient on seizure precautions, and anticipate hypertonic saline for severe symptomatic hyponatremia per order. Maintain strict intake and output in all of these states.

Mind the pearls. Do not start an insulin infusion when potassium is critically low; correct potassium first and monitor continuously. Avoid external warming devices that can burn cold skin in myxedema; use passive warming. Do not give aspirin in thyroid storm because it can increase free thyroid hormone. In SIADH, avoid hypotonic fluids and excess free water intake.

Renal/Fluid-Electrolyte. The renal system's red flags are arrhythmogenic electrolytes, rapid volume shifts, and access complications. Acute kidney injury with hyperkalemia shows weakness, paresthesias, nausea, and on EKG, peaked T waves, PR prolongation, QRS widening, and potentially sine-wave. Fluid overload and pulmonary edema in chronic kidney disease or dialysis patients surface as dyspnea, crackles, hypoxemia, edema, and rising blood pressure. Dialysis complications include hypotension during treatment, bleeding from the access site, and dialysis disequilibrium syndrome post-treatment with headache, nausea, confusion, and in severe cases seizures.

Take decisive first actions. Place the patient on a cardiac monitor and quickly verify the potassium level when hyperkalemia is suspected. Stop all potassium sources (infusions, supplements, high-K diet). Prepare to administer calcium gluconate to stabilize the myocardium, insulin with dextrose to shift potassium intracellularly, and nebulized albuterol; sodium bicarbonate may be used if acidotic. Remove potassium with loop diuretics, potassium binders, or dialysis per order. For fluid overload or pulmonary edema, enforce strict intake and output, obtain daily weights, elevate the head of bed, apply oxygen, and prepare IV diuretics; if diuretics are ineffective or contraindicated, anticipate dialysis. Protect the vascular access: assess for thrill and bruit; if absent, notify the provider immediately; never take blood pressure, perform venipuncture, or insert IVs in the fistula arm. If the fistula or graft bleeds, apply firm direct pressure and monitor for hemodynamic compromise. If hypotension occurs during or after dialysis, position the patient supine, check the access, and give fluids per order.

Avoid preventable harm. Do not administer potassium-containing fluids or medications to a patient with hyperkalemia. Renally dose medications and hold nephrotoxins when acute kidney injury is suspected. Check for and manage post-dialysis heparin effects if procedures are planned.

Evaluate and escalate. After every intervention, reassess vital signs, mental status, work of breathing, SpO2, rhythm, and pain; trend changes, not single numbers. If there is no improvement or deterioration continues, escalate: call Rapid Response, anticipate definitive therapies (e.g., thrombolysis, cath lab, chest tube, intubation, dialysis). Document the cues you recognized, the actions you took, exact times, and the patient's responses. Handoff succinctly using SBAR, highlighting instability, what has been tried, and what is pending.

NGN/CJMM tie-in: think cue to action and partial credit. Crushing chest pain with diaphoresis and new ST elevation means you put the patient on oxygen, get a 12-lead EKG now, give chewable aspirin if not contraindicated, start an IV, place on a monitor, and notify the provider or activate the cath lab pathway—points for each correct step. A suddenly dyspneic, tachycardic postoperative patient with pleuritic chest pain cues suspected PE; you elevate the head of bed, apply oxygen, keep the patient on bedrest, place on a monitor, start an IV, and notify the provider for imaging and anticoagulation—do not massage the calves. A seizing patient for more than five minutes with continued altered consciousness triggers status epilepticus management: position side-lying, protect the airway with suction and oxygen, time the seizure, obtain IV access, administer a benzodiazepine per order, and check glucose—each safe step earns credit and demonstrates clinical judgment.

5.5 Knowledge check

Clinical Vignette 1

A 72-year-old man is admitted from a surgical ward with increased ileostomy output and acute shortness of breath during a morning bolus enteral feeding. He has colon cancer with ileostomy created 6 days ago, seizure disorder on phenytoin 300 mg daily via NG tube, and hypertension on lisinopril; no drug allergies. His wife reports large-volume ileostomy output (~1.5 L/24 hr), poor oral intake, and lightheadedness on standing. Exam: thin, BP 100/56, HR 110, RR 24, T 37.4°C, SpO_2 88% RA; coarse crackles and decreased breath sounds in the right lower lobe. During observation, he coughed with a wet voice while a 250 mL bolus was delivered via NG tube; tube length was unchanged. Stoma: beefy red, moist, watery output, with early mucocutaneous redness. Labs: Na 146, K 3.2, Cl 110, HCO_3 22; glucose 150. Feeding record: bolus every 4 hours around the clock; phenytoin given 30 minutes post-bolus. He wants to go home today and is anxious about delaying discharge.

Question 1: Based on the vignette, which of the following is the most likely immediate clinical problem the nurse should recognize?

[A] Pulmonary embolism from postoperative immobility
[B] Acute myocardial ischemia presenting with dyspnea
[C] Ileostomy ischemia causing systemic sepsis and hypoxia
[D] Aspiration of enteral feeding leading to impaired oxygenation

Question 2: Given the events in the vignette (coughing and desaturation during a bolus enteral feed), what is the nurse's best immediate action?

[A] Suction the airway and continue the bolus feed to finish on schedule
[B] Stop the feeding, raise the head of bed to 30–45 degrees, and assess airway and oxygenation
[C] Flush the feeding tube with water, then resume the bolus at a slower rate
[D] Check the ileostomy output and call the provider only if output increases further

Question 3: What pathophysiologic mechanism best explains the drop in oxygen saturation after aspiration of enteral formula in this patient?

[A] Aspiration causes direct myocardial suppression leading to decreased cardiac output and hypoxemia
[B] Enteral formula embolizes pulmonary vessels causing large-vessel occlusion and abrupt arterial desaturation
[C] Instilled gastric contents obstruct airways and trigger local inflammation, producing ventilation–perfusion mismatch and shunt physiology
[D] Aspiration increases venous return and precipitates pulmonary edema from fluid overload

Question 4: The patient is on phenytoin given via the enteral tube. Which is the most appropriate nursing action regarding phenytoin administration to reduce the risk of subtherapeutic levels?

[A] Crush the sustained-release phenytoin tablet and give with the next bolus feed to improve tolerance
[B] Hold feeds for 15 minutes before and after phenytoin dosing and flush with 5 mL of water
[C] Mix phenytoin with a full bolus of formula to ensure consistent absorption
[D] Stop the enteral feed 1–2 hours before and after phenytoin administration and flush tube with 15–30 mL water before and after

Question 5: The patient insists on discharge today despite ongoing large-volume ileostomy output, lightheadedness, and the recent aspiration event. Which action best reflects the nurse's ethical and clinical responsibility?

[A] Delay discharge, notify the provider about high ostomy output and recent aspiration, begin oral rehydration and closer monitoring, and reinforce teaching until stable
[B] Provide written ostomy homecare instructions and schedule a home health visit without delaying discharge
[C] Offer reassurance and discharge with oral antidiarrheal medication to reduce stomal output at home
[D] Honor his autonomy and prepare discharge teaching since he remains alert and oriented

ANSWERS

1. Correct Answer: D

Rationale: The vignette documents coughing and a wet-sounding voice during a bolus enteral feed with an acute drop in SpO2 and focal crackles—classic cues for aspiration of enteral formula causing impaired oxygenation. A pulmonary embolism (A) usually presents with sudden pleuritic chest pain, tachycardia, and hypoxia but is less linked to an immediate cough during feeding. Acute myocardial ischemia (B) would have ischemic chest pain, ECG changes, or troponin elevation—not the feeding-related cough/wet voice. Ileostomy ischemia (C) would present with a dusky or black stoma and abdominal findings; the stoma here is beefy red, making ischemia unlikely.

2. Correct Answer: B

Rationale: The chapter emphasizes the airway is priority for aspiration risk: stop the feed, elevate the head of bed to reduce further aspiration (30–45° for enteral feeds), then suction and assess oxygenation and breath sounds. Suctioning and continuing the feed (A) risks further aspiration. Flushing and resuming the bolus (C) is unsafe during suspected aspiration. Checking ileostomy output and only calling the provider later (D) delays urgent airway-focused care.

3 Correct Answer: C

Rationale: Aspirated gastric or enteral contents obstruct airways and provoke inflammatory response, causing alveolar collapse and ventilation–perfusion mismatch (shunt physiology) leading to hypoxemia—this fits the immediate desaturation after a witnessed aspiration. Myocardial suppression (A) is not the primary mechanism for post-aspiration hypoxia. Enteral formula does not embolize pulmonary vessels as a typical mechanism (B). While severe aspiration can contribute to pulmonary edema in some settings, increased venous return from aspiration (D) is not the typical pathophysiology.

4. Correct Answer: D

Rationale: Phenytoin interacts with enteral feeds; best practice is to hold enteral feedings 1–2 hours before and after phenytoin dosing and flush the tube with 15–30 mL of water before and after to reduce binding and ensure absorption. Crushing sustained- or extended-release formulations (A) is contraindicated. Holding feeds only 15 minutes (B) is insufficient to prevent binding and reduced absorption. Mixing phenytoin with formula (C) increases interaction risk and variability in absorption.

5. Correct Answer: A

Rationale: The nurse must prioritize safety (beneficence/nonmaleficence) over an early discharge when the patient has high ostomy output with lightheadedness (dehydration risk) and a recent aspiration event. Delaying discharge, notifying the provider, initiating rehydration, and providing targeted teaching and monitoring is appropriate. Simply honoring autonomy without addressing risks (D) neglects duty to protect. Sending him home with only written instructions and a home visit (B) or discharging with an antidiarrheal (C) without clinical stabilization and provider involvement is unsafe given current signs.

Clinical Vignette 2

A 72-year-old woman is 24 hours post–total hip arthroplasty reporting increased groin pain; her chart lists a patient-controlled analgesia (PCA) pump delivering hydromorphone with a 0.5 mg demand dose and a 0.5 mg/hr basal rate. Her past medical history includes chronic obstructive pulmonary disease (COPD), obstructive sleep apnea treated with nighttime CPAP, and osteoarthritis; she takes inhaled tiotropium and a nightly zolpidem as needed. Allergies: none. The nurse reports the patient received 0.5 mg IV lorazepam 30 minutes earlier for anxiety while still on the PCA. Focused exam shows somnolence with a sedation score of 4, respiratory rate 8 breaths/min, shallow respirations, oxygen saturation 86% on 2 L nasal cannula, blood pressure 90/56 mm Hg, and pinpoint pupils; lung sounds are diminished bilaterally without wheeze. Capillary glucose is 112 mg/dL. Arterial blood gas on 2 L nasal cannula shows pH 7.25, PaCO2 62 mm Hg, PaO2 58 mm Hg, HCO3- 26 mEq/L. The PCA infusion is visible at the bedside; pump logs show multiple recent demand doses and a basal infusion. The patient's family states she uses CPAP at home but has not used it since surgery.

Question 1: Based on the vignette, which condition is the most likely cause of the patient's acute deterioration?

[A] Acute myocardial infarction from perioperative stress
[B] Acute pulmonary embolism from postoperative immobility
[C] Medication-induced hypoventilation from combined opioid and sedative effects
[D] Hypoglycemia causing decreased level of consciousness

Question 2: What is the nurse's best immediate action for this patient referenced in the vignette?

[A] Increase the nasal cannula flow to 6 L/min and reassess in 10 minutes
[B] Stop the PCA and any sedatives, call for help/rapid response, support airway/ventilation, and administer naloxone per protocol
[C] Administer flumazenil to reverse benzodiazepine effects and observe for improvement
[D] Reduce the PCA basal rate by half and document the change on the MAR

Question 3: Which pharmacologic explanation best describes why this patient is experiencing severe respiratory depression?

[A] Benzodiazepines increase histamine release causing bronchospasm that leads to hypoxia
[B] Pharmacodynamic synergism: concurrent opioids and benzodiazepines produce additive CNS and respiratory depression
[C] Impaired renal clearance of hydromorphone caused accumulation due to elevated creatinine alone
[D] Hydromorphone interacts with tiotropium to produce anticholinergic respiratory suppression

Question 4: How should the arterial blood gas (pH 7.25, PaCO2 62 mm Hg, PaO2 58 mm Hg) be interpreted and what monitoring or next steps are indicated per the vignette context?

[A] Primary metabolic acidosis with respiratory compensation; obtain lactate and hold opioids pending results
[B] Hypoxemic respiratory alkalosis from hyperventilation; increase pain control to reduce tachypnea
[C] Normal postoperative ABG for a patient with COPD; continue current therapy and reassess in 2 hours
[D] Acute respiratory acidosis with hypoxemia consistent with hypoventilation; immediately support ventilation/oxygenation, reverse opioids per protocol, monitor for renarcotization, and perform frequent sedation and respiratory assessments

Question 5: After the patient is stabilized, which action best reflects safe practice and professional responsibility in response to this event?

[A] Omit documentation of the naloxone dose to avoid disciplinary review but inform the provider verbally
[B] Chart the naloxone and interventions before giving them in order to maintain a complete MAR record
[C] Remove the PCA pump and discard its records to prevent confusion during handoff
[D] Notify the provider and leadership per policy, complete an incident/variance report objectively, document assessments/interventions and patient response, and participate in education to prevent recurrence

ANSWERS

1. Correct Answer: C

Rationale: The vignette shows classic signs of medication-induced hypoventilation—marked sedation, respiratory rate 8, pinpoint pupils, low SpO_2, and ABG with elevated $PaCO_2$—occurring while the patient is receiving an opioid PCA plus recent lorazepam, supporting combined sedative-opioid effects. A and B are less likely because MI or pulmonary embolism more commonly cause chest pain, tachycardia, pleuritic pain, or sudden hypoxia without pinpoint pupils or high $PaCO_2$ from hypoventilation. D is unlikely because capillary glucose is normal.

2. Correct Answer: B

Rationale: Chapter guidance: immediately stop the offending medication(s), maintain airway and breathing, call for help, and administer naloxone per protocol for opioid-related respiratory depression. A is insufficient alone given severe hypoventilation. C (flumazenil) is not first-line when opioids are involved and may precipitate seizures in benzodiazepine-dependent or at-risk patients; naloxone addresses opioid effect. D (simply reducing basal rate) is too slow and does not address current respiratory compromise.

3. Correct Answer: B

Rationale: The vignette demonstrates pharmacodynamic synergism: opioids and benzodiazepines both depress central respiratory drive, producing additive respiratory depression—this is emphasized in the chapter as a high-risk interaction. A is incorrect: benzodiazepines do not cause histamine-mediated bronchospasm as a primary mechanism. C may contribute in some cases but the ABG and timing after lorazepam point to acute CNS depression rather than chronic renal accumulation alone. D is incorrect; tiotropium is anticholinergic bronchodilator and does not produce the observed central respiratory suppression.

4. Correct Answer: D

Rationale: The ABG shows acute respiratory acidosis (low pH, elevated $PaCO_2$) with hypoxemia—findings consistent with hypoventilation from sedative/opioid effect. Chapter guidance directs immediate support of ventilation/oxygenation, reversal of opioids per protocol, and close monitoring for renarcotization and recurrent respiratory depression with frequent sedation/respiratory checks. A is incorrect because the primary disturbance is respiratory, not metabolic. B misinterprets as alkalosis. C is unsafe: these values are not normal and require immediate intervention.

5. Correct Answer: D

Rationale: After stabilization, best practice per the chapter is to notify the provider and leadership, complete an objective incident/variance report, and document assessments/interventions and patient response; this supports a just culture and patient safety. A and C are unethical and violate policy—concealing events or records is impermissible. B is incorrect procedure: you must document what was actually done after the fact, not fabricate prior documentation; the chapter stresses accurate, timely, and objective documentation and appropriate reporting of errors or adverse events.

Clinical Vignette 3

A 28-year-old man presents to the ED with 2 days of nausea, vomiting, abdominal pain, polyuria, polydipsia, and increasing drowsiness. He has a history of type 1 diabetes mellitus and reports he missed his insulin doses for 24 hours after losing his pump battery; he takes no other daily medications and has no known drug allergies. On exam he is ill-appearing, tachycardic (HR 112), hypotensive 96/58 mm Hg, with deep, rapid respirations and dry mucous membranes; capillary refill is delayed. Initial fingerstick glucose is 520 mg/dL; serum chemistry shows Na 130 mEq/L, K 4.2 mEq/L, bicarbonate 10 mEq/L, and venous blood gas pH 7.18; urine dipstick is positive for large ketones. He weighs 90 kg; a standardized insulin infusion concentration (100 units regular insulin in 100 mL normal saline) is available on the unit. The physician orders an insulin infusion at 0.1 units/kg/hr and hourly glucose checks, and notifies nursing that cardiac monitoring will be applied. Family at bedside asks whether treatment can wait while they fetch identification and financial documents.

Question 1: Based on the vignette, which is the most likely primary diagnosis?

[A] Diabetic ketoacidosis (DKA)
[B] Hyperosmolar hyperglycemic state (HHS)
[C] Lactic acidosis from sepsis
[D] Alcoholic ketoacidosis

Question 2: The physician orders insulin 0.1 units/kg/hr. Using the available bag (100 units regular insulin in 100 mL NS) and the patient weight in the vignette, what is the correct pump rate in mL/hr?

[A] 1.0 mL/hr
[B] 90 mL/hr
[C] 9 mL/hr
[D] 0.9 mL/hr

Question 3: Which mechanism best explains why serum potassium often falls after insulin therapy is started in this patient?

[A] Increased renal excretion of potassium due to osmotic diuresis induced by hyperglycemia
[B] Insulin-induced renal loss of potassium via increased aldosterone secretion
[C] Loss of potassium from vomiting and poor intake only
[D] Insulin stimulates Na+/K+ ATPase activity, driving potassium into cells and lowering serum potassium

Question 4: Before initiating the prescribed insulin infusion for this high-alert medication, which is the most important laboratory value or preparation the nurse should confirm per safe-practice guidelines in the vignette?

[A] Serum potassium is ≥3.3 mEq/L and dextrose is immediately available per protocol
[B] Hemoglobin A1c is within target range before infusion
[C] The patient has eaten a full meal to prevent hypoglycemia after starting the infusion
[D] An order to discontinue all cardiac monitoring once infusion begins

Question 5: Which immediate nursing action best follows high-alert medication safety principles before starting the insulin infusion described in the vignette?

[A] Start the infusion now because hyperglycemia is severe and time is critical
[B] Rely only on barcode scanning of the bag to verify correct drug and rate
[C] Perform an independent double-check with another licensed nurse confirming drug, concentration, calculation, and pump settings before initiation
[D] Request family consent to proceed with the infusion because this is a high-risk medication

ANSWERS

1. Correct Answer: A

Rationale: The vignette shows hyperglycemia (glucose 520 mg/dL), metabolic acidosis (pH 7.18, HCO3 10), and large urinary ketones in a patient with type 1 diabetes and missed insulin—classic for DKA. B is less likely because HHS typically occurs in type 2 diabetes with minimal ketosis and much higher osmolality; C is unlikely because there are specific hyperglycemia and ketone findings; D is unlikely without history of heavy alcohol use and the presence of severe hyperglycemia and ketoacidosis points to DKA.

2. Correct Answer: C

Rationale: Calculate: 0.1 units/kg/hr × 90 kg = 9 units/hr. Bag concentration is 100 units/100 mL = 1 unit/mL, so 9 units/hr = 9 mL/hr. A (1.0 mL/hr) and D (0.9 mL/hr) reflect decimal-place errors; B (90 mL/hr) is a tenfold error. The estimate-before-calc step (about 9 units/hr) helps catch those unit/decimal errors.

3. Correct Answer: D

Rationale: Insulin promotes cellular uptake of potassium by stimulating Na+/K+ ATPase, shifting potassium intracellularly and lowering serum potassium—this is the principal mechanism after insulin therapy in DKA. A and C are contributing factors to overall potassium balance but do not explain the rapid post-insulin fall; B incorrectly assigns the primary effect to aldosterone.

4. Correct Answer: A

Rationale: Chapter guidance specifies confirming serum K ≥3.3 mEq/L before starting insulin (risk of hypokalemia with insulin-driven potassium shift) and having dextrose available for hypoglycemia management. Hemoglobin A1c (B) is not required acutely; expecting the patient to have eaten (C) is inappropriate in DKA management and may be unsafe; stopping cardiac monitoring (D) would contradict monitoring needs for electrolyte shifts.

5. Correct Answer: C

Rationale: Insulin infusions are high-alert; the recommended safety action is an independent double-check with another licensed nurse confirming correct drug, concentration, dose, calculation, and pump programming before initiation. A bypasses safety checks; B over-relies on technology—barcode scanning supports but does not replace independent verification; D is incorrect because routine treatment does not require family consent before emergent, clinician-ordered life-saving therapy and consent cannot substitute for safety verification.

Clinical Vignette 4

A 72-year-old woman presents to the emergency department with sudden swelling of her lips and tongue that began one hour after taking her morning medications; she reports mild shortness of breath but no urticaria or known insect bite. Her medical history includes hypertension, heart failure with reduced ejection fraction, type 2 diabetes, and chronic kidney disease stage 3. Home medications listed by the patient are lisinopril, spironolactone, furosemide, metformin, and an over-the-counter potassium supplement she "sometimes" takes; she is allergic to penicillin (rash). On exam she is alert, BP 88/54 mm Hg, HR 96/min, RR 20/min, SpO2 94% on room air; her tongue and perioral tissues are edematous, with mild inspiratory wheeze but no skin rash. Labs show potassium 5.8 mEq/L and creatinine 1.9 mg/dL (baseline ~1.3), and a bedside ECG demonstrates peaked T waves. She declines invasive procedures initially and asks what caused the swelling; family is en route. The nurse prepares for possible airway compromise while gathering supplies and notifying the provider.

Question 1: Based on the vignette, which is the most likely explanation for this patient's sudden lip and tongue swelling?

[A] IgE-mediated anaphylaxis to an unknown food allergen
[B] Allergic reaction to penicillin causing angioedema
[C] Urticarial reaction from a viral illness causing facial edema
[D] Angioedema associated with an ACE inhibitor

Question 2: Given the patient's presentation in the vignette, what is the nurse's highest priority immediate action?

[A] Assess and monitor the airway; stop lisinopril and notify the provider while preparing for possible airway support
[B] Administer intramuscular epinephrine for anaphylaxis and then obtain labs
[C] Give IV diphenhydramine and wait for swelling to decrease before further intervention
[D] Encourage the patient to take oral antihistamine and observe vital signs every 30 minutes

Question 3: Which pathophysiologic mechanism best explains ACE inhibitor–associated angioedema described in the vignette?

[A] Accumulation of bradykinin due to inhibition of its degradation by ACE
[B] IgE-mediated mast cell degranulation with histamine release
[C] Immune complex deposition in submucosal tissues causing complement activation
[D] Increased aldosterone secretion causing mucosal edema

Question 4: The nurse notes the potassium is 5.8 mEq/L with peaked T waves on ECG as in the vignette. Which nursing action is most appropriate immediately?

[A] Administer oral sodium polystyrene sulfonate (kayexalate) and discharge the patient when asymptomatic
[B] Hold lisinopril and spironolactone, place the patient on continuous cardiac monitoring, and prepare IV calcium gluconate while notifying the provider
[C] Give IV insulin with dextrose only and continue all home medications as prescribed
[D] Encourage the patient to drink grapefruit juice to lower serum potassium and monitor repeat labs in 24 hours

Question 5: The alert patient refuses transfer to the ICU and possible intubation despite progressive tongue swelling. Which action best reflects appropriate ethical and nursing practice?

[A] Honor the refusal and document that the patient declined transfer without further discussion
[B] Assess the patient's decision-making capacity, explain risks/benefits, notify the provider, and document an informed refusal if capacity is intact
[C] Restrain the patient to prevent agitation and move her to the ICU for airway protection against her wishes
[D] Immediately arrange involuntary admission because airway compromise is life-threatening

ANSWERS

1. Correct Answer: D
Rationale: The vignette lists lisinopril (an ACE inhibitor) and acute isolated orofacial swelling without urticaria—classic for ACE inhibitor–associated angioedema. Her presentation lacks the multisystem features (hypotension, widespread rash, bronchospasm) typical of IgE-mediated anaphylaxis (A), and she denies recent penicillin exposure making B unlikely; urticaria from viral illness (C) usually includes rash and a more gradual onset.

2. Correct Answer: A
Rationale: Airway assessment and readiness to secure the airway are highest priority when angioedema threatens the oropharynx; stopping the offending ACE inhibitor and quickly notifying the provider are appropriate immediate steps. IM epinephrine (B) is first-line for anaphylaxis but ACE inhibitor angioedema is bradykinin-mediated and may not respond predictably; IV diphenhydramine alone (C) or oral antihistamine/observation (D) are inadequate when airway compromise is possible.

3. Correct Answer: A
Rationale: ACE inhibitors reduce breakdown of bradykinin, leading to its accumulation and non–IgE-mediated angioedema. IgE-mediated histamine release (B) describes classic allergic anaphylaxis rather than ACE inhibitor angioedema; immune complex (C) and aldosterone-related (D) mechanisms are not responsible for this presentation.

4. Correct Answer: B
Rationale: Peaked T waves indicate potentially life-threatening hyperkalemia; immediate steps include cardiac monitoring and administration of IV calcium to stabilize the myocardium, and holding medications that raise potassium (ACE inhibitors, potassium-sparing diuretics). Kayexalate alone and discharge (A) is inappropriate acutely; IV insulin with dextrose (part of potassium-shifting therapy) may be used but continuing potassium-raising home meds (as implied in C) is contraindicated; grapefruit juice (D) is ineffective and can cause drug interactions.

5. Correct Answer: B
Rationale: If a patient refuses recommended treatment, the nurse should assess capacity, provide clear information about risks/benefits, notify the provider, and document informed refusal—respecting autonomy while ensuring safety and communication. Simply honoring refusal without discussion (A) neglects assessment of capacity and informed decision-making; restraining (C) or involuntary admission without assessment (D) are coercive and violate ethical and legal standards unless the patient lacks capacity or is imminently dangerous and legal criteria are met.

Clinical Vignette 5

A 72-year-old woman is postoperative day 2 following a left total knee arthroplasty and reports new right calf pain and swelling that began this morning. Her past medical history includes hypertension and osteoarthritis; home medication lisinopril; she was started on enoxaparin 40 mg subcutaneously nightly for DVT prophylaxis after surgery. She has no medication allergies and lives alone. On assessment she is alert; vital signs: HR 110 bpm, BP 130/78 mm Hg, RR 20/min, SpO_2 95% on room air, temperature 37.8°C. The right calf measures 3 cm larger than the left, is warm and tender to palpation, and dorsalis pedis pulses are palpable and symmetric. Urine output has decreased over the past 4 hours; the left knee incision is clean with minimal serosanguinous drainage. Laboratory results show hemoglobin 9.0 g/dL (preop 11.0), platelets 110,000/µL, and aPTT within reference range. She is using a patient-controlled analgesia pump for pain and received a bolus 30 minutes ago.

Question 1: Based on the vignette, which condition is the most likely cause of the new right calf pain and swelling?

[A] Cellulitis
[B] Deep vein thrombosis (DVT)
[C] Lymphedema from chronic venous insufficiency
[D] Compartment syndrome

Question 2: Given the current assessment findings in the vignette, what is the nurse's most appropriate immediate action?

[A] Encourage the client to ambulate to promote venous return.
[B] Gently massage the calf to reduce pain and swelling.
[C] Apply warm compresses and have the client dangle the leg to assess relief.
[D] Keep the client on bed rest, avoid calf massage, elevate the leg, and notify the provider while preparing for duplex ultrasonography.

Question 3: Which pathophysiologic factor best explains why a postoperative, immobile client in the vignette is at increased risk for the suspected condition?

[A] Venous stasis due to decreased calf-muscle pump activity
[B] Arterial vasospasm causing distal ischemia
[C] Increased platelet production from surgical stress
[D] Decreased synthesis of clotting factors in the liver

Question 4: Enoxaparin, the prophylactic agent the client is receiving, exerts its primary anticoagulant effect by which mechanism?

[A] Potentiation of antithrombin III leading to inhibition of factor Xa
[B] Direct inhibition of thrombin (factor IIa) independent of antithrombin
[C] Inhibition of vitamin K–dependent gamma-carboxylation of clotting factors II, VII, IX, and X
[D] Activation of plasminogen to increase fibrinolysis

Question 5: Considering the vignette shows hemoglobin 9.0 g/dL and platelets 110,000/µL in a client receiving enoxaparin with new unilateral calf swelling, which nursing action is most appropriate?

[A] Continue scheduled enoxaparin and encourage ambulation to reduce stasis.
[B] Remove the PCA access and send blood cultures before notifying the provider.
[C] Apply sequential compression devices (SCDs) and have the client ambulate now.
[D] Hold the next enoxaparin dose and notify the provider for further orders and diagnostic testing.

ANSWERS

1. Correct Answer: B
Rationale: The vignette describes new unilateral calf swelling, warmth, and tenderness in a postoperative immobile client—classic cues for DVT. Cellulitis (A) often includes more systemic infection signs and skin erythema with diffuse tenderness rather than a unilateral enlarged calf immediately after joint surgery. Lymphedema (C) is typically chronic and non-tender and less likely to present acutely after surgery. Compartment syndrome (D) causes severe, disproportionate pain, tense swelling, and neurovascular compromise (pain with passive stretch, pulselessness), which are not described here.

2. Correct Answer: D
Rationale: For suspected DVT, the chapter emphasizes prevention-first and safety: keep the client on bed rest, avoid massage (which can dislodge a clot), elevate the extremity, and notify the provider while preparing for diagnostic testing (duplex ultrasound). Encouraging ambulation (A) or applying SCDs/ambulating (C) are inappropriate if DVT is suspected because they may increase embolization risk. Massaging the calf (B) is contraindicated due to risk of clot dislodgement.

3. Correct Answer: A
Rationale: Venous stasis from decreased calf-muscle pumping in immobilized postoperative clients is a primary element of Virchow's triad and explains increased DVT risk. Arterial vasospasm (B) relates to arterial ischemia, not venous thrombosis. Increased platelet production (C) is not the predominant mechanism in postoperative venous thrombosis. Decreased hepatic synthesis of clotting factors (D) would cause bleeding tendency rather than promote venous thrombus formation.

4. Correct Answer: A
Rationale: Enoxaparin (a low–molecular-weight heparin) potentiates antithrombin III, primarily inhibiting factor Xa (and to a lesser extent IIa), which is its main anticoagulant action. Direct thrombin inhibitors (B) describe agents such as dabigatran. Vitamin K antagonists (C) describe warfarin. Activation of plasminogen (D) describes fibrinolytic agents (e.g., tPA).

5. Correct Answer: D
Rationale: The chapter advises stopping a suspected harmful therapy and notifying the provider when complications are possible. With new unilateral calf swelling suggestive of DVT plus a drop in hemoglobin and platelets that may alter bleeding risk, the safest immediate action is to hold the next enoxaparin dose and notify the provider while preparing diagnostic testing and labs. Continuing enoxaparin and ambulation (A) risks bleeding or embolization without confirmation. Removing PCA and sending cultures (B) is unrelated to the current problem. Applying SCDs and ambulating now (C) is contraindicated if DVT is suspected and could precipitate embolization.

Clinical Vignette 6

A 68-year-old man presents to the emergency department with one hour of worsening generalized weakness and a sensation of "pressure" in the chest; he also reports nausea and lightheadedness. Past medical history includes atrial fibrillation on warfarin, chronic kidney disease stage 3 (baseline creatinine ~1.3 mg/dL), and hypertension treated with lisinopril and spironolactone; he takes no over-the-counter potassium supplements and has no known drug allergies. On exam he is alert but somewhat diaphoretic, BP 96/58 mm Hg, HR irregular at 110/min, RR 18, SpO2 94% on room air; cardiac exam reveals irregular rhythm without murmurs and no focal neuro deficits. A stat basic metabolic panel shows potassium 6.2 mEq/L and creatinine 2.2 mg/dL; INR is 3.5, hemoglobin 13.2 g/dL, and lactate 1.6 mmol/L. A 12-lead ECG demonstrates tall, peaked T waves and a slightly widened QRS. There is no external bleeding, and the patient denies melena or hematuria; he is worried and asks whether dialysis will be needed. He is NPO in anticipation of possible procedures, and the nurse prepares cardiac monitoring and IV access while notifying the provider.

Question 1: Based on the vignette, which condition is the most likely immediate threat accounting for the ECG changes and the patient's weakness?

[A] Acute ST-elevation myocardial infarction causing ischemic ECG changes
[B] Hyperkalemia causing peaked T waves and conduction widening
[C] Intracranial hemorrhage presenting with altered mental status and ECG changes
[D] Active gastrointestinal bleed with hypovolemia causing ECG abnormalities

Question 2: Given the ECG findings and the laboratory value in the vignette, what is the nurse's best immediate action while awaiting further orders?

[A] Administer oral sodium polystyrene sulfonate (kayexalate) to remove potassium
[B] Give IV calcium gluconate to stabilize cardiac membranes
[C] Start an insulin-dextrose infusion to shift potassium intracellularly
[D] Place the patient on high-flow nasal oxygen to improve tissue perfusion

Question 3: Which pathophysiologic explanation best accounts for this patient's hyperkalemia in the context of his history and labs?

[A] Excess dietary potassium intake from supplements producing acute elevation
[B] Hemolysis of the blood sample causing a spurious elevation in measured potassium
[C] Massive cellular release of potassium from rhabdomyolysis after recent trauma
[D] Reduced renal potassium excretion due to acute kidney injury on chronic CKD compounded by ACE inhibitor and spironolactone therapy

Question 4: The patient's INR is 3.5 and there is no active bleeding. According to best practice described in the vignette context, what is the most appropriate initial nursing action regarding his warfarin therapy?

[A] Hold the warfarin dose and notify the provider to reassess anticoagulation and interactions
[B] Give IV vitamin K immediately to reverse anticoagulation
[C] Continue the current warfarin dosing because INR is within therapeutic range for all indications
[D] Prepare fresh frozen plasma (FFP) for immediate infusion to normalize INR

Question 5: The provider indicates dialysis may be required but the patient becomes increasingly confused and is unable to provide informed consent; no surrogate is immediately available. What is the most appropriate ethical/legal action to take next?

[A] Wait until written consent from a surrogate or family member is obtained before proceeding
[B] Refuse dialysis because the patient cannot provide consent and there is no surrogate present
[C] Proceed with emergent life-saving dialysis under implied consent for an incapacitated patient in a life-threatening emergency
[D] Contact the hospital ethics committee and delay treatment until they issue guidance

ANSWERS

1. Correct Answer: B

Rationale: The vignette shows serum potassium 6.2 mEq/L with ECG findings of tall, peaked T waves and a widened QRS—classic signs of hyperkalemia causing conduction abnormalities and muscle weakness. A STEMI would typically show regional ST elevations and chest pain patterns; the ECG description indicates peaked T waves rather than ST elevations, making A less likely. Intracranial hemorrhage (C) would present with focal neuro signs or severe headache and not produce peaked T waves from hyperkalemia. An active GI bleed (D) could cause hypotension and tachycardia but would not explain a markedly elevated potassium with peaked T waves.

2. Correct Answer: B

Rationale: With ECG changes from hyperkalemia, IV calcium gluconate is the immediate priority to stabilize cardiac myocyte membranes while definitive potassium-lowering measures are arranged; the vignette explicitly notes peaked T waves and widened QRS, which warrant calcium first. Insulin-dextrose (C) shifts potassium intracellularly and is important but comes after membrane stabilization; delaying calcium risks arrhythmia. Kayexalate (A) removes potassium more slowly and is not first-line for immediate ECG changes. High-flow oxygen (D) is not the priority intervention for hyperkalemia unless hypoxemia is present.

3. Correct Answer: D

Rationale: The patient has CKD with an acute rise in creatinine (from baseline ~1.3 to 2.2 mg/dL) and is on lisinopril and spironolactone—both reduce aldosterone activity or its effects and impair renal potassium excretion, making reduced renal excretion the most likely mechanism for hyperkalemia. Excess dietary intake (A) is less likely to produce such a rapid, high potassium level without renal impairment. Hemolysis (B) can artifactually raise potassium but the ECG changes and clinical picture support a true hyperkalemia rather than a lab artifact. Rhabdomyolysis (C) would have additional clues (muscle pain, dark urine, very elevated CK) not present here.

4. Correct Answer: A

Rationale: An INR of 3.5 is mildly supratherapeutic for most indications (typical goal 2.0–3.0); in the absence of bleeding, holding warfarin and notifying the provider to reassess dosing and interacting medications is appropriate initial management. Immediate vitamin K (B) or FFP (D) is reserved for significant/symptomatic bleeding or very high INR per institutional protocols. Continuing warfarin unchanged (C) risks further anticoagulation without addressing the supratherapeutic INR.

5. Correct Answer: C

Rationale: In life-threatening emergencies where delay would likely result in significant harm and the patient lacks capacity with no surrogate available, implied consent allows clinicians to provide emergent, potentially life-saving treatment—here, dialysis for refractory, dangerous hyperkalemia. Waiting for surrogate consent (A) or refusing treatment (B) could cause harm. Contacting an ethics committee (D) is appropriate for non-urgent dilemmas but would unacceptably delay emergent care.

Clinical Vignette 7

A 68-year-old male arrives to the PACU after an elective total hip arthroplasty for osteoarthritis. His history includes atrial fibrillation (warfarin stopped 4 days ago), hypertension, type 2 diabetes, and obstructive sleep apnea treated with home CPAP; he reports taking aspirin and an herbal supplement (ginkgo) the night before surgery. Current medications listed include lisinopril and metformin; no known drug allergies. On assessment he is somnolent and intermittently snoring, respiratory rate 8 breaths/min, SpO2 88% on room air, blood pressure 88/52 mmHg, heart rate 120 bpm, skin cool and clammy. The surgical dressing is noticeably saturated with bright red blood and the surgical drain has collected ~150 mL in the past 15 minutes; urinary output has been <10 mL in the past hour. Pre-op labs showed Hgb 12.5 g/dL and INR 1.9; a stat postoperative Hgb return is 8.2 g/dL. ECG shows sinus tachycardia; anesthesia handed off opioid-based PCA use in the OR.

Question 1: Based on the vignette, which postoperative complication is the MOST likely cause of the patient's acute deterioration?

[A] Pulmonary embolism
[B] Malignant hyperthermia
[C] Postoperative hemorrhage
[D] Acute myocardial infarction

Question 2: What is the nurse's most appropriate immediate action for this patient in the PACU?

[A] Apply direct pressure to the saturated dressing, call the surgeon/anesthesia immediately, and prepare for IV fluid resuscitation and type & cross.
[B] Obtain an arterial blood gas and portable chest x-ray to evaluate the low SpO2 before intervening.
[C] Administer intravenous furosemide to reduce fluid overload and improve oxygenation.
[D] Encourage incentive spirometry and deep breathing exercises to improve SpO2.

Question 3: The patient's low SpO2 and intermittent snoring are most likely explained by which mechanism in this clinical context?

[A] Large ventilation–perfusion mismatch from pulmonary embolism.
[B] Aspiration of gastric contents causing acute hypoxemia.
[C] Upper airway obstruction and hypoventilation from residual opioids compounded by obstructive sleep apnea.
[D] Postoperative atelectasis alone from shallow breathing.

Question 4: If the nurse suspects opioid-induced respiratory depression is contributing to hypoventilation, which pharmacologic intervention is most appropriate to administer per protocol?

[A] Naloxone IV titrated to effect.
[B] Dantrolene IV.
[C] Flumazenil IV.
[D] Protamine sulfate IV.

Question 5: How should the nurse interpret the change from preoperative Hgb 12.5 g/dL to postoperative Hgb 8.2 g/dL with an INR of 1.9 in this patient?

[A] Findings most suggest acute hemolytic transfusion reaction requiring exchange transfusion.
[B] Laboratory pattern diagnostic of disseminated intravascular coagulation requiring immediate heparin.
[C] INR of 1.9 indicates no anticoagulation concern and no need to involve the surgeon.
[D] Significant acute blood loss likely worsened by residual anticoagulant effect and antiplatelet/herbal agents; urgent surgical control and blood product support should be anticipated.

ANSWERS

1. Correct Answer: C
Rationale: The vignette documents a rapidly saturated dressing, large drain output (150 mL/15 min), hypotension, tachycardia, cool clammy skin, oliguria, and a marked drop in hemoglobin from 12.5 to 8.2 g/dL — a classic pattern of acute postoperative hemorrhage. A pulmonary embolism (A) can cause sudden hypoxemia and tachycardia but would not explain active external bleeding and rapid Hgb loss. Malignant hyperthermia (B) presents with hypercarbia, rigidity, and hyperthermia (not described). Acute MI (D) may cause hypotension/tachycardia but does not account for overt bleeding and Hgb drop.

2. Correct Answer: A
Rationale: Immediate actions for suspected hemorrhage are to assess and control bleeding (apply direct pressure if accessible), notify the surgeon/anesthesia, and begin resuscitation (IV fluids, prepare type & cross) — all time-sensitive, airway/circulation-first steps per the chapter. Waiting for ABG and chest x-ray (B) delays life-saving hemorrhage control. Diuresis with furosemide (C) is contraindicated in hypovolemia. Incentive spirometry (D) is appropriate for preventing atelectasis but is not the priority when active hemorrhage and hemodynamic instability are present.

3. Correct Answer: C
Rationale: The patient is somnolent with RR 8, snoring, low SpO2, and has received opioids (PCA); combined with known OSA, this strongly indicates upper airway obstruction and opioid-induced hypoventilation. PE (A) and aspiration (B) can cause hypoxemia but do not explain the snoring and hypoventilation pattern paired with opioid exposure and OSA. Atelectasis (D) contributes to hypoxemia later but is less likely to produce acute snoring and very low RR immediately post-op.

4. Correct Answer: A
Rationale: Naloxone IV titrated to effect is the appropriate reversal agent for opioid-induced respiratory depression. Dantrolene (B) treats malignant hyperthermia, not opioid overdose. Flumazenil (C) reverses benzodiazepines. Protamine (D) reverses heparin and is not used for opioid respiratory depression.

5. Correct Answer: D
Rationale: A rapid fall in Hgb coupled with active bleeding and an elevated INR (1.9) — plus reported aspirin and ginkgo use — indicates significant acute blood loss worsened by residual anticoagulant/antiplatelet effects; this situation warrants urgent surgical control and blood product support. Acute hemolytic transfusion reaction (A) is unlikely without recent transfusion and would have hemolysis markers. DIC (B) has additional coagulopathy and fibrinogen/D-dimer abnormalities not presented. Saying the INR indicates no anticoagulation concern (C) is incorrect: an INR of 1.9 in the postoperative bleeding patient is clinically significant and should prompt discussion about reversal/management.

Clinical Vignette 8

A 29-year-old G2P1 woman at 38 weeks gestation presents to triage complaining of severe headache and visual blurring for 2 hours; she was diagnosed with preeclampsia and received a loading dose of IV magnesium sulfate in the labor unit 45 minutes ago. Her past medical history is otherwise unremarkable; she takes no home meds, has no known drug allergies, and lives with her partner. On exam she is somnolent but arousable, BP 162/108 mm Hg, RR 10 breaths/min, SpO2 94% on room air, heart rate 98 bpm; deep tendon reflexes are absent bilaterally and she has scant urine output of 20 mL in the past hour. Continuous fetal heart monitoring shows baseline 135 bpm with moderate variability. Point-of-care labs return serum magnesium 5.6 mg/dL (reference 1.5–2.5 mg/dL) and a bedside ABG: pH 7.25, PaCO2 60 mm Hg, HCO3- 26 mEq/L. The IV magnesium infusion pump is running per protocol and a standing order for IV labetalol is available on the chart. The labor nurse calls for assistance.

Question 1: Based on the vignette, which is the most likely cause of the patient's current deterioration?

[A] Progression to eclampsia with impending seizure
[B] Opioid-induced respiratory depression from analgesia given in labor
[C] Magnesium sulfate toxicity causing neuromuscular and respiratory depression
[D] Pulmonary embolism causing hypoventilation and low urine output

Question 2: What is the nurse's best immediate action for this patient while additional help is arriving?

[A] Stop the magnesium infusion and prepare IV calcium gluconate; support airway and monitor respirations
[B] Administer the standing order of IV labetalol to lower blood pressure immediately
[C] Intubate the patient now for airway protection without stopping the infusion
[D] Increase the IV fluid rate and continue the magnesium infusion per protocol

Question 3: How should the bedside ABG (pH 7.25, PaCO2 60, HCO3- 26) be interpreted in this context?

[A] Metabolic acidosis with respiratory compensation
[B] Mixed metabolic and respiratory acidosis
[C] Acute respiratory acidosis from hypoventilation (acute ventilatory failure)
[D] Chronic respiratory acidosis with renal compensation

Question 4: Which statement best describes the mechanism by which elevated magnesium causes the patient's absent reflexes and respiratory depression?

[A] Magnesium increases central GABAergic activity, leading to generalized CNS depression and apnea
[B] Magnesium antagonizes presynaptic calcium entry, reducing acetylcholine release and impairing neuromuscular transmission
[C] Magnesium upregulates neuromuscular junction acetylcholine receptors, causing depolarization block
[D] Magnesium acts like a beta-adrenergic agonist causing muscle weakness and hypoventilation

Question 5: Which action best reflects appropriate professional practice and delegation for the RN caring for this patient?

[A] Ask the LPN to titrate the magnesium infusion while the RN calls the provider for orders
[B] Instruct a nursing assistant to perform the neurological assessment while the RN goes to consult the obstetrician
[C] Remain at the bedside, stop the magnesium, call for calcium gluconate and anesthesia/OB assistance, and continuously monitor respirations and urine output
[D] Transfer the patient immediately to the post-partum unit where continuous fetal monitoring is available

ANSWERS

1. Correct Answer: C

Rationale: The vignette shows recent magnesium sulfate administration, absent deep tendon reflexes, depressed respiratory rate (RR 10), oliguria, and an elevated serum magnesium (5.6 mg/dL), all classic for magnesium toxicity causing neuromuscular and respiratory depression. A (eclampsia) is less likely because there is no seizure activity—current signs point to drug toxicity rather than imminent seizure. B (opioid overdose) is unlikely because there is no documentation of opioid administration and physical findings (absent DTRs, high Mg level) point elsewhere. D (pulmonary embolism) would more commonly present with sudden hypoxia, tachycardia, pleuritic chest pain and would not explain high serum magnesium or absent reflexes.

2. Correct Answer: A

Rationale: Stopping the magnesium infusion and giving IV calcium gluconate (antidote) while supporting airway/respirations is the immediate priority for suspected magnesium toxicity; the vignette documents toxicity signs and a high serum magnesium. B (administer labetalol) addresses hypertension but does not treat the life-threatening respiratory depression. C (immediate intubation without stopping magnesium) ignores treating the reversible cause and gives avoidable sedation risk—stopping the offending agent and antidote first is appropriate while preparing advanced airway if needed. D (increase fluids and continue magnesium) would worsen toxicity by continuing the offending agent.

3. Correct Answer: C

Rationale: The ABG shows low pH with an elevated PaCO2 and normal HCO3-, indicating primary acute respiratory acidosis from hypoventilation (acute ventilatory failure), consistent with the low RR and decreasing mental status. A (metabolic acidosis) would show low HCO3- as the primary disturbance. B (mixed) would require abnormal HCO3- in addition to the high PaCO2. D (chronic respiratory acidosis with renal compensation) would show elevated HCO3- reflecting compensation; here HCO3- is near normal, consistent with an acute process.

4. Correct Answer: B

Rationale: Magnesium toxicity impairs neuromuscular transmission primarily by antagonizing presynaptic calcium entry, decreasing acetylcholine release at the neuromuscular junction, which leads to reduced reflexes and respiratory muscle weakness. A (increased GABAergic activity) is not the primary peripheral mechanism responsible for absent DTRs in magnesium toxicity. C (upregulation of ACh receptors causing depolarization block) is inconsistent with the known action of magnesium. D (beta-adrenergic agonist effect) is incorrect—magnesium does not act via beta-adrenergic pathways to cause these findings.

5. Correct Answer: C

Rationale: The patient is unstable (airway/respiratory compromise, absent DTRs, oliguria); the RN must remain at bedside, stop the offending infusion, call for antidote and additional help, and continuously monitor—these are nondelegable, time-sensitive responsibilities. A (ask LPN to titrate magnesium) is inappropriate because titration of a high-alert infusion in an unstable patient should not be delegated. B (delegate neuro assessment to nursing assistant) is inappropriate because unstable assessments require RN judgment. D (transfer to postpartum unit) is unsafe—the patient needs immediate bedside stabilization and escalation, not transfer.

Clinical Vignette 9

A 68-year-old man 24 hours after elective exploratory laparotomy reports lightheadedness and increasing abdominal tenderness; his wife states the surgical dressing is soaked with bright red fluid. Past medical history includes atrial fibrillation on warfarin, hypertension, and type 2 diabetes; medications: warfarin, lisinopril, metformin; no known drug allergies. On exam he is pale and diaphoretic, RR 22/min, HR 128/min, BP 86/50 mm Hg, SpO2 96% on room air, cool clammy extremities, capillary refill >4 seconds, and abdominal dressing saturated with sanguineous drainage; surgical drain output is documented as ~400 mL in the last hour. Foley catheter shows urine output 15 mL/hr since surgery. Labs: hemoglobin 7.8 g/dL (preop 11.5 g/dL), INR 3.0, lactate 4.2 mmol/L; bedside ECG shows sinus tachycardia. The patient is alert but anxious and able to answer questions briefly. The surgeon is currently in another unit; the wife asks staff to "do everything" to help him.

Question 1: Based on the vignette, which condition is the most likely cause of this patient's acute instability?

[A] Cardiogenic shock due to acute myocardial dysfunction
[B] Hypovolemic shock from acute hemorrhage
[C] Septic shock from intra-abdominal infection
[D] Obstructive shock from pulmonary embolism

Question 2: What is the nurse's best immediate action for this patient while calling for help?

[A] Elevate the head of bed and administer high-flow oxygen via nonrebreather mask
[B] Activate the rapid response team, place supine with legs elevated, obtain two large-bore IVs and begin isotonic fluid bolus while applying pressure to the dressing and calling the surgeon
[C] Administer IV furosemide to reduce presumed fluid overload and pulmonary edema
[D] Start peripheral vasopressor infusion through the existing small-bore IV to raise blood pressure immediately

Question 3: Which physiologic mechanism best explains this patient's hypotension and tachycardia?

[A] Acute decrease in myocardial contractility leading to reduced stroke volume and compensatory tachycardia
[B] Systemic vasodilation causing a drop in systemic vascular resistance with reflex tachycardia
[C] Acute right ventricular outflow obstruction decreasing left-sided preload and causing compensatory tachycardia
[D] Loss of circulating intravascular volume (hemorrhage) causing decreased venous return (preload), decreased cardiac output, and reflex tachycardia

Question 4: The patient has an INR of 3.0 and active surgical bleeding. Which pharmacologic intervention most appropriately addresses the coagulopathy for rapid reversal?

[A] Transfuse packed red blood cells only to correct anemia
[B] Simply hold warfarin and observe overnight for INR normalization
[C] Give fresh frozen plasma alone for reversal of anticoagulation
[D] Administer prothrombin complex concentrate (PCC) for rapid factor replacement and IV vitamin K for sustained reversal

Question 5: After initiating the recommended immediate interventions, which clinical improvement best indicates restoration of adequate tissue perfusion?

[A] Urine output increases from 15 mL/hr to 35 mL/hr
[B] Heart rate decreases from 128 to 100 beats per minute
[C] Hemoglobin rises from 7.8 to 9.0 g/dL on the first post-intervention lab
[D] INR decreases from 3.0 to 1.5 within 30 minutes

ANSWERS

1. Correct Answer: B

Rationale: The vignette shows acute blood loss: saturated dressing, 400 mL drain output in one hour, falling hemoglobin from 11.5 to 7.8 g/dL, hypotension, tachycardia, cool clammy extremities, low urine output, and elevated lactate — all classic for hypovolemic shock from hemorrhage. A: Cardiogenic shock would more likely have signs of cardiac ischemia or pulmonary edema, jugular venous distention, and not an acute drop in hemoglobin with external bleeding. C: Septic shock typically presents with fever or warm skin in early distributive phase and an infectious source; here there is obvious external bleeding and rapid Hgb drop. D: Pulmonary embolism commonly causes sudden hypoxia, pleuritic chest pain, and often right-heart strain on ECG; the key features here point to hemorrhage.

2. Correct Answer: B

Rationale: Immediate priorities are to support circulation and stop ongoing blood loss: activate rapid response, place supine with legs elevated to improve venous return, obtain two large-bore IVs, begin isotonic fluid bolus (unless cardiogenic signs), apply direct pressure to the dressing/drain site, and notify the surgeon — all per the chapter's ABC-focused first actions. A: Elevating the head and giving oxygen may be appropriate for respiratory compromise, but this patient's primary problem is hypovolemia and hypotension; upright positioning would worsen venous return. C: IV furosemide would worsen hypovolemia and is contraindicated with active hemorrhagic shock. D: Vasopressors should not be the first step in hypovolemia before attempting volume resuscitation and controlling bleeding; peripheral vasopressors through a small-bore IV are also unsafe.

3. Correct Answer: D

Rationale: Active hemorrhage reduces circulating blood volume, lowering venous return (preload), reducing stroke volume and cardiac output, which produces hypotension and a compensatory tachycardia — the central mechanism in hypovolemic shock. A: Decreased myocardial contractility is the mechanism in cardiogenic shock, which is not supported here by the acute external blood loss and hemoglobin drop. B: Systemic vasodilation is typical of distributive (septic/anaphylactic) shock; the vignette points to volume loss rather than primary vasodilation. C: Obstructive shock (e.g., massive PE, tamponade) impairs filling or outflow, but there is clear ongoing external hemorrhage making intravascular volume loss the primary problem.

4. Correct Answer: D

Rationale: With active bleeding and an elevated INR from warfarin, rapid reversal is required: prothrombin complex concentrate (PCC) provides immediate clotting factors and IV vitamin K restores synthesis for sustained reversal; this is preferred for urgent surgical/bleeding scenarios. A: PRBCs address oxygen-carrying capacity and anemia but do not correct coagulopathy; both transfusion and factor reversal may be needed. B: Simply holding warfarin is too slow when there is active hemorrhage and INR 3.0. C: Fresh frozen plasma can reverse anticoagulation but requires larger volumes and longer preparation; PCC is faster and more concentrated for rapid reversal.

5. Correct Answer: A

Rationale: Urine output increasing to ≥30 mL/hr is a reliable, real-time indicator of restored renal pefusion and improved end-organ perfusion after resuscitation and is specifically listed as a key sign of successful interventions. B: A decrease in heart rate toward normal may occur but is nonspecific and can lag or be influenced by pain, medications, or vagal tone. C: Hemoglobin rise reflects transfusion effect but is not an immediate measure of tissue perfusion and may take lab confirmation. D: INR reduction indicates correction of coagulopathy, important for bleeding control, but it does not by itself demonstrate restored tissue perfusion; laboratory reversal may also take time.

Clinical Vignette 10

A 68-year-old man presents to the emergency department with progressive shortness of breath and vague chest pressure that began several hours ago; his wife reports increasing fatigue and lightheadedness. Past medical history includes hypertension, congestive heart failure, and end-stage renal disease on hemodialysis (he missed his last scheduled dialysis), and atrial fibrillation treated with warfarin; he takes lisinopril and metoprolol and has no known drug allergies. On arrival he is pale and diaphoretic; vital signs are T 37.2°C, HR 110 irregular, RR 24, BP 86/58, SpO2 92% on room air. Exam reveals jugular venous distention, distant/muffled heart sounds, mild peripheral edema, lungs clear to auscultation, and a palpable decrease in systolic blood pressure of approximately 16 mm Hg during inspiration. A bedside 12-lead ECG shows low-voltage QRS complexes with electrical alternans; portable chest x-ray demonstrates an enlarged cardiac silhouette. His most recent basic metabolic panel (drawn in triage) shows K+ 5.8 mEq/L and creatinine consistent with his ESRD. His chart has no documented advance directive; his wife says he had mentioned previously that he "would not want heroic measures" but did not complete paperwork.

Question 1: Based on the vignette, which is the most likely cause of this patient's current hemodynamic instability?

[A] Acute ST-elevation myocardial infarction (STEMI)
[B] Cardiac tamponade from pericardial effusion
[C] Tension pneumothorax
[D] Massive pulmonary embolism

Question 2: Referencing the vignette, what is the nurse's most appropriate immediate action?

[A] Place the patient on continuous cardiac monitoring, establish at least one large-bore IV, give oxygen, and notify the provider to prepare for emergent pericardiocentesis.
[B] Administer sublingual nitroglycerin to relieve chest pressure and reassess blood pressure in 5 minutes.
[C] Prepare the patient for emergent chest tube insertion at bedside.
[D] Begin systemic thrombolytic therapy while arranging CT pulmonary angiography.

Question 3: Which physiologic mechanism best explains the greater-than-normal drop in systolic blood pressure with inspiration noted in the vignette?

[A] Inspiratory increase in left ventricular afterload from increased systemic vascular resistance.
[B] Elevated intrapericardial pressure limiting ventricular filling during inspiration, causing an exaggerated fall in systolic pressure (pulsus paradoxus).
[C] Acute obstruction of the pulmonary artery increasing right ventricular afterload and decreasing left ventricular preload.
[D] Severe bronchospasm causing dynamic hyperinflation and reduced venous return.

Question 4: Which medication or intervention listed would be least appropriate for this patient at this time?

[A] Supplemental oxygen to maintain adequate saturation.
[B] Rapid infusion of isotonic crystalloid if ordered to support perfusion.
[C] Preparation for urgent pericardiocentesis by notifying the provider and assembling equipment.
[D] Administration of sublingual or IV nitroglycerin to lower cardiac preload.

Question 5: The patient's wife states he had said he "would not want heroic measures," but there is no written advance directive in the chart. If the patient becomes pulseless and unresponsive in the ED, what should the nurse do?

[A] Honor the wife's statement and withhold CPR immediately.
[B] Ask the wife to sign a do-not-resuscitate order before initiating any resuscitation.
[C] Delay CPR while the physician attempts to locate a legal document or contact family.
[D] Initiate high-quality CPR and activate the Code team, while notifying the provider and attempting to clarify the patient's wishes and locate documentation.

ANSWERS

1. Correct Answer: B

Rationale: The vignette demonstrates Beck's triad (hypotension, JVD, muffled heart sounds), electrical alternans and low-voltage QRS on ECG, and an enlarged cardiac silhouette—classic clues for pericardial effusion with cardiac tamponade. A (STEMI) often has chest pain with ischemic ECG changes rather than electrical alternans; C (tension pneumothorax) typically produces unilateral absent breath sounds and tracheal deviation, which are not present; D (massive PE) would more commonly cause sudden hypoxemia, pleuritic pain, and right-sided strain on ECG, but the exam and ECG findings here favor tamponade.

2. Correct Answer: A

Rationale: Immediate priorities are airway/oxygenation, continuous cardiac monitoring, IV access, hemodynamic support, and urgent provider notification to prepare for definitive decompression (pericardiocentesis). This follows ABC order and escalation principles. B (nitroglycerin) is unsafe in hypotension and could worsen shock; C (chest tube) is for pneumothorax and not indicated here; D (thrombolytics) is for massive PE and inappropriate without confirming diagnosis and in a patient on warfarin/ESRD without clear indication.

3. Correct Answer: B

Rationale: Pulsus paradoxus in tamponade occurs because increased intrapericardial pressure restricts cardiac chamber filling, accentuating the normal inspiratory decrease in left ventricular stroke volume and causing an exaggerated (>10 mm Hg) fall in systolic BP. A is incorrect because afterload changes do not explain the inspiratory drop; C describes PE physiology but does not account for electrical alternans or muffled heart sounds; D (bronchospasm) can affect venous return but the vignette lacks wheeze or asthma history.

4. Correct Answer: D

Rationale: Nitrates reduce preload and can precipitously lower blood pressure—contraindicated in hypotensive patients and may worsen perfusion in tamponade. A (oxygen) supports oxygenation and is appropriate; B (IV isotonic fluids if ordered) can transiently improve preload in tamponade as a bridge if hypotensive; C (preparing for pericardiocentesis) is the definitive, appropriate intervention to relieve tamponade.

5. Correct Answer: D

Rationale: In the absence of a documented advance directive or physician DNR order, the nurse must initiate resuscitation for a pulseless patient, activate the Code team, and promptly notify the provider while attempting to locate documentation or clarify the patient's wishes—verbal family statements alone do not legally substitute for a documented DNR. A and B are incorrect because family statements or signatures do not replace proper documentation and physician orders; C is unsafe because delaying CPR while searching for paperwork violates resuscitation standards and patient safety.

CHAPTER 6

Mock Exams

6.1 Exam 1

6.1.1 Management of Care

Question 1: A 65-year-old client scheduled for laparoscopic cholecystectomy says, "I'm not sure why the surgeon chose the laparoscopic approach and what the risks are. I don't want to sign until I understand." What is the nurse's best action?

[A] Explain the risks and benefits of laparoscopic versus open surgery and obtain the signature.
[B] Notify the surgeon to return and answer the client's questions before obtaining the signature.
[C] Encourage the client to sign the consent form now and assure them the surgeon will explain before the procedure.
[D] Ask a family member to explain what the surgeon said previously to help the client decide.

Question 2: You are the charge nurse receiving morning report. Which client should you assess first?

[A] A 58-year-old, post–total knee replacement, reporting pain 8/10 and due for analgesic in 15 minutes.
[B] A 34-year-old, 2 hours post-thyroidectomy, with new hoarseness and inspiratory stridor.
[C] A 72-year-old with pneumonia, O2 saturation 92% on 2 L nasal cannula, productive cough of yellow sputum.
[D] A 26-year-old with Crohn's disease reporting 6/10 cramping and requesting assistance to the bathroom.

Question 3: The RN is determining which tasks to delegate to an experienced unlicensed assistive personnel (UAP). Which task is appropriate?

[A] Reinforce teaching on timing and technique for NPH insulin administration.
[B] Monitor effects of a newly prescribed antihypertensive and titrate dose at the bedside.
[C] Perform a sterile dressing change on a postoperative wound.
[D] Assist a stable client 1 day post–hip arthroplasty to the bathroom using a gait belt.

Question 4: The charge nurse is assigning clients. Which client is most appropriate for an experienced LPN/VN under RN supervision?

[A] A client with stable heart failure receiving routine oral diuretics and daily weights.
[B] A client with an active upper GI bleed receiving a blood transfusion.
[C] A client 2 hours post–carotid endarterectomy requiring frequent neurologic checks.
[D] A client newly diagnosed with type 1 diabetes needing initial insulin teaching.

Question 5: Unit data show a rise in catheter-associated urinary tract infections (CAUTIs) over the last quarter. What is the nurse manager's first step in the quality improvement process?

[A] Provide an immediate unit-wide in-service on catheter care.
[B] Implement a nurse-driven protocol for early catheter removal starting today.
[C] Form an interprofessional QI team to define the problem using baseline data and map the current catheter-care process.
[D] Report the unit to the state health department and initiate disciplinary actions.

Question 6: Which nursing action violates client confidentiality (HIPAA)?

[A] Displaying a whiteboard inside the client's room that lists the client's first name and daily mobility goal.
[B] Discussing a client's medication allergies with the pharmacist to clarify a prescription.
[C] Leaving printed shift-report sheets with client names and diagnoses on the nurses' station counter after handoff.
[D] Calling the lab for a critical potassium value using two client identifiers.

Question 7: A 54-year-old client with an active GI bleed refuses blood products due to religious beliefs. The client is alert and oriented. What is the nurse's best action?

[A] Notify the provider, verify the client's understanding of risks/benefits, document informed refusal, and explore acceptable alternatives (e.g., volume expanders).
[B] Call the ethics committee to override the refusal due to life-threatening circumstances.
[C] Obtain consent from the client's spouse to proceed with transfusion.
[D] Administer blood emergently as a life-saving measure under implied consent.

Question 8: Which discharge action best promotes continuity of care for an older adult with heart failure who lives alone and was hospitalized for fluid overload?

[A] Provide a printed brochure on low-sodium diets and ask the client to call with questions.
[B] Instruct the client to schedule a cardiology follow-up within 1–2 weeks.
[C] Arrange a home health nursing visit within 48 hours and send a detailed handoff (medication reconciliation, weight parameters, diet, follow-up appointments) to the agency and PCP.
[D] Teach daily weights and assume understanding because the client correctly repeats back the steps.

Question 9: The RN delegates pre-meal capillary blood glucose checks to a trained UAP. Which follow-up demonstrates appropriate supervision?

[A] Verifying that results are documented, confirming critical values are reported immediately, and reassessing any abnormal findings.
[B] Assuming competency and not verifying performance or outcomes.
[C] Allowing the UAP to decide when to hold insulin based on readings.
[D] Providing corrective feedback in the hallway where other staff can hear.

Question 10: As charge nurse on a medical-surgical unit, which assignment is safest for a float RN from an outpatient clinic with minimal recent inpatient experience?

[A] A client day 0 post–total hip arthroplasty with epidural analgesia requiring frequent neurovascular checks, plus a client with suspected hip dislocation.
[B] A client with septic shock on norepinephrine via central line in step-down, plus a client with DKA on an insulin infusion.
[C] A client admitted 2 hours ago with acute stroke requiring q15-minute neurologic checks and dysphagia screening, plus a client with a tracheostomy needing frequent suctioning.
[D] Two stable clients: one with cellulitis receiving scheduled IV antibiotics via peripheral IV and one on day 3 of community-acquired pneumonia requiring routine assessment, oral meds, and 2 L/min nasal cannula.

ANSWERS

1. Correct Answer: B

Rationale: The provider is responsible for explaining the procedure, risks, benefits, and alternatives; the nurse advocates by ensuring informed consent and can witness the signature only after questions are answered. A and C inappropriately place the teaching burden on the nurse and pressure signing. D is inappropriate; family should not provide the explanation.

2. Correct Answer: B

Rationale: New hoarseness and inspiratory stridor after thyroidectomy suggest airway compromise from laryngeal edema or hematoma (ABCs). A is important but not life-threatening. C is expected with pneumonia and currently stable. D is non-urgent.

3. Correct Answer: D

Rationale: UAPs may assist with ADLs and safe ambulation of stable clients. A (teaching), B (assessment/titration), and C (sterile procedures) require licensed personnel.

4. Correct Answer: A

Rationale: LPNs manage stable clients with predictable outcomes (routine meds, weights). B (active bleed/transfusion), C (frequent neuro checks), and D (initial teaching) require an RN.

5. Correct Answer: C

Rationale: QI begins by defining the problem with data and mapping current processes via an interprofessional team (Plan phase of PDSA). A and B implement changes without understanding root issues. D is punitive and not part of standard QI initiation.

6. Correct Answer: C

Rationale: Leaving identifiable client information in a public area breaches HIPAA. A is permissible when limited and privacy is maintained. B and D are appropriate for treatment/operations with safeguards (two identifiers).

7. Correct Answer: A

Rationale: Respect autonomy and advocate by ensuring informed refusal, notifying the provider, and exploring acceptable alternatives. B and D disregard autonomy; C is invalid because the competent client's decision prevails.

8.Correct Answer: C

Rationale: Coordinated handoff with home health and the PCP plus timely follow-up supports continuity, safety, and adherence. A and D are insufficient alone. B shifts responsibility without ensuring linkage.

9. Correct Answer: A

Rationale: Supervision includes clear expectations, verification of completion, evaluation of outcomes, and feedback. B abdicates responsibility. C exceeds the UAP scope. D is unprofessional; feedback should be private and constructive.

10. Correct Answer: D

Rationale: Assign stable clients with predictable needs within the float RN's skill set. A, B, and C involve higher acuity (epidural, vasoactive drips, insulin infusions, frequent neuro checks, tracheostomy care) inappropriate for a minimally experienced float.

6.1.2 Safety & Infection Prevention and Control

Question 1: The nurse is prioritizing isolation precautions for four clients. Which client requires contact precautions?

[A] Adult with measles (rubeola) confirmed by PCR
[B] Child with pertussis and copious nasal secretions
[C] Older adult with profuse diarrhea due to Clostridioides difficile
[D] Teen with suspected pulmonary tuberculosis awaiting AFB smear results

Question 2: You are preparing to enter the room of a patient with pulmonary tuberculosis. What is the correct order for donning PPE?

[A] Hand hygiene → gown → N95 respirator → goggles/face shield → gloves
[B] Hand hygiene → N95 respirator → gloves → gown → goggles/face shield
[C] Hand hygiene → goggles/face shield → gloves → gown → N95 respirator
[D] Hand hygiene→ gown → gloves→ goggles/face shield → N95 respirator

Question 3: During a sterile dressing change of a central line, which action maintains surgical asepsis?

[A] Turning away briefly to reach for additional supplies as long as sterile gloves remain on
[B] Pouring sterile saline directly onto the center of the sterile field to moisten gauze
[C] Keeping the sterile field in constant view at or above waist level and opening the first package flap away from the body
[D] Reaching over the sterile field with gloved hands to reposition a sterile drape

Question 4: The provider orders bilateral soft wrist restraints for a confused patient pulling at tubes after less-restrictive measures failed. Which action by the nurse is appropriate?

[A] Tying the restraints to the side rails using a double knot for security
[B] Applying the restraints PRN based on nursing judgment without a time-limited provider order
[C] Securing restraints to the bed frame with a quick-release knot, allowing two fingers under the cuff, and assessing skin, circulation, and range of motion at least every 2 hours
[D] Using the same restraint for both wrists to keep arms together and limit movement

Question 5: An 82-year-old postoperative patient with intermittent confusion is identified as high fall risk. Which intervention is best to prevent falls?

[A] Raise all four side rails and keep the door closed to minimize stimulation
[B] Administer a PRN sedative at bedtime to promote uninterrupted sleep
[C] Place the bed in the lowest position with wheels locked, activate the bed alarm, ensure non-skid footwear, keep the call light and personal items within reach, and implement scheduled toileting and hourly rounding
[D] Keep the IV pole and pump positioned away from the patient to reduce tampering

Question 6: You encounter a large blood spill on the unit hallway. What is the safest initial action to manage this hazardous material according to infection prevention and control policy?

[A] Place dry towels over the spill and notify housekeeping; no PPE is required if you do not touch the blood
[B] Don appropriate PPE (gloves, and gown/face protection if splash risk), contain and absorb the spill, clean visible organic material, then disinfect the area with an approved EPA-registered disinfectant (e.g., 1:10 bleach for large spills) and dispose of waste in biohazard receptacles
[C] Quickly mop the area with hot water to dilute the blood, then apply alcohol-based gel
[D] Put the blood-soaked materials in a standard trash bag and double-bag to prevent leakage

Question 7: Which assignment reflects correct isolation for a patient with active pulmonary tuberculosis?

[A] Private, positive-pressure room with the door open; staff wear surgical masks
[B] Airborne infection isolation room (negative pressure) with the door closed; staff wear fit-tested N95 respirators; patient wears a surgical mask during transport
[C] Shared room with a patient with bacterial pneumonia; staff use droplet masks and gloves
[D] Standard precautions only; airborne masks are not needed after 48 hours of therapy

Question 8: You see flames in a trash can in a semi-private room. What is your first action?

[A] Attempt to extinguish the fire using PASS with the nearest fire extinguisher
[B] Close all doors on the unit to contain smoke and fire
[C] Pull the fire alarm to activate the emergency response
[D] Remove clients in immediate danger from the room to a safe area

Question 9: What PPE is recommended when caring for a patient with confirmed influenza receiving nebulized treatments?

[A] Fit-tested N95 respirator; no need for a surgical mask
[B] No mask is required; influenza is contact only
[C] Surgical mask only if within 1 foot of the patient; no other precautions
[D] Droplet precautions: wear a surgical mask upon entry (especially within 3–6 feet), add eye protection during aerosol-generating procedures, use gloves and gown when contact with secretions is anticipated, and dedicate equipment

Question 10: After providing care to a patient on contact precautions, what is the correct sequence for doffing PPE before leaving the room?

[A] Gown → gloves → mask/respirator → goggles/face shield → hand hygiene
[B] Gloves → goggles/face shield → gown → mask/respirator → hand hygiene
[C] Mask/respirator → gloves → gown → goggles/face shield → hand hygiene
[D] Goggles/face shield → mask/respirator → gloves → gown → hand hygiene

ANSWERS

1. Correct Answer: C
Rationale: C. difficile requires contact precautions (gloves and gown; dedicated equipment). Measles and TB are airborne; pertussis is droplet.

2. Correct Answer: A
Rationale: Donning sequence: hand hygiene → gown → mask/respirator → eye protection → gloves. For airborne, an N95 is required before entry.

3. Correct Answer: C
Rationale: Surgical asepsis requires maintaining the sterile field in view and above waist level; opening the first flap away prevents contamination. Turning away, reaching over the field, or wetting the center of the field break sterility.

4. Correct Answer: C
Rationale: Restraints are secured to the bed frame with quick-release knots, allow two fingers under the cuff, and require frequent assessment and release for care. Side rails and PRN use are inappropriate.

5. Correct Answer: C
Rationale: A fall-prevention bundle (low bed, alarm, non-skid footwear, accessible call light, scheduled toileting, rounding) is evidence-based. Four side rails and sedatives increase fall risk.

6. Correct Answer: B
Rationale: Blood spills are hazardous. Use PPE, contain/absorb, clean organic material, then disinfect with an EPA-registered product (e.g., 1:10 bleach for large spills), and discard waste in biohazard containers.

7. Correct Answer: B
Rationale: TB requires airborne isolation: negative-pressure room, closed door, N95 for staff, surgical mask for patient during transport. Positive pressure and droplet-only precautions are incorrect.

8. Correct Answer: D
Rationale: Follow RACE: Rescue, Alarm, Contain, Extinguish/Evacuate. The first action is to remove anyone in immediate danger.

9. Correct Answer: D
Rationale: Influenza is droplet spread. Use a surgical mask upon entry (especially within 3–6 feet), add eye protection for aerosol-generating procedures, and wear gown/gloves if contact with secretions is likely.

10. Correct Answer: B
Rationale: Doffing sequence minimizes self-contamination: remove the most contaminated items first (gloves), then eye protection, gown, mask/respirator, and perform hand hygiene.

6.1.3 Health Promotion & Maintenance

Question 1: At a 12-month well-child visit, which finding indicates the child is meeting expected developmental milestones?

[A] Stacks four blocks and uses two-word phrases
[B] Uses a pincer grasp to pick up small objects and feeds self finger foods
[C] Walks up stairs alternating feet without support
[D] Names colors and counts to three

Question 2: A client planning pregnancy asks about nutrition to reduce birth defects. Which teaching is correct?

[A] Begin 400–800 mcg of folic acid daily before conception and continue through the first trimester
[B] Increase vitamin A supplements substantially to support fetal eye development
[C] Avoid all fish during pregnancy to eliminate mercury exposure
[D] Limit iron intake during the first trimester unless anemia is diagnosed

Question 3: The nurse teaches new parents about safe sleep for their newborn. Which parent statement indicates correct understanding?

[A] "We'll place the baby on the side to sleep and use soft bumper pads to prevent injury."
[B] "We'll put the baby on the back on a firm mattress in a separate sleep space with no loose bedding or toys."
[C] "We'll share our adult bed to promote bonding as long as we don't smoke."
[D] "We'll use a space heater near the crib to keep the room very warm at night."

Question 4: A 52-year-old adult at average risk asks about colorectal cancer screening. Which plan is appropriate?

[A] Begin screening at age 55 because risk is still low at 52
[B] Order a yearly carcinoembryonic antigen (CEA) blood test for screening
[C] Defer screening until gastrointestinal symptoms develop
[D] Begin screening now with options such as annual FIT or colonoscopy every 10 years, per guidelines

Question 5: A 2-month-old infant presents for routine immunizations. Which vaccine set is appropriate today for an infant with no contraindications?

[A] MMR, varicella, and hepatitis A
[B] DTaP, MMR, and HPV
[C] Hepatitis B only, and only if the mother is HBsAg-positive
[D] DTaP, Hib, IPV, PCV, rotavirus, and hepatitis B per schedule

Question 6: A client on postpartum day 3 calls the clinic. Which symptom requires immediate follow-up?

[A] Mild uterine cramping that increases during breastfeeding
[B] Saturating a perineal pad in 15 minutes with passage of large (golf ball–sized) clots
[C] Lochia changing from bright red to pink/brown
[D] Full, tender breasts as milk production increases

Question 7: A client at 26 weeks' gestation calls the nurse. Which symptom requires urgent evaluation?

[A] Nasal stuffiness and occasional nosebleeds
[B] Mild ankle edema that improves with rest and elevation
[C] Irregular, painless uterine tightening that resolves with hydration
[D] Severe headache with visual disturbances and right upper quadrant/epigastric pain

Question 8: The nurse is teaching parents how to assess adequate intake in an exclusively breastfed newborn by the end of the first week. Which finding indicates adequate intake?

[A] Six or more wet diapers daily and 3–4 yellow, seedy stools per day with good tone and activity
[B] Two wet diapers per day and dark green meconium stools for the first 7 days
[C] Sleeping more than 6 hours between feeds with fewer than five wet diapers daily
[D] No more than 1% weight loss in the first 3 days of life

Question 9: A 52-year-old sedentary client asks how to reduce cardiovascular risk through exercise. Which counseling is best?

[A] Do vigorous exercise only on weekends for a total of 60 minutes; strength training is unnecessary
[B] Eliminate all dietary sodium and fats; begin exercise only after losing 10 pounds
[C] Aim for at least 150 minutes/week of moderate-intensity aerobic activity (or 75 minutes vigorous) plus muscle-strengthening on 2 or more days; increase gradually
[D] Focus solely on flexibility and yoga; aerobic activity is optional

Question 10: A 30-week pregnant client has not yet received a flu shot this season and last received Tdap 2 years ago. Which immunization plan is appropriate today?

[A] Defer all vaccines until after delivery to avoid fetal exposure
[B] Administer Tdap now (at 27–36 weeks) and inactivated influenza vaccine if in season; avoid live vaccines
[C] Administer MMR and varicella vaccines now to protect maternal immunity
[D] Give the live attenuated intranasal influenza vaccine for stronger respiratory protection

ANSWERS

1. Correct Answer: B
Rationale: By 12 months, infants typically have a mature pincer grasp and can pick up small objects and self-feed finger foods. Options A, C, and D reflect skills of older toddlers/preschoolers (18 months to 3+ years).

2. Correct Answer: A
Rationale: Folic acid 400–800 mcg daily started preconception and continued through the first trimester reduces neural tube defects. Excess vitamin A is teratogenic (B). Low-mercury fish provide beneficial omega-3s and need not be completely avoided (C). Routine prenatal vitamins include iron; limiting iron is not recommended (D).

3. Correct Answer: B
Rationale: Safe sleep includes supine positioning, a firm mattress, and an empty crib (no soft objects or loose bedding). Side/prone sleep and soft bedding increase SIDS risk (A). Bed-sharing increases suffocation risk (C). Overheating is a SIDS risk; avoid space heaters near the crib (D).

4. Correct Answer: D
Rationale: Average-risk adults begin colorectal cancer screening at age 45; at 52, screening should occur now. Acceptable options include annual FIT or colonoscopy every 10 years. CEA is not a screening test (B). Delaying until symptoms (C) or to age 55 (A) is inappropriate.

5. Correct Answer: D
Rationale: At 2 months, recommended vaccines include DTaP, Hib, IPV, PCV, rotavirus, and the next dose of hepatitis B (if not already given at 1 month). MMR, varicella, and hepatitis A are first given at 12 months or later (A). HPV is for adolescents (B). Hep B is not limited to infants of HBsAg-positive mothers (C).

6. Correct Answer: B
Rationale: Soaking a pad in 15 minutes with large clots suggests postpartum hemorrhage and requires urgent evaluation. Mild cramping with breastfeeding (A), lochia transitioning to serosa (C), and breast engorgement as milk increases (D) are expected findings on day 3.

7. Correct Answer: D
Rationale: Severe headache, visual changes, and RUQ/epigastric pain suggest preeclampsia with severe features and require immediate evaluation. Nasal stuffiness (A), mild dependent edema (B), and Braxton Hicks contractions (C) are common/benign pregnancy symptoms.

8. Correct Answer: A
Rationale: By the end of the first week, adequate breastfeeding is indicated by ≥6 wet diapers and several yellow, seedy stools daily, with normal activity/tone. Persistent meconium (B), prolonged sleep with low output (C), and minimal expected weight loss (D) are inconsistent with typical patterns; up to 7–10% weight loss in the first 3–5 days is common, with regain by 10–14 days.

9. Correct Answer: C
Rationale: National guidelines call for ≥150 min/week moderate (or 75 min vigorous) activity plus 2+ days of strength training. Sixty minutes of weekend-only vigorous activity is insufficient (A). Extreme dieting or delaying exercise is inappropriate (B). Flexibility alone is inadequate for cardiometabolic health (D).

10. Correct Answer: B
Rationale: Pregnant clients should receive Tdap during each pregnancy at 27–36 weeks for passive neonatal pertussis protection and the inactivated influenza vaccine during flu season. Live vaccines (MMR, varicella, live nasal influenza) are contraindicated in pregnancy (C, D). Vaccines should not be deferred if indicated (A).

6.1.4 Psychosocial Integrity

Question 1: A client with major depressive disorder states, "Sometimes I think everyone would be better off if I weren't here." What is the nurse's best initial response?

[A] "Are you thinking about harming or killing yourself?"
[B] "You have so much to live for; your family needs you."
[C] "Let's distract you with a walk; that usually helps."
[D] "You shouldn't say that; things will get better soon."

Question 2: A client reports, "When I'm furious after a bad shift, I go to the gym and box until I'm exhausted." Which defense mechanism is the client using?

[A] Displacement
[B] Sublimation
[C] Projection
[D] Rationalization

Question 3: Eight hours after last drink, a hospitalized client is tremulous, diaphoretic, anxious, with HR 112 and BP 168/96. Which prescription should the nurse implement first?

[A] Haloperidol 5 mg PO for agitation as needed
[B] Thiamine 100 mg IM before glucose administration
[C] Lorazepam per CIWA-Ar protocol for symptom-triggered dosing
[D] Intravenous fluids with dextrose at 125 mL/hr

Question 4: An adult client seen in the ED for a fractured wrist quietly says, "My partner gets rough sometimes. Please don't tell." Which nursing action is most appropriate?

[A] Encourage the client to immediately leave the relationship and call the police
[B] Inform the client that reporting intimate partner violence is legally mandatory for all adults
[C] Provide a private setting to assess immediate safety and lethality, validate concerns, document objectively, and offer safety-planning resources while respecting autonomy
[D] Invite the partner into the room to get "both sides" and clarify what happened

Question 5: A client with schizophrenia says, "Voices are telling me I'm worthless and should be punished." What is the nurse's best response?

[A] "Those voices aren't real, so you should ignore them."
[B] "Take your medication now, and the voices will go away."
[C] "I don't hear any voices, but I can see you're upset. What are the voices saying right now?"
[D] "Let's turn up the TV so you can't hear the voices."

Question 6: A family member at the bedside after a client's death is tearful and says, "I don't know how I'm going to get through this." What is the nurse's best action?

[A] Provide pamphlets on grief support groups and then allow privacy
[B] Sit with the family member and say, "I'm here with you. Would you like to tell me about your loved one?"
[C] Explain the stages of grief and that the feelings will pass with time
[D] Suggest calling the hospital chaplain immediately, regardless of the family's preference

Question 7: In a bereavement support group, a new member says, "No one understands what I'm going through." Which leader statement best uses a therapeutic group factor to help this client?

[A] "Let's focus on coping skills rather than how you feel right now."
[B] "I'll meet with you alone so you don't have to share with the group."
[C] "We will assign you a worksheet to complete before next session."
[D] "Many people here have had similar experiences and feelings—you are not alone."

Question 8: A client experiencing a panic attack is hyperventilating and says, "I'm going to die." What is the nurse's priority intervention?

[A] Teach progressive muscle relaxation and assign a journaling exercise
[B] Provide detailed education about the physiology of panic to reduce fear
[C] Move the client to a quiet space and coach slow, paced breathing using short, simple statements
[D] Encourage the client to explore childhood origins of anxiety to gain insight

Question 9: Following a community tornado, the nurse provides psychological first aid (PFA) to survivors at a shelter. Which action aligns best with PFA principles?

[A] Facilitate an immediate group debriefing where survivors recount traumatic details
[B] Encourage survivors to discuss their deepest feelings to achieve catharsis
[C] Screen everyone on arrival for PTSD using a standardized diagnostic tool
[D] Ensure safety and basic needs, offer calm practical support, provide brief factual information, and connect survivors with social supports and services

Question 10: A school-age child presents with bruises in different stages of healing and a vague explanation. What is the nurse's priority action?

[A] Report suspected abuse immediately to child protective services per mandatory reporting laws
[B] Ask the parent to explain in detail how the child was injured before deciding to report
[C] Confront the child directly and demand the truth to obtain a clear disclosure
[D] Wait for diagnostic imaging results to confirm abuse before taking further action

ANSWERS

1. Correct Answer: A
Rationale: The priority is direct suicide risk assessment. Asking plainly about intent and plan is therapeutic, does not increase risk, and guides immediate safety interventions. Options B, C, and D minimize or dismiss risk and are nontherapeutic.

2. Correct Answer: B
Rationale: Sublimation channels unacceptable impulses into socially acceptable activities (eg, boxing instead of aggressive behavior toward others). Displacement redirects feelings to a safer target; projection attributes one's feelings to others; rationalization provides justifying explanations.

3. Correct Answer: C
Rationale: Benzodiazepines are first-line for alcohol withdrawal to prevent seizures and delirium tremens; symptom-triggered dosing via CIWA-Ar is evidence-based. Thiamine (B) is important but not the immediate priority to control escalating withdrawal. Haloperidol (A) may worsen withdrawal seizures, and fluids (D) are supportive but not definitive.

4. Correct Answer: C
Rationale: Best practice for IPV includes private assessment for safety/lethality, validation, objective documentation, and providing safety-planning resources while respecting autonomy. Mandatory reporting typically applies to children, elders, or vulnerable adults, not all IPV cases (B). A and D can increase danger and are not trauma-informed.

5. Correct Answer: C
Rationale: This response presents reality without arguing, acknowledges distress, and assesses command hallucination content for safety. A dismisses the experience, B is directive and premature, and D uses distraction alone without assessment or validation.

6. Correct Answer: B
Rationale: Presence, empathy, and an open invitation to share are therapeutic in acute grief. A with pamphlets alone is distancing; C is didactic and may invalidate feelings; D imposes spiritual care without consent.

7. Correct Answer: D
Rationale: Universality (recognizing others share similar experiences) is a curative factor in group therapy and reduces isolation. A, B, and C bypass group therapeutic processes.

8. Correct Answer: C
Rationale: During a panic attack, reduce stimuli and use calm, simple coaching for paced breathing to lower physiologic arousal. A and B are not appropriate during acute panic; D explores insight, which is not effective in crisis.

9. Correct Answer: D
Rationale: Psychological first aid emphasizes safety, comfort, stabilization, practical assistance, and linkage to supports, avoiding forced recounting of trauma. A and B can retraumatize; C is not the immediate focus in acute disaster response.

10. Correct Answer: A
Rationale: Nurses are mandated reporters for suspected child abuse; report immediately without requiring proof. B and D delay safety actions; C is coercive and inappropriate.

6.1.5 Basic Care & Comfort

Question 1: A bedbound client with limited mobility is at high risk for pressure injuries. Which positioning strategy is most appropriate to reduce sacral pressure while maintaining spinal alignment?

[A] Elevate the head of bed to 60 degrees and place a foam ring (donut) under the coccyx
[B] Use a 30-degree lateral tilt with pillows to protect bony prominences and keep the head of bed at or below 30 degrees unless contraindicated
[C] Massage any reddened areas over the sacrum to promote circulation every 2 hours
[D] Place the client in high-Fowler's position continuously to relieve sacral pressure

Question 2: A client receives continuous enteral tube feedings via a nasogastric tube. Which nursing intervention best reduces the risk of aspiration pneumonia?

[A] Maintain the head of the bed at 30–45 degrees during feeding and for at least 30–60 minutes after
[B] Verify placement once per shift by auscultation of air insufflation into the stomach
[C] Place the client supine if coughing occurs to reduce reflux
[D] Hold oral care to twice weekly to avoid dislodging the tube

Question 3: The nurse is caring for a client with an indwelling urinary catheter. Which action is appropriate to prevent catheter-associated urinary tract infection (CAUTI)?

[A] Irrigate the catheter with sterile normal saline every shift to maintain patency
[B] Secure the catheter to the thigh and keep the drainage bag below bladder level at all times
[C] Apply antibiotic ointment to the meatus twice daily as routine care
[D] Obtain urine specimens from the drainage bag sampling port at the end of the shift

Question 4: A client presents with an acute ankle sprain sustained 2 hours ago. Which nursing intervention is most appropriate for comfort and to minimize swelling?

[A] Apply a moist heating pad for 30 minutes every 2 hours during the first 24 hours
[B] Alternate heat and cold every 5 minutes during the first hour post-injury
[C] Place crushed ice directly on the skin for prolonged periods for maximum effect
[D] Apply a cold pack for 20 minutes on, 20 minutes off for the first 24–48 hours and elevate the limb

Question 5: A client receiving palliative care reports distressing dyspnea at rest. Which intervention best promotes comfort?

[A] Administer a prescribed low-dose opioid, elevate the head of the bed, and use a fan for cool airflow to the face
[B] Withhold opioids due to the risk of respiratory depression and offer high-flow oxygen to allay anxiety
[C] Encourage deep suctioning every 2 hours to remove secretions even if it causes discomfort
[D] Restrict fluids to reduce pulmonary congestion as a first-line measure

Question 6: The nurse performs passive range-of-motion (ROM) exercises for a client with left-sided hemiplegia. Which technique reflects correct practice?

[A] Perform ROM once or twice weekly to avoid fatigue and joint irritation
[B] Move each joint to the point of pain to maximize stretch of tendons and ligaments
[C] Support the joint above and below, move slowly to the point of resistance (not pain), and perform ROM 1–2 times daily as tolerated
[D] Keep the knee brace locked and force full extension to prevent contractures

Question 7: The nurse is teaching a client with a new ileostomy about stoma and pouch care. Which statement indicates correct understanding?

[A] "If my stoma looks pale or bluish, that means it's healing well."
[B] "I'll clean the stoma with alcohol-based wipes to ensure it is disinfected."
[C] "I will only change the pouching system weekly regardless of leakage to maintain skin integrity."
[D] "My stoma should be moist and beefy red; I'll cut the wafer opening about 1/8 inch larger than the stoma and empty the pouch when it's one-third to one-half full."

Question 8: A client is unconscious and NPO. Which oral care technique is safest and most appropriate?

[A] Use a syringe to flush the mouth with copious water to remove debris
[B] Place the client supine with the chin up to facilitate access to the oral cavity
[C] Position side-lying with the head turned, use a suction toothbrush or Yankauer, and avoid excessive fluids
[D] Use a tongue depressor as a bite block and place fingers between the teeth to keep the mouth open

Question 9: A client with neurogenic bowel is beginning a bowel training program. Which instruction is essential for success?

[A] Schedule toileting at the same time each day, preferably 20–30 minutes after meals; ensure adequate fluid and fiber intake
[B] Use stimulant laxatives daily at varying times to trigger a bowel movement
[C] Delay attempts to defecate until a strong urge is present to strengthen reflexes
[D] Restrict fluids to firm stool and reduce incontinence

Question 10: A post-stroke client has oropharyngeal dysphagia. Which dietary plan is most appropriate to reduce aspiration risk?

[A] Regular diet with thin liquids and mixed textures to encourage appetite
[B] Pureed solids with nectar-thick liquids, small bites/sips, upright positioning, and chin-tuck technique as ordered
[C] Dry, crumbly foods like crackers to stimulate saliva and facilitate swallowing
[D] Encourage use of a straw for faster intake and less fatigue

ANSWERS

1. Correct Answer: B

Rationale: A 30-degree lateral tilt reduces sacral pressure and protects bony prominences; keeping HOB ≤30° also reduces shear. Donut devices, high-Fowler's, and massaging reddened areas increase risk of injury.

2. Correct Answer: A

Rationale: Elevating the HOB 30–45° during and after feeding reduces aspiration risk. Auscultation is not reliable for tube placement; supine position and limiting oral care increase aspiration risk.

3. Correct Answer: B

Rationale: Securing the catheter and keeping the bag below bladder level maintain a closed system and prevent reflux. Routine irrigation, meatal ointments, and sampling from the bag are not recommended and increase infection risk.

4. Correct Answer: D

Rationale: Cold therapy (RICE) in the first 24–48 hours reduces pain and swelling. Heat early post-injury and direct prolonged ice contact are unsafe; alternating modalities immediately is not evidence-based.

5. Correct Answer: A

Rationale: Low-dose opioids relieve the sensation of breathlessness; elevating HOB and fan therapy enhance comfort. Withholding opioids and unnecessary aggressive suctioning increase distress; high-flow oxygen is not always beneficial.

6. Correct Answer: C

Rationale: Proper ROM supports joints, moves slowly to resistance (not pain), and is done regularly as tolerated to prevent contractures. Forcing movement or infrequent ROM is unsafe/ineffective.

7. Correct Answer: D

Rationale: A healthy stoma is moist and beefy red; cutting 1/8 inch larger protects skin, and emptying at 1/3–1/2 full prevents leaks. Pale/blue indicates ischemia; alcohol irritates; leaking pouches must be changed promptly.

8. Correct Answer: C

Rationale: Side-lying with suction reduces aspiration risk during oral care. Copious water and supine positioning increase aspiration; placing fingers between teeth is unsafe.

9. Correct Answer: A

Rationale: Consistent timing after meals leverages the gastrocolic reflex; adequate fiber and fluids promote regularity. Routine stimulants, delaying defecation, and fluid restriction undermine training.

10. Correct Answer: B

Rationale: Pureed solids with nectar-thick liquids and compensatory strategies (upright posture, chin tuck) reduce aspiration in dysphagia. Thin liquids, mixed textures, dry crumbly foods, and straws generally increase risk.

6.1.6 Pharmacological & Parenteral Therapies

Question 1: During a medication pass, the nurse prepares to administer IV morphine sulfate 2 mg to a postoperative patient. Which action best demonstrates adherence to safe medication administration rights?

[A] Scan the medication barcode, verify one patient identifier, and administer the dose quickly to provide prompt relief.
[B] Ask the LPN to give the medication while the RN completes other tasks, then cosign the documentation.
[C] Verify the provider order, compare the medication label to the MAR three times, and document after administration.
[D] Confirm two patient identifiers, assess pain and respiratory rate, verify allergies and indication, explain the medication, administer via the correct route and rate per policy, then document and evaluate the response within the appropriate timeframe.

Question 2: A patient started on warfarin for atrial fibrillation requires discharge teaching. Which patient statement indicates a need for further instruction?

[A] "I will keep my intake of leafy greens consistent rather than eliminating them."
[B] "I can take ibuprofen as needed for headaches because it's over the counter."
[C] "I'll have my INR checked regularly and will report unusual bruising or bleeding."
[D] "I'll use a soft-bristled toothbrush and an electric razor."

Question 3: The provider orders 1,000 mL of 0.9% sodium chloride to infuse over 8 hours. The IV tubing has a drop factor of 15 gtt/mL. What is the correct drip rate in gtt/min?

[A] 31 gtt/min
[B] 21 gtt/min
[C] 38 gtt/min
[D] 19 gtt/min

Question 4: Fifteen minutes after initiating a unit of PRBCs, a patient develops chills, a temperature of 38.9°C (102°F), and low back pain. What is the nurse's priority action?

[A] Slow the transfusion rate and reassess in 15 minutes.
[B] Notify the provider and await further orders.
[C] Stop the transfusion immediately and keep the IV line open with normal saline using new tubing; notify the provider and blood bank.
[D] Administer acetaminophen and continue the transfusion if symptoms improve.

Question 5: A patient receiving total parenteral nutrition (TPN) via a central line has nearly completed the current bag, and the next TPN bag is not yet available from the pharmacy. What is the best nursing action?

[A] Hang D10W at the same rate as the TPN and notify the pharmacy.
[B] Hang 0.9% normal saline until the TPN arrives.
[C] Stop the infusion and wait for the TPN to arrive to avoid fluid overload.
[D] Hang only the lipid emulsion to prevent hypoglycemia.

Question 6: A patient is receiving IV vancomycin. When should the nurse draw the trough level to appropriately monitor therapy?

[A] One hour after the infusion is complete.
[B] Within 30 minutes before the next scheduled dose.
[C] Any time prior to the third dose.
[D] Immediately after initiating the infusion.

Question 7: Which is the correct technique when preparing to mix NPH insulin and regular insulin in one syringe?

[A] Withdraw the cloudy insulin first, then the clear insulin, to avoid contaminating the regular insulin.
[B] Do not mix these insulins in the same syringe because they are incompatible.
[C] Inject air into NPH, then into regular; withdraw regular (clear) first, then withdraw NPH (cloudy).
[D] Vigorously shake both vials to ensure proper mixing before drawing up the doses.

Question 8: Ten minutes after receiving 2 mg IV hydromorphone, a postoperative patient is difficult to arouse, with a respiratory rate of 8/min and SpO2 of 86% on 2 L/min O2. What is the nurse's priority action?

[A] Place the patient NPO and obtain an arterial blood gas sample.
[B] Increase oxygen to 6 L/min via nasal cannula and reassess in 30 minutes.
[C] Document the sedation level and continue to monitor every 15 minutes.
[D] Stop opioid infusion, stimulate patient, support ventilation, and give naloxone per protocol.

Question 9: A patient on an IV heparin infusion for DVT has an aPTT of 120 seconds (control 30 seconds) and oozing at the IV site. What is the nurse's first action?

[A] Stop the heparin infusion and notify the provider; anticipate administering protamine sulfate.
[B] Continue the heparin and recheck the aPTT in 6 hours.
[C] Administer vitamin K as the antidote for heparin.
[D] Decrease the heparin infusion rate by 2 units/kg/hr and reassess bleeding.

Question 10: While administering a vesicant chemotherapeutic agent via a peripheral IV, the patient reports burning at the site and swelling is noted. What is the immediate nursing action?

[A] Remove the IV catheter and apply warm compresses to disperse the drug.
[B] Elevate the extremity and restart the infusion at a new site proximal to the infiltration.
[C] Stop the infusion, leave the catheter in place, attempt to aspirate residual drug, and follow facility protocol for antidote and compress application; notify the provider.
[D] Flush the line with 10 mL normal saline to clear the irritation and resume the infusion.

ANSWERS

1. Correct Answer: D

Rationale: D integrates the core medication rights: right patient, drug, dose, route, time, indication, assessment, education, documentation, and evaluation. A uses only one identifier and unsafe rapid administration. B violates delegation and documentation standards. C omits full assessment, patient education, and evaluation of response.

2. Correct Answer: B

Rationale: NSAIDs like ibuprofen increase bleeding risk with warfarin. A is correct (maintain consistent vitamin K intake). C and D reflect appropriate safety and monitoring behaviors.

3. Correct Answer: A

Rationale: gtt/min = (volume mL × drop factor) ÷ minutes = (1000 × 15) ÷ 480 = 31.25 ≈ 31 gtt/min. Other options reflect miscalculations.

4. Correct Answer: C

Rationale: Signs suggest an acute hemolytic or febrile transfusion reaction. Priority is to stop the transfusion and maintain IV access with NS using new tubing, then notify the provider and blood bank. A and D inappropriately continue the transfusion. B is not the first action.

5. Correct Answer: A

Rationale: If TPN is temporarily unavailable, infuse D10W at the same rate to prevent hypoglycemia and rebounds; notify pharmacy. NS (B) and stopping TPN (C) risk hypoglycemia. Lipids alone (D) do not provide needed dextrose.

6. Correct Answer: B

Rationale: Vancomycin trough levels are drawn within 30 minutes before the next dose to assess lowest serum concentration. A and D capture peaks/early levels. C is nonspecific and may be inaccurate.

7. Correct Answer: C

Rationale: Correct sequence: inject air into NPH, then regular; withdraw regular (clear) first, then NPH (cloudy). A reverses the order and risks contaminating regular insulin. B is incorrect; they are compatible. D: do not shake insulin vials; roll NPH gently.

8. Correct Answer: D

Rationale: The patient has opioid-induced respiratory depression. Priority is to support airway/breathing and administer naloxone per protocol. A and B delay definitive treatment. C is unsafe without intervention.

9. Correct Answer: A

Rationale: Excess anticoagulation with bleeding warrants stopping heparin and notifying the provider; protamine sulfate reverses heparin. B delays care. C is the antidote for warfarin, not heparin. D insufficiently addresses active bleeding and excessive aPTT.

10. Correct Answer: C

Rationale: Suspected vesicant extravasation requires stopping the infusion, leaving the catheter to aspirate drug and administer antidote per protocol, and applying appropriate compresses. A removes access needed for aspiration/antidote. B and D risk worsening tissue injury.

6.1.7 Reduction of Risk Potential

Question 1: The nurse reviews morning labs for four clients. Which result requires immediate intervention to reduce risk of life-threatening complications?

[A] Potassium 6.4 mEq/L in a client with chronic kidney disease
[B] Sodium 131 mEq/L in a client on a thiazide diuretic
[C] Hemoglobin 10.8 g/dL in a client with iron-deficiency anemia
[D] INR 2.2 in a client taking warfarin for atrial fibrillation

Question 2: A client is 24 hours post–total hip arthroplasty. Which assessment finding most strongly suggests development of a deep vein thrombosis (DVT)?

[A] Oral temperature 99.1°F (37.3°C) without chills
[B] Bilateral pedal pulses 2+ and equal
[C] Unilateral calf swelling, warmth, and tenderness with palpation
[D] Incisional pain improved with elevation and rest

Question 3: In the preoperative holding area, which finding requires immediate nursing action before the client is transported to surgery?

[A] Client reports past lip swelling and itching after using latex gloves; no allergy band is applied
[B] Blood pressure 148/88 mm Hg; baseline yesterday 140/84 mm Hg
[C] Client NPO since midnight and took morning beta-blocker with a sip of water as prescribed
[D] A wedding ring is taped and covered per policy

Question 4: The nurse teaches a client with a new arteriovenous (AV) fistula for hemodialysis. Which statement indicates correct understanding?

[A] "I'll take my blood pressure pill right before dialysis so I don't get a headache."
[B] "If I don't feel the vibration in my fistula one morning, I'll just recheck it later."
[C] "I'll check for a bruit and thrill each day and avoid blood draws, IVs, and blood pressures in this arm."
[D] "Once it heals, I can carry heavy grocery bags with my fistula arm."

Question 5: The nurse is preparing to suction a client with a mature tracheostomy. Which action is appropriate to reduce complications?

[A] Insert the catheter until resistance is met, then apply suction while advancing
[B] Use clean technique at the bedside because the tracheostomy is established
[C] Apply suction continuously for 20–30 seconds to fully clear secretions
[D] Pre-oxygenate with 100% oxygen, suction for no more than 10 seconds, and allow re-oxygenation between passes using sterile technique

Question 6: A client with septic shock has received fluid resuscitation. Which finding best indicates adequate tissue perfusion at this time?

[A] Mean arterial pressure (MAP) of 70 mm Hg with warm, dry skin
[B] Central venous pressure (CVP) 12 mm Hg with new bibasilar crackles
[C] Urine output 15 mL/hour for the last two hours
[D] Systolic blood pressure 88 mm Hg with alert mentation

Question 7: Four hours after an open abdominal procedure, which postoperative finding requires immediate intervention to reduce risk of deterioration?

[A] Incisional pain rated 7/10 despite use of PCA
[B] Oral temperature 100.4°F (38.0°C)
[C] Small amount of serosanguineous drainage on the surgical dressing
[D] Heart rate 124/min, blood pressure 86/52 mm Hg, cool clammy skin

Question 8: A client with a traumatic brain injury is undergoing hourly neurologic checks. Which finding is the earliest indicator of increased intracranial pressure (ICP)?

[A] Positive Babinski reflex bilaterally
[B] Increasing restlessness and confusion from baseline
[C] Unilateral dilated, nonreactive pupil
[D] Bradycardia with widened pulse pressure and irregular respirations

Question 9: The nurse is administering a bolus feeding via nasogastric tube. Which action is the priority to reduce the risk of aspiration?

[A] Check gastric residual volume every 6 hours and hold feeding for a single residual >250 mL
[B] Place the client supine for comfort during and after the feeding
[C] Add blue food coloring to the formula to help detect aspiration
[D] Maintain the head of bed at 30–45 degrees during the feeding and for at least 30–60 minutes afterward

Question 10: A client with type 1 diabetes becomes diaphoretic and shaky; fingerstick glucose is 54 mg/dL. The client is awake and able to swallow. What is the nurse's first action?

[A] Give 15 grams of fast-acting carbohydrate (e.g., 4 oz fruit juice), then recheck glucose in 15 minutes
[B] Administer 1 mg glucagon IM immediately
[C] Start an IV and begin a dextrose 10% infusion per protocol
[D] Notify the provider and document the event prior to intervention

ANSWERS

1. Correct Answer: A

Rationale: Potassium >6.0 mEq/L is a critical value due to risk of lethal dysrhythmias; treat urgently. Mild hyponatremia (131), mild anemia (Hgb 10.8), and therapeutic INR for AF (≈2–3) are not immediately life-threatening.

2. Correct Answer: C

Rationale: Unilateral calf swelling, warmth, and tenderness are classic for DVT after orthopedic surgery. Equal pulses are normal, low-grade fever is nonspecific, and incisional pain improved with elevation is expected.

3. Correct Answer: A

Rationale: Suspected latex allergy without allergy identification poses high risk for anaphylaxis in the OR; implement latex precautions and notify the team before transport. The other findings are not immediate safety threats.

4. Correct Answer: C

Rationale: Correct fistula care includes daily assessment for bruit/thrill and avoiding venipuncture/BP on the access arm. Antihypertensives are often held before dialysis to prevent hypotension; absence of thrill requires immediate reporting; heavy lifting should be avoided.

5. Correct Answer: D

Rationale: Best practice: hyperoxygenate, limit each suction pass to ≤10 seconds, allow re-oxygenation between passes, and use sterile technique. Suctioning while advancing, clean technique in acute care, and prolonged suctioning increase complications.

6. Correct Answer: A

Rationale: A MAP ≥65–70 mm Hg suggests adequate perfusion. Elevated CVP with crackles indicates fluid overload, urine output <0.5 mL/kg/hr indicates poor renal perfusion, and SBP 88 is hypotensive.

7. Correct Answer: D

Rationale: Tachycardia, hypotension, and cool clammy skin indicate potential hemorrhage/hypovolemic shock and require immediate intervention. Pain, mild fever early postop, and small serosanguineous drainage are expected findings.

8. Correct Answer: B

Rationale: The earliest sign of rising ICP is a change in level of consciousness (restlessness, confusion). Fixed/dilated pupil and Cushing's triad are late signs; Babinski is abnormal in adults but not the earliest deterioration indicator.

9. Correct Answer: D

Rationale: Elevating the head of bed 30–45 degrees during and after enteral feeding is the priority to prevent aspiration. Routine residual checks have evolving guidance; supine positioning and dye in formula are contraindicated.

10. Correct Answer: A

Rationale: For conscious hypoglycemia, give 15 g rapid-acting carbohydrate and recheck in 15 minutes (15/15 rule). IM glucagon or IV dextrose are for patients who are unconscious, seizing, or unable to swallow.

6.1.8 Physiological Adaptation

Question 1: A client with end-stage renal disease presents with serum potassium 6.7 mEq/L and new-onset palpitations. Which electrocardiographic change is most consistent with this electrolyte abnormality?

[A] Tall, narrow, peaked T waves with possible widening of the QRS and prolonged PR interval
[B] Prominent U waves with ST-segment depression and flattened T waves
[C] Shortened QT interval with widened, tall P waves
[D] Diffuse ST-segment elevation with PR-segment depression

Question 2: A client with COPD exacerbation is somnolent and has the following ABG: pH 7.28, PaCO2 60 mm Hg, HCO3– 26 mEq/L, PaO2 58 mm Hg on 2 L/min nasal cannula. Which priority intervention should the nurse anticipate?

[A] Increase IV fluids to 200 mL/hr to improve perfusion
[B] Administer IV sodium bicarbonate to correct the acidosis
[C] Titrate oxygen to maintain SpO2 ≥ 98%
[D] Initiate noninvasive positive-pressure ventilation (BiPAP) as prescribed to improve alveolar ventilation

Question 3: A febrile client with suspected sepsis has BP 82/46, HR 124, RR 28, lactate 5.2 mmol/L, and warm, flushed skin. Orders include: draw blood cultures x2, administer 30 mL/kg lactated Ringer's, start broad-spectrum antibiotics, insert Foley catheter. Which order has the highest immediate priority?

[A] Draw blood cultures x2 from two sites
[B] Start broad-spectrum antibiotics
[C] Administer 30 mL/kg crystalloid bolus rapidly
[D] Insert Foley catheter for strict I&O

Question 4: Thirty minutes after receiving IV ampicillin, a client develops wheezing, stridor, hives, swelling of the lips, and BP 78/42. What is the nurse's priority action?

[A] Elevate the head of bed and apply cool compresses to hives
[B] Administer IV diphenhydramine as prescribed
[C] Apply high-flow oxygen via nonrebreather mask
[D] Administer intramuscular epinephrine in the lateral thigh immediately

Question 5: A client with a left-sided chest tube to water-seal suction for a pneumothorax is being assessed. Which finding requires immediate intervention?

[A] Drainage of 120 mL serosanguinous fluid in the first postoperative hour
[B] Intermittent bubbling in the water-seal chamber during exhalation and coughing
[C] Continuous bubbling in the water-seal chamber
[D] Gentle continuous bubbling in the suction control chamber

Question 6: Two hours after abdominal surgery, a client is restless and pale with HR 132/min, BP 80/50 mm Hg, RR 28/min, cool clammy skin, UOP 10 mL over the last hour, and a rapidly saturating abdominal dressing. MAP is 60 mm Hg. What is the nurse's priority action?

[A] Notify the surgeon of possible postoperative bleeding
[B] Assess pain level and administer prescribed opioid analgesic
[C] Reinforce the dressing and reassess in 30 minutes
[D] Activate the rapid response team, apply high-flow oxygen, and begin rapid infusion of isotonic crystalloid via large-bore IV

Question 7: A 68-year-old with sudden right-sided weakness and aphasia arrived 45 minutes after symptom onset. BP is 176/98 mm Hg, glucose 112 mg/dL, and NIH Stroke Scale is 12. Which order should the nurse implement first to determine eligibility for reperfusion therapy?

[A] Administer aspirin 325 mg orally
[B] Obtain a stat non-contrast head CT
[C] Start IV heparin infusion per stroke protocol
[D] Administer alteplase (tPA) within 60 minutes of arrival

Question 8: Which ABG is most consistent with metabolic alkalosis?

[A] pH 7.30, $PaCO_2$ 50 mm Hg, HCO_3^- 24 mEq/L
[B] pH 7.50, $PaCO_2$ 30 mm Hg, HCO_3^- 23 mEq/L
[C] pH 7.50, $PaCO_2$ 44 mm Hg, HCO_3^- 32 mEq/L
[D] pH 7.30, $PaCO_2$ 28 mm Hg, HCO_3^- 14 mEq/L

Question 9: A client with chronic heart failure calls the clinic reporting new symptoms. Which report requires immediate evaluation for potential acute decompensation?

[A] Bilateral 2+ ankle edema by evening that improves overnight
[B] Weight gain of 2 lb over the last 2 days
[C] Increased nocturia over the last week
[D] Sudden onset of pink, frothy sputum with severe dyspnea and crackles

Question 10: A hospitalized client is found unresponsive, not breathing, and pulseless. The code blue has been activated and the defibrillator is en route. What is the nurse's next action?

[A] Check the monitor leads and obtain a 12-lead ECG
[B] Deliver one rescue breath and then reassess the pulse
[C] Call the provider to obtain CPR orders
[D] Begin high-quality chest compressions at 100–120/min with a depth of at least 2 inches and allow full recoil

ANSWERS

1. Correct Answer: A
Rationale: Hyperkalemia classically produces tall, peaked T waves and may progress to PR prolongation and QRS widening. B reflects hypokalemia; C suggests hypercalcemia; D is more consistent with pericarditis.

2. Correct Answer: D
Rationale: The ABG indicates acute respiratory acidosis from hypoventilation. Noninvasive positive-pressure ventilation (BiPAP) improves alveolar ventilation and CO_2 clearance. IV fluids (A) do not address hypoventilation; bicarbonate (B) is not indicated for respiratory acidosis; targeting $SpO_2 \geq 98\%$ (C) may worsen CO_2 retention—COPD targets are typically 88–92%.

3. Correct Answer: C
Rationale: In septic shock with hypotension and elevated lactate, rapid 30 mL/kg crystalloid resuscitation is the immediate priority to restore perfusion. Cultures (A) and antibiotics (B) are urgent but fluid resuscitation treats life-threatening hypotension. Foley insertion (D) is supportive.

4. Correct Answer: D
Rationale: Anaphylaxis is treated first with intramuscular epinephrine in the lateral thigh to reverse airway edema, bronchospasm, and hypotension. Oxygen (C), antihistamines (B), and positioning (A) are adjuncts but not the priority.

5. Correct Answer: C
Rationale: Continuous bubbling in the water-seal chamber indicates an air leak and requires immediate troubleshooting to prevent loss of negative pressure and recurrent pneumothorax. Intermittent bubbling (B) can be expected with a pneumothorax; gentle bubbling in suction control (D) is expected. Drainage of 120 mL in the first hour (A) may be acceptable depending on surgery and trend.

6. Correct Answer: D
Rationale: Findings indicate hemorrhagic shock. Priority is to support airway/breathing/circulation: activate rapid response, provide high-flow oxygen, and start rapid isotonic crystalloid infusion via large-bore IVs while preparing for definitive hemorrhage control. Notifying the surgeon (A) occurs after stabilization. Analgesia (B) is not priority. Simply reinforcing the dressing (C) delays resuscitation.

7. Correct Answer: B
Rationale: A non-contrast head CT must be obtained rapidly to rule out hemorrhage before thrombolysis in acute ischemic stroke. Aspirin (A) is deferred until after hemorrhage is excluded; heparin (C) is not routinely indicated; alteplase (D) cannot be given before CT confirmation.

8. Correct Answer: C
Rationale: Elevated pH with elevated HCO_3^- and normal $PaCO_2$ is metabolic alkalosis. A indicates respiratory acidosis; B indicates respiratory alkalosis; D indicates metabolic acidosis (with respiratory compensation).

9. Correct Answer: D
Rationale: Pink, frothy sputum with severe dyspnea and crackles indicates acute pulmonary edema, a medical emergency. Edema (A), 2-lb weight gain (B), and nocturia (C) reflect chronic fluid overload but are less emergent.

10. Correct Answer: D
Rationale: In a pulseless, apneic patient, start high-quality chest compressions immediately while awaiting the defibrillator and additional help. ECG acquisition (A) and rescue breaths alone (B) are not the first step. No provider order (C) is needed to begin CPR.

6.2 Exam 2

6.2.1 Management of Care

Question 1: A client scheduled for elective surgery has already received IV midazolam for anxiety when the provider arrives and asks the nurse to obtain the client's informed consent for the procedure. Which action is most appropriate by the nurse?

[A] Ask the client's spouse to sign the consent form as the next of kin since the client has been sedated
[B] Notify the provider that informed consent must be obtained before sedation; if sedation has been given, request that the procedure be delayed until the client regains decision-making capacity
[C] Explain the procedure and risks and obtain the client's verbal consent, then have the client sign when more alert
[D] Proceed with the procedure because the client verbally agreed earlier in the day and implied consent applies

Question 2: The nurse is receiving morning report. Which client should the nurse see first?

[A] A client 2 days after total knee arthroplasty reporting pain 8/10 with heart rate 110/min
[B] A client 1 hour after thyroidectomy with new-onset hoarseness, drooling, and difficulty swallowing
[C] A client with heart failure with 2+ bilateral leg edema and a 2-kg (4.4-lb) overnight weight gain, scheduled for IV furosemide
[D] A client with community-acquired pneumonia reporting fever of 38.3°C (100.9°F) and productive cough

Question 3: The RN is delegating tasks to an experienced unlicensed assistive personnel (UAP). Which task is appropriate to delegate?

[A] Assess the character and amount of drainage from a new chest tube insertion site and document the findings
[B] Provide initial teaching on ostomy care to a client newly post-op from a colostomy
[C] Titrate supplemental oxygen to maintain SpO2 92% to 96% per sliding-scale protocol
[D] Obtain a postprandial capillary blood glucose and report the numeric value to the RN

Question 4: A 68-year-old client with COPD is being discharged on home oxygen and scheduled nebulizer treatments. The client has limited finances and lives alone. Which case management action best promotes continuity of care?

[A] Coordinate durable medical equipment delivery for home oxygen, verify insurance coverage, arrange a home health RN visit within 24–48 hours, and schedule pulmonology follow-up before discharge
[B] Instruct the client to call a local oxygen company to arrange equipment after arriving home
[C] Provide a pamphlet about COPD and encourage the client to pick up prescriptions at a convenient pharmacy
[D] Ask a family member to set up follow-up appointments after the client is discharged

Question 5: A hospitalized adult client asks to review their electronic health record (EHR). What is the nurse's best response?

[A] Inform the client that only the provider can grant access and discourage review to avoid confusion
[B] Print the entire chart and give it to the client without documenting the request to protect privacy
[C] Follow facility policy to facilitate access via Health Information Management; verify the client's identity, provide assistance in reviewing the record as appropriate, and document the request and access provided
[D] Instruct the client to obtain a court order to view their medical record after discharge

Question 6: The nurse manager notes an increase in catheter-associated urinary tract infections (CAUTIs) on the unit over the past quarter. Which initial quality improvement (QI) action is most appropriate?

[A] Send a reminder email to all staff to "avoid CAUTIs" and re-educate during annual competencies only
[B] Identify individual nurses linked to infections and provide punitive write-ups to deter future errors
[C] Convene an interprofessional team to conduct a root cause analysis, review evidence-based CAUTI bundles, audit current practices, pilot targeted interventions, and track outcomes
[D] Immediately remove all indwelling catheters from clients on the unit to reduce infection risk

Question 7: Which action by the nurse best upholds HIPAA and confidentiality standards when communicating about a client?

[A] Conduct a private, face-to-face bedside handoff with the oncoming nurse, verify the recipient's identity, share only minimum necessary information, and ensure doors/curtains are closed
[B] Discuss the client's condition using initials in the hospital cafeteria to avoid revealing full identity
[C] Text the client's lab results to the provider using the nurse's personal smartphone to expedite care
[D] Provide an update to a neighbor who states they are a "close friend," as long as no written documents are shared

Question 8: The charge nurse is making assignments for one RN, one LPN/VN, and one UAP. Which client is most appropriate to assign to the LPN/VN?

[A] A newly admitted client with hematemesis requiring initial assessment and stabilization
[B] A client with unstable angina receiving a heparin infusion and titrated nitroglycerin
[C] A postoperative day 2 client after laparoscopic cholecystectomy with stable vital signs who needs wound care and scheduled oral medications
[D] A client requiring initial discharge teaching for a new colostomy and ostomy equipment

Question 9: A competent adult client with gastrointestinal bleeding who is hemodynamically stable refuses a blood transfusion due to religious beliefs. The family insists the transfusion be given. What is the nurse's best action?

[A] Honor the refusal; assess the client's understanding, notify the provider, document the refusal and teaching provided, and explore acceptable alternatives
[B] Ask the family to persuade the client to accept the transfusion because the situation could become emergent
[C] Administer the transfusion under implied consent because the client's life may be at risk
[D] Seek a court order to override the client's refusal in the interest of preserving life

Question 10: In the emergency department, a police officer asks the nurse to disclose a conscious adult client's blood alcohol concentration (BAC) following a motor vehicle collision. What is the most appropriate response by the nurse?

[A] Provide the BAC result because law enforcement has requested it as part of an investigation
[B] Confirm that the client is currently in the ED but decline to share details about test results
[C] Provide de-identified clinical information so long as the client's name is not used
[D] Decline to disclose any protected health information without patient authorization, a valid warrant/subpoena, or a law requiring reporting; refer the officer to Health Information Management per facility policy

ANSWERS

1. Correct Answer: B
Rationale: Informed consent must be obtained by the provider before sedation. After midazolam, the client lacks capacity, so the nurse should notify the provider. A spouse cannot sign unless legal surrogate, nurses cannot obtain consent, and prior discussion or implied consent does not apply here.

2. Correct Answer: B
Rationale: After thyroidectomy, airway compromise from edema/hematoma is the greatest risk; hoarseness, drooling, and dysphagia suggest obstruction (ABC priority). A: Pain with mild tachycardia isn't life-threatening. C: Fluid overload needs care but not immediate airway support. D: Pneumonia with fever isn't immediately life-threatening.

3. Correct Answer: D
Rationale: UAPs can perform routine tasks with predictable outcomes, such as capillary glucose testing, and report numeric values. A: Assessing/evaluating chest tube drainage requires RN assessment. B: Initial teaching is an RN role. C: Titrating oxygen per protocol requires nursing judgment and is not appropriate for UAP.

4. Correct Answer: A
Rationale: Case management promotes continuity by arranging needed services before discharge—equipment delivery, coverage verification, home health referral, and follow-up appointments. B, C, D: Placing responsibility solely on the client/family risks gaps in care and readmissions and does not ensure coordination.

5. Correct Answer: C
Rationale: Clients have the right to access their medical records. The nurse facilitates access per policy, verifies identity, assists as appropriate, and documents. A: Incorrect—provider permission is not required. B: Printing the entire chart without process breaches policy and may compromise privacy. D: A court order is not required for client access.

6. Correct Answer: C
Rationale: Effective QI begins with a systems approach: root cause analysis, evidence-based bundles, auditing, piloting, and measurement. A: Reminders alone are insufficient. B and D: Punitive approaches or blanket removal are unsafe and do not address system contributors.

7. Correct Answer: A
Rationale: HIPAA permits sharing PHI with providers involved in care using reasonable safeguards and minimum necessary information; private bedside handoff with identity verification is appropriate. B: Public spaces risk incidental disclosure. C: Personal devices and unsecured texting violate policy. D: Friends/neighbors are not authorized recipients.

8. Correct Answer: C
Rationale: LPN/VNs care for stable clients with predictable outcomes and can perform wound care and administer routine oral meds. A: New admissions require RN assessment. B: Unstable clients on titrated IV anticoagulants/vasodilators require RN care. D: Initial discharge teaching is an RN responsibility.

9. Correct Answer: A
Rationale: Respect for autonomy and informed refusal require honoring a competent client's decision. The nurse verifies understanding, informs the provider, documents, and explores acceptable alternatives (e.g., volume expanders, iron therapy). B, C, D: Coercion, implied consent in non-emergency, and court orders are inappropriate and violate patient rights.

10. Correct Answer: D
Rationale: HIPAA prohibits disclosure of PHI to law enforcement without patient authorization, a valid warrant/subpoena, or a specific law mandating disclosure. The nurse should not release information and should refer the request per policy. A–C: Providing results, confirming presence, or sharing "de-identified" details in response to a law enforcement request without proper authority violates HIPAA and facility policy.

6.2.2 Safety & Infection Prevention and Control

Question 1: A client with suspected pulmonary tuberculosis is being admitted from the emergency department. Which initial infection-control action is most appropriate?

[A] Place the client in a private room with the door open and require staff to wear surgical masks.
[B] Implement droplet precautions and require staff to wear a surgical mask within 3 feet of the client.
[C] Place the client in an airborne infection isolation room (negative-pressure) and require staff to wear a fit-tested N95 or PAPR; keep the door closed and have the client wear a surgical mask during transport.
[D] Implement contact precautions only and require staff to wear gown and gloves.

Question 2: A nurse prepares to enter the room of a patient on droplet and contact precautions. What is the correct sequence for donning PPE?

[A] Gown → mask/respirator → goggles/face shield → gloves
[B] Mask/respirator → gloves → gown → goggles/face shield
[C] Gloves → gown → mask/respirator → goggles/face shield
[D] Gown → gloves → mask/respirator → goggles/face shield

Question 3: Which action best maintains surgical asepsis when preparing a sterile field for a central line dressing change?

[A] Holding the solution bottle with the label in the palm, "lipping" if previously opened, and pouring 4–6 inches above a sterile receptacle without splashing.
[B] Placing the bottle cap face-down on the sterile field while pouring sterile solution.
[C] Reaching over the sterile field to adjust a sterile drape.
[D] Turning your back briefly on the sterile field to obtain additional supplies.

Question 4: Which action demonstrates correct management of non-violent medical restraints for a patient pulling at IV lines despite alternatives?

[A] Securing restraints to the side rails with a double-knot to prevent escape.
[B] Applying four-point restraints per nurse judgment without a provider order for up to 48 hours.
[C] Obtaining a time-limited provider order; using the least restrictive device with a quick-release tie to the bed frame; ensuring two-finger spacing; assessing/documenting skin, circulation, and need at least every 2 hours with ROM, fluids, toileting; and removing one restraint at a time for care.
[D] Using bed sheets as makeshift restraints if commercial devices are unavailable.

Question 5: A client is admitted with confirmed influenza A. Which is the best infection-control plan?

[A] Airborne precautions in a negative-pressure room with a fit-tested N95.
[B] Private room with the door open; no mask required if the nurse is vaccinated.
[C] Droplet precautions: private room (or cohort), staff wear a surgical mask within 3–6 feet of the client, the client wears a mask during transport, and use gloves/gown if contact with secretions is anticipated.
[D] Standard precautions only, as influenza is community-acquired.

Question 6: An 82-year-old postoperative client receiving opioids is confused and repeatedly tries to get out of bed. Which fall-prevention plan is most appropriate?

[A] Raise all four side rails and apply a vest restraint until sedation wears off.
[B] Keep the bed in the lowest position with wheels locked, activate bed/chair alarms, provide non-skid footwear, keep the call light and belongings within reach, perform scheduled rounding/toileting, and use a gait belt for assisted ambulation.
[C] Keep the room dark to promote sleep and reduce agitation.
[D] Instruct unlicensed assistive personnel to ambulate the client as needed without a gait belt to encourage independence.

Question 7: While handling a chemical disinfectant, a nurse experiences a splash to the eyes. What is the priority action?

[A] Notify the supervisor and wait for instructions before rinsing to preserve evidence.
[B] Immediately flush eyes at an eyewash station for at least 15 minutes, remove contact lenses, then notify the supervisor, consult the Safety Data Sheet (SDS), and complete an incident report.
[C] Rinse for 30 seconds, apply a neutralizing agent, and return to work.
[D] Call poison control before rinsing to determine the appropriate antidote.

Question 8: After caring for a patient on contact and droplet precautions, what is the correct sequence for removing PPE before leaving the room?

[A] Mask → goggles/face shield → gown → gloves → hand hygiene
[B] Goggles/face shield → mask → gloves → gown → hand hygiene
[C] Gown and gloves together → mask → goggles/face shield → hand hygiene
[D] Gloves → goggles/face shield → gown → mask → hand hygiene (remove respirator after exiting if airborne precautions were used)

Question 9: You enter a room, see flames in a trash can, and the patient is on oxygen therapy. What is your first action following fire response protocols?

[A] Pull the fire alarm and then determine who needs evacuation.
[B] Turn off the oxygen wall supply and remove all oxygen tanks.
[C] Attempt to extinguish the fire using PASS before moving the patient.
[D] Rescue the patient from immediate danger and close the door to contain smoke, then activate the alarm.

Question 10: A patient has profuse watery diarrhea and tests positive for Clostridioides difficile. Which action is essential to prevent transmission?

[A] Use alcohol-based hand sanitizer after removing gloves.
[B] Perform hand hygiene with soap and water after removing gloves.
[C] Place the patient on droplet precautions and wear a surgical mask only.
[D] Dispose of sharps used for this patient in a red biohazard bag.

ANSWERS

1. Correct Answer: C
Rationale: TB requires airborne precautions: a negative-pressure (AIIR) room with the door closed, and staff wear a fit-tested N95/PAPR. Mask the patient with a surgical mask during transport. Options A/B reflect droplet-level protection and are insufficient; D omits respiratory protection.

2. Correct Answer: A
Rationale: Correct donning sequence: gown → mask/respirator → goggles/face shield → gloves. This reduces self-contamination risk. Other sequences place gloves too early or misorder mask/eye protection.

3. Correct Answer: A
Rationale: Maintaining sterility includes holding the bottle with the label in the palm, lipping if previously opened, and pouring 4–6 inches above to avoid splashing. Reaching over the field, placing caps on the field, or turning your back contaminates the sterile field.

4. Correct Answer: C
Rationale: Restraints require a time-limited provider order, least restrictive use, quick-release tie to bed frame (not rails), frequent assessments (at least q2h for non-violent), and care (ROM, fluids, toileting). A and D are unsafe; B lacks a provider order and misstates time frames.

5. Correct Answer: C
Rationale: Influenza requires droplet precautions: surgical mask within 3–6 feet, mask the patient for transport, and add gloves/gown if contact with secretions is likely. Airborne (A) is unnecessary; B and D under-protect.

6. Correct Answer: B
Rationale: Evidence-based fall prevention includes low/locked bed, alarms, non-skid footwear, call light within reach, scheduled rounding/toileting, and gait belt. A uses restraints inappropriately; C increases risk; D is unsafe.

7. Correct Answer: B
Rationale: Immediate copious irrigation (≥15 minutes) is the priority, followed by removing contacts, notifying a supervisor, consulting the SDS, and documenting. Delaying irrigation (A, D) or brief rinsing/neutralizers (C) is unsafe.

8. Correct Answer: D
Rationale: Standard doffing: gloves → goggles/face shield → gown → mask → hand hygiene. For airborne, remove the respirator after exiting the AIIR. Other sequences increase self-contamination risk.

9. Correct Answer: D
Rationale: RACE: Rescue, Alarm, Contain, Extinguish. The first action is to remove the patient from danger and close the door. Then activate the alarm. A/C misprioritize; B may follow but is not first.

10. Correct Answer: B
Rationale: C. difficile spores are not killed by alcohol; soap-and-water hand hygiene is essential after glove removal. Contact precautions with gown/gloves and sporicidal cleaning are also required. A is inadequate; C misapplies droplet precautions; D misstates sharps disposal (use puncture-resistant sharps containers).

6.2.3 Health Promotion & Maintenance

Question 1: A parent of a 9-month-old infant asks the nurse which developmental milestone is expected at this age. Which response is most accurate?

[A] Walks independently without support and stacks two blocks
[B] Uses a crude pincer grasp to pick up small objects like a cereal puff
[C] Speaks in two-word phrases and follows two-step commands
[D] Sits independently by 4 months and crawls by 5 months

Question 2: A pregnant client at 16 weeks' gestation asks which vaccines she should receive during pregnancy. Which recommendation is appropriate?

[A] Inactivated influenza vaccine during flu season and a Tdap dose between 27–36 weeks' gestation
[B] Live-attenuated intranasal influenza vaccine any time in pregnancy and Tdap postpartum
[C] MMR vaccine now if nonimmune and varicella vaccine at 28 weeks
[D] HPV vaccine series during the second trimester to maximize antibody response

Question 3: The nurse provides safe sleep education to new parents of a healthy term newborn. Which statement indicates correct understanding?

[A] We will place the baby prone for sleep to reduce spit-up and choking
[B] The baby should sleep on the back on a firm mattress with no pillows, blankets, or toys in the crib
[C] We'll elevate the head of the mattress slightly and use a small infant pillow
[D] Co-sleeping in our bed is safest because we can monitor the baby closely

Question 4: Which screening plan best reflects current preventive care guidelines for average-risk clients?

[A] A 25-year-old woman: cervical cancer screening with Pap plus HPV co-test every 5 years
[B] A 42-year-old woman: start screening mammograms at age 50 unless a lump is found
[C] A 65-year-old man who never smoked: annual low-dose CT scan for lung cancer
[D] A 45-year-old adult at average risk: begin colorectal cancer screening

Question 5: A patient smokes one pack per day and says, "I'm not ready to quit right now." What is the nurse's best next step?

[A] Prescribe varenicline immediately and schedule a quit date this week
[B] Advise the patient to reduce smoking to fewer than 10 cigarettes per day
[C] Use motivational interviewing to explore ambivalence and increase readiness to quit
[D] Provide pamphlets only and plan to revisit quitting in one year U

Question 6: A healthy 67-year-old with no documented pneumococcal vaccination asks about vaccines. What is the best recommendation?

[A] Give PPSV23 only today; no additional doses are needed
[B] Administer a single dose of PCV20 today (or PCV15 today followed by PPSV23 in 1 year)
[C] No pneumococcal vaccine is needed if the client has no chronic illnesses
[D] Give PCV13 and PPSV23 on the same day in opposite arms

Question 7: An Rh-negative gravida at 28 weeks with a negative antibody screen asks about Rho(D) immune globulin. Which teaching is correct?

[A] You receive Rho(D) immune globulin once at 20 weeks; no further doses are needed
[B] Because your indirect Coombs test is negative, you do not need Rho(D) immune globulin
[C] Rho(D) is only needed after procedures like amniocentesis, not routinely
[D] You receive Rho(D) at 28 weeks and again within 72 hours postpartum if the infant is Rh-positive

Question 8: The school nurse reviews immunizations for an 11-year-old with up-to-date childhood vaccines. Which action is appropriate?

[A] Delay HPV vaccination until the adolescent is sexually active
[B] Administer Tdap booster, start the HPV vaccine series, and give the meningococcal ACWY vaccine
[C] Give routine MMR and varicella boosters at this age even if fully immunized at 4–6 years
[D] Provide pneumococcal conjugate vaccine to all healthy 11-year-olds

Question 9: The nurse provides postpartum discharge education. Which client report requires immediate follow-up?

[A] Lochia rubra with occasional small clots on day 2
[B] Perineal soreness relieved by sitz baths and ibuprofen
[C] Feeling tearful on day 3 but improved with rest and support
[D] Severe headache with blurry vision 5 days after delivery

Question 10: Which preventive service is most appropriate at a routine 3-year-old well-child visit?

[A] Routine fasting lipid panel for early cholesterol screening in all children
[B] Vision screening to detect amblyopia risk factors and decreased visual acuity
[C] Annual pure-tone audiometry for hearing at age 3
[D] Universal hemoglobin screening for iron deficiency anemia at age 3

ANSWERS

1. Answer: B
Rationale: By about 9 months, infants typically develop a crude pincer grasp, enabling them to pick up small items. Walking independently usually occurs around 12–15 months; two-word phrases emerge closer to 18–24 months; unsupported sitting typically occurs around 7–8 months.

2. Correct Answer: A
Rationale: Pregnant clients should receive the inactivated influenza vaccine (any trimester during flu season) and Tdap during 27–36 weeks each pregnancy. Live vaccines (MMR, varicella, live-attenuated intranasal influenza) and HPV are not recommended during pregnancy.

3. Correct Answer: B
Rationale: Safe sleep includes supine positioning on a firm mattress without pillows, blankets, bumper pads, or toys; room-sharing without bed-sharing is recommended. Prone positioning and soft bedding increase SIDS risk.

4. Correct Answer: D
Rationale: Colorectal cancer screening begins at age 45 for average-risk adults. For cervical cancer, ages 21–29 should have cytology alone every 3 years; routine mammography now begins at age 40; lung cancer screening is for adults 50–80 with significant smoking history.

5. Correct Answer: C
Rationale: When a patient is not ready to quit, motivational interviewing and the 5 R's (Relevance, Risks, Rewards, Roadblocks, Repetition) help enhance readiness. Pharmacotherapy without readiness, cutting down without a plan, or handing out pamphlets alone are less effective.

6. Correct Answer: B
Rationale: For adults 65+ with unknown/no pneumococcal vaccination, give either a single dose of PCV20 or PCV15 followed by PPSV23 one year later. PPSV23 alone or co-administering PCV and PPSV23 the same day is not recommended for vaccine-naïve older adults.

7. Correct Answer: D
Rationale: Rh-negative clients receive Rho(D) immune globulin at 28 weeks and within 72 hours postpartum if the newborn is Rh-positive. It's also indicated after potential fetomaternal hemorrhage (e.g., amniocentesis, trauma). A negative antibody screen does not negate routine prophylaxis.

8. Correct Answer: B
Rationale: At 11–12 years, adolescents should receive Tdap, initiate the HPV series, and get the meningococcal ACWY vaccine. HPV should not be delayed until sexual activity. Routine MMR/varicella boosters at this age are not indicated if the childhood series is complete; pneumococcal vaccine is not routinely given to healthy adolescents.

9. Correct Answer: D
Rationale: Severe headache and visual changes postpartum are red flags for postpartum preeclampsia and warrant urgent evaluation. Lochia rubra with small clots early postpartum, perineal soreness relieved by measures, and transient "baby blues" are expected findings.

10. Correct Answer: B
Rationale: Vision screening at ages 3–5 helps detect amblyopia and refractive errors. Routine universal lipid screening is not recommended at age 3; pure-tone audiometry typically begins around age 4; hemoglobin screening is recommended at 12 months, with later testing based on risk.

6.2.4 Psychosocial Integrity

Question 1: A client with major depressive disorder says, "Nothing will ever get better; I can't do this anymore." Which response by the nurse is most therapeutic?

[A] "You're feeling overwhelmed right now. I'm here with you. Can you tell me more about what feels hardest today?"
[B] "You shouldn't think that way. Try focusing on the positives in your life."
[C] "If you don't try harder to change your thinking, you won't improve."
[D] "Let's distract you with a game so you don't dwell on those thoughts."

Question 2: A family caregiver for a client with Alzheimer disease says, "I'm exhausted and I can't keep up. I feel like I'm failing." What is the most appropriate nursing intervention to promote adaptive coping?

[A] Encourage the caregiver to "push through" and suppress feelings to avoid upsetting the client.
[B] Teach the caregiver to schedule regular respite breaks, use problem-solving strategies, and connect with community resources and caregiver support groups.
[C] Suggest increasing caffeine intake to maintain alertness during caregiving tasks.
[D] Advise the caregiver to confront the client about difficult behaviors to regain control.

Question 3: An inpatient with major depressive disorder states, "I have a plan to take all the pills I've been hoarding so I won't wake up," and shows the nurse a bag of medications taken from other clients. What is the nurse's priority action?

[A] Document the statement and notify the provider at the end of the shift.
[B] Ask the client to sign a "no-suicide" contract as reassurance.
[C] Stay with the client, remove the medications, initiate suicide precautions with one-to-one observation, and notify the provider immediately.
[D] Encourage the client to attend group therapy and discuss feelings later.

Question 4: A client with schizophrenia says, "The voices say I'm evil and must be punished." Which response best demonstrates therapeutic communication?

[A] "The voices are not real, so you need to stop listening to them."
[B] "You're hearing voices because you missed your medication again."
[C] "I don't hear the voices, but I can see they're scary for you. Let's talk about how to help you feel safe right now."
[D] "Why do you think you deserve punishment?"

Question 5: A 48-year-old client with heavy alcohol use reports last drink 8 hours ago. The client is anxious, diaphoretic, has tremors, HR 120/min, and BP 160/94 mm Hg. Which prescription should the nurse anticipate to manage withdrawal safely?

[A] Haloperidol PO PRN for agitation
[B] Naloxone IM now
[C] Lorazepam IV per CIWA-Ar protocol
[D] Disulfiram PO now

Question 6: In the emergency department, a client presents with vague injuries and limited eye contact. The client's partner answers most questions and refuses to leave the bedside. The nurse suspects intimate partner violence. What is the nurse's best initial action?

[A] Ask screening questions in front of the partner to obtain corroboration.
[B] Request to speak with the client alone in a private, safe setting and use a validated IPV screening tool, explaining confidentiality within legal limits.
[C] Immediately call law enforcement to report IPV without assessing the client's wishes.
[D] Provide printed IPV resources directly to the client while the partner watches to ensure transparency.

Question 7: A hospice client with end-stage lung cancer is restless, anxious, and reports "air hunger." RR is 26/min with accessory muscle use; SpO2 is 85% on room air. Orders include: low-dose oral morphine, PRN lorazepam, oxygen via non-rebreather at 10 L/min PRN, and suction PRN. What is the most appropriate intervention to promote comfort?

[A] Apply a non-rebreather mask at 10 L/min as the primary intervention.
[B] Coach deep breathing and incentive spirometry to improve ventilation.
[C] Perform nasopharyngeal suctioning to remove possible secretions.
[D] Administer the prescribed low-dose morphine to decrease dyspnea and air hunger.

Question 8: During an inpatient anxiety-management group, one client repeatedly interrupts and speaks at length, leaving little time for others. Which group-leadership response is most appropriate?

[A] Allow the client to continue to promote catharsis and self-expression.
[B] Use sarcasm to confront the behavior and discourage further interruptions.
[C] Acknowledge the client's contribution, set a limit, and invite quieter members to share: "Thank you for sharing. Let's hear from others who haven't spoken yet."
[D] End the group session early to prevent escalating conflict.

Question 9: After a mass-casualty event, the nurse uses START triage. Which victim should be tagged as Immediate (red)?

[A] 26-year-old who is walking with superficial abrasions and is oriented
[B] Unresponsive adult who is not breathing after airway repositioning and remains apneic
[C] 45-year-old with RR 24/min, capillary refill 1 second, follows commands, and has a closed femur deformity
[D] 60-year-old with RR 36/min, capillary refill 3 seconds, and follows simple commands

Question 10: A daughter at the bedside of her actively dying mother says, "I feel terrible for thinking this, but I just want it to be over. I'm so tired." What is the nurse's best response?

[A] "Many caregivers feel that way when they're exhausted and watching someone they love suffer. It's okay to have these feelings. Can you tell me more?"
[B] "You shouldn't say that. Your mother needs you to stay positive."
[C] "Let's focus on planning the funeral so you have something concrete to do."
[D] "You need to go home and rest now; that will fix how you feel."

ANSWERS

1. Correct Answer: A
Rationale: Reflecting feelings, offering presence, and inviting elaboration are therapeutic techniques that validate the client's experience and promote further communication. The other options minimize, judge, or deflect feelings.

2. Correct Answer: B
Rationale: Evidence-based stress management for caregivers includes planned respite, problem-solving, and linkage to social support/resources. The other options are maladaptive or inappropriate.

3. Correct Answer: C
Rationale: Imminent suicide risk with plan and means requires immediate safety measures: remain with the client, remove lethal means, initiate one-to-one observation, and notify the provider. Documentation alone or no-suicide contracts are insufficient.

4. Correct Answer: C
Rationale: Presenting reality without arguing, acknowledging the client's feelings, and refocusing on safety are therapeutic responses to hallucinations. The other options invalidate, blame, or explore delusional content.

5. Correct Answer: C
Rationale: Benzodiazepines (e.g., lorazepam) are first-line for acute alcohol withdrawal to prevent seizures and delirium tremens. Haloperidol may be adjunctive; naloxone treats opioid overdose; disulfiram is not used during acute withdrawal.

6. Correct Answer: B
Rationale: Best practice is private screening using validated tools, ensuring safety and confidentiality within legal limits. Screening in front of the partner may increase danger; mandatory reporting varies and assessment comes first; handing materials openly may escalate risk.

7. Correct Answer: D
Rationale: Low-dose opioids effectively reduce the sensation of dyspnea (air hunger) in end-of-life care. Oxygen may be considered but is less effective for subjective dyspnea; suctioning and incentive spirometry are not indicated for comfort-focused care without secretion burden.

8. Correct Answer: C
Rationale: Limit-setting with respectful acknowledgment and facilitation of broader participation supports group process and safety. Allowing monopolizing, sarcasm, or ending the session are non-therapeutic.

9. Correct Answer: D
Rationale: START triage assigns Immediate (red) to RR >30/min, cap refill >2 seconds, or inability to follow commands. The client in option D meets two criteria. A is Minor (green), B is Deceased/expectant (black), and C is Delayed (yellow).

10. Correct Answer: A
Rationale: Normalizing and validating anticipatory grief while inviting further exploration exemplifies therapeutic communication. The other responses are judgmental, prematurely directive, or dismissive of the daughter's emotions.

6.2.5 Basic Care & Comfort

Question 1: A nurse is teaching a client with left-sided weakness after a stroke how to use a standard cane for ambulation on a flat surface. Which instruction is correct?

[A] Hold the cane on the weaker side; move the stronger leg forward first, then the cane, then the weaker leg.
[B] Hold the cane on the stronger side; move the cane forward, then the weaker leg to the level of the cane, followed by the stronger leg past the cane.
[C] Hold the cane on the stronger side; move the stronger leg first, then the cane, then the weaker leg.
[D] Hold the cane on the weaker side; move the cane and stronger leg forward together, then the weaker leg.

Question 2: Before initiating the first feeding through a newly placed nasogastric tube for enteral nutrition, which verification method is required to confirm correct tube placement?

[A] Obtain radiographic (X-ray) confirmation of tube placement.
[B] Auscultate over the stomach while injecting 20 mL of air into the tube.
[C] Check for a pH of 6–8 from aspirated gastric contents.
[D] Observe for the absence of coughing or respiratory distress during insertion.

Question 3: Which nursing action best prevents catheter-associated urinary tract infection (CAUTI) in a client with an indwelling urinary catheter?

[A] Perform routine catheter irrigation every shift to prevent obstruction.
[B] Apply povidone-iodine around the meatus at least twice per shift.
[C] Disconnect the catheter from the drainage tubing to obtain a sterile urine specimen.
[D] Keep the drainage bag below bladder level and off the floor; maintain a closed drainage system.

Question 4: The nurse is assessing a client who had a new end colostomy created 24 hours ago. Which finding requires immediate provider notification?

[A] Stoma is moist, shiny, and red.
[B] Stoma appears dusky/purple with minimal output.
[C] Small amount of bleeding noted when cleansing the stoma.
[D] Mild edema present around the stoma.

Question 5: Which intervention is most effective for promoting sleep and rest for a hospitalized older adult with frequent nighttime awakenings?

[A] Cluster nursing care to minimize nighttime interruptions; dim lights and reduce noise after 2200.
[B] Offer a caffeinated beverage with dinner to prevent nighttime hunger.
[C] Encourage daytime napping for several hours to "catch up" on rest.
[D] Schedule routine vital signs and medication administration every 2 hours at night.

Question 6: A client with an acute ankle sprain is prescribed cold therapy. Which instruction should the nurse provide?

[A] Apply the cold pack directly to the skin continuously for 60 minutes.
[B] Use cold therapy only after the first 48 hours to prevent swelling.
[C] Wrap the cold pack in a towel; apply for about 20 minutes on, then off for at least 20 minutes during the first 24–48 hours.
[D] Alternate cold and heat every 10 minutes for the first hour after injury.

Question 7: What is the priority nursing action when providing oral care to an unconscious client to reduce aspiration risk?

[A] Place the client supine with a small pillow under the neck.
[B] Use lemon-glycerin swabs to moisten the mucosa.
[C] Position the client side-lying with head turned and use suction as needed during oral care.
[D] Insert a large oral airway and pour water gently into the mouth to rinse.

Question 8: A client is receiving continuous enteral feeding via a nasogastric tube. Which nursing action best reduces the risk of aspiration?

[A] Stop the feeding if gastric residual volume is greater than 100 mL once.
[B] Lay the client flat for comfort during feeding, then raise the head of bed afterward.
[C] Maintain the head of bed at 30–45 degrees during feeding and for 30–60 minutes afterward.
[D] Add blue dye to the enteral formula to detect aspiration.

Question 9: The nurse is developing a bowel training program for a client with neurogenic bowel after spinal cord injury. Which strategy is most appropriate?

[A] Schedule toileting 20–30 minutes after breakfast daily to utilize the gastrocolic reflex.
[B] Alternate random toileting times to avoid dependence on a routine.
[C] Restrict fluids to decrease stool frequency and promote continence.
[D] Use a stimulant laxative every night regardless of stool pattern.

Question 10: A hospice client is actively dying and has noisy respiratory secretions ("death rattle") and intermittent dyspnea. Which nursing action is most appropriate?

[A] Perform deep oropharyngeal suctioning every hour to clear secretions.
[B] Reposition laterally, provide gentle oral care, and use anticholinergic drops if prescribed; avoid aggressive suctioning.
[C] Initiate continuous pulse oximetry and titrate oxygen to maintain $SpO_2 > 98\%$.
[D] Bolus IV fluids to thin secretions and reduce noise.

ANSWERS

1. Correct Answer: B
Rationale: Proper cane use on a level surface is to hold the cane on the stronger side, move the cane forward, advance the weaker leg to the level of the cane, then move the stronger leg past the cane. This widens the base of support and transfers weight safely. A and D place the cane on the weaker side, which reduces stability. C advances the stronger leg first, which does not provide adequate support for the weaker side.

2. Correct Answer: A
Rationale: Radiographic confirmation is the gold standard for verifying initial nasogastric tube placement before the first feeding or medication administration. Air auscultation is unreliable; gastric pH testing can be helpful but is not definitive for initial placement; absence of coughing does not confirm gastric placement and is unsafe.

3. Correct Answer: D
Rationale: Keeping the drainage bag below bladder level, off the floor, and maintaining a closed system are key CAUTI prevention measures. Routine irrigation (A) increases infection risk. Disconnecting the system (C) breaks sterility; specimens should be obtained from the sampling port. Routine antiseptic meatal care (B) is not recommended; use routine hygiene with soap and water.

4. Correct Answer: B
Rationale: A dusky/purple or black stoma indicates compromised perfusion/ischemia and requires immediate notification. A moist, red stoma (A) is normal. Small bleeding with cleaning (C) and mild edema (D) are expected in the early postoperative period.

5. Correct Answer: A
Rationale: Clustering care and reducing environmental stimuli at night best promote sleep in hospitalized adults. Caffeine (B) disrupts sleep. Long daytime naps (C) worsen nighttime insomnia. Frequent nighttime interruptions (D) fragment sleep.

6. Correct Answer: C
Rationale: Cold therapy should be applied with a barrier for about 20 minutes on and 20 minutes off for the first 24–48 hours to reduce pain and swelling. Direct application (A) risks tissue injury; waiting 48 hours (B) is not appropriate. Alternating heat and cold immediately after injury (D) is not recommended.

7. Correct Answer: C
Rationale: Side-lying positioning with the head turned and using suction as needed minimizes aspiration risk during oral care in an unconscious client. Supine positioning (A) increases aspiration risk. Lemon-glycerin swabs (B) can dry mucosa. Pouring water into the mouth (D) is unsafe and may cause aspiration.

8. Correct Answer: C
Rationale: Elevating the head of bed to 30–45 degrees during and after enteral feedings reduces aspiration risk. Single residual values (A) are not by themselves an indication to stop feedings; thresholds vary by policy. Lying flat (B) increases aspiration risk. Adding blue dye (D) is unsafe and not recommended.

9. Correct Answer: A
Rationale: Scheduling toileting after breakfast leverages the gastrocolic reflex to promote bowel evacuation and consistency. Random schedules (B) hinder training. Fluid restriction (C) can worsen constipation. Routine stimulant laxatives (D) risk dependence; bowel regimens should be individualized.

10. Correct Answer: B
Rationale: In end-of-life care, managing terminal secretions focuses on comfort: lateral positioning, gentle oral care, and anticholinergic agents as prescribed. Aggressive deep suctioning (A) is uncomfortable and ineffective. Continuous monitoring and high oxygen targets (C) do not enhance comfort. IV fluids (D) can worsen secretions and discomfort.

6.2.6 Pharmacological & Parenteral Therapies

Question 1: A postoperative adult client has an order for morphine sulfate 2 mg IV every 2 hours PRN for pain. On assessment, the client is difficult to arouse, has shallow respirations at 8/min, SpO2 88% on 2 L/min via nasal cannula, and a sedation score of 3 (frequently drowsy, arousable). What is the nurse's priority action?

[A] Administer the morphine as ordered and recheck sedation in 30 minutes
[B] Reduce the morphine dose to 1 mg IV and administer now
[C] Document the findings and reassess in 15 minutes
[D] Withhold morphine, support respirations, and prepare to administer naloxone; notify the provider

Question 2: A client with systolic heart failure is taking lisinopril. The provider adds spironolactone to improve morbidity. Which laboratory result should the nurse report to the provider before administering the first dose of spironolactone?

[A] Sodium 134 mEq/L
[B] Potassium 5.8 mEq/L
[C] Creatinine 1.0 mg/dL
[D] BUN 18 mg/dL

Question 3: The provider orders lactated Ringer's at 125 mL/hr via gravity to an adult client. The tubing has a drop factor of 60 gtt/mL. What is the correct drip rate in gtt/min?

[A] 125 gtt/min
[B] 60 gtt/min
[C] 31 gtt/min
[D] 250 gtt/min

Question 4: Fifteen minutes into a transfusion of packed red blood cells (PRBCs), a client reports chills, back pain, and feels "very anxious." Vital signs show T 38.9°C (102°F), BP 88/52, HR 124, RR 26. What is the nurse's priority action?

[A] Slow the transfusion rate and reassess in 10 minutes
[B] Administer acetaminophen for fever and continue the transfusion
[C] Stop the transfusion immediately, maintain IV access with normal saline using new tubing, and notify the provider and blood bank
[D] Obtain a urine sample to test for hemoglobin before stopping the transfusion

Question 5: A client is receiving total parenteral nutrition (TPN) via a central line. The TPN bag is nearly empty, and the pharmacy informs the nurse the next bag will be delayed. Which solution should the nurse hang to prevent hypoglycemia until the next TPN bag arrives?

[A] Dextrose 10% in water (D10W) at the previous TPN rate
[B] 0.9% sodium chloride at keep-vein-open rate
[C] Lactated Ringer's at the previous TPN rate
[D] Dextrose 5% in water (D5W) at 50 mL/hr

Question 6: The nurse is preparing to administer the next scheduled dose of warfarin to a client with atrial fibrillation. Which finding requires immediate intervention before administration?

[A] INR 2.4
[B] INR 4.5
[C] aPTT 30 seconds
[D] Platelets 140,000/mm^3

Question 7: Which action best reduces central line-associated bloodstream infection (CLABSI) risk during a routine transparent dressing change for a tunneled central venous catheter?

[A] Cleanse the site with alcohol and apply dry gauze using clean gloves
[B] Have only the client wear a mask; the nurse may speak during the procedure without a mask
[C] Perform hand hygiene; don a mask and sterile gloves; scrub with chlorhexidine in a back-and-forth motion for at least 30 seconds and allow it to dry completely before applying a sterile transparent dressing
[D] Use povidone-iodine, then blow on the site to speed drying before replacing the dressing

Question 8: The nurse is teaching a family caregiver about handling chemotherapy excreta after the client receives an IV vesicant agent. Which statement indicates correct understanding?

[A] "I can flush urine and stool without gloves after 12 hours."
[B] "If the client can't swallow the oral chemo pill, I can crush it and mix it with applesauce."
[C] "Pregnant caregivers can handle chemotherapy waste with standard gloves as long as they wash hands after."
[D] "I will wear double gloves and a disposable chemotherapy-rated gown when handling body fluids for at least 48 hours after treatment."

Question 9: A client on digoxin for heart failure presents for routine labs. Which finding places the client at greatest risk for digoxin toxicity?

[A] Potassium 3.0 mEq/L
[B] Apical heart rate 68/min
[C] Digoxin level 1.4 ng/mL
[D] Creatinine 0.9 mg/dL

Question 10: Heparin 18 units/kg/hr is prescribed for a client weighing 70 kg. The pharmacy dispenses heparin 25,000 units in 250 mL D5W. What infusion rate (mL/hr) should the nurse set on the IV pump?

[A] 8 mL/hr
[B] 11 mL/hr
[C] 13 mL/hr
[D] 21 mL/hr

ANSWERS

1. Correct Answer: D

Rationale: The client shows opioid-induced respiratory depression (RR 8/min, sedation). The priority is to withhold the opioid, support respirations (increase O2, prepare to ventilate if needed), and prepare to administer naloxone; notify the provider. Administering or reducing the dose (A, B) is unsafe; delaying action (C) risks deterioration.

2. Correct Answer: B

Rationale: ACE inhibitors (lisinopril) plus potassium-sparing diuretics (spironolactone) increase hyperkalemia risk; K^+ 5.8 mEq/L is dangerous. The other labs are acceptable for initiation.

3. Correct Answer: A

Rationale: Microdrip tubing is 60 gtt/mL. gtt/min = (125 mL/hr × 60 gtt/mL) ÷ 60 min/hr = 125 gtt/min.

4. Correct Answer: C

Rationale: Suspected acute hemolytic transfusion reaction requires stopping the transfusion immediately, keeping the line open with normal saline using new tubing, and notifying the provider/blood bank. Slowing (A) or treating symptoms while continuing (B) is unsafe. Labs (D) are obtained after stopping.

5. Correct Answer: A

Rationale: If TPN is interrupted, hang D10W at the same rate to prevent rebound hypoglycemia. NS or LR (B, C) lack dextrose; D5W (D) may be insufficient depending on the prior TPN dextrose concentration.

6. Correct Answer: B

Rationale: For most indications, therapeutic INR is 2.0–3.0. INR 4.5 indicates supratherapeutic anticoagulation—hold dose and notify the provider. INR 2.4 is therapeutic (A). aPTT (C) monitors heparin, not warfarin. Platelets 140k (D) is low-normal.

7. Correct Answer: C

Rationale: CLABSI prevention includes hand hygiene, mask for nurse (and client if possible), sterile gloves, chlorhexidine scrub with friction for ≥30 seconds, and allowing it to dry before applying a sterile transparent dressing. The other options break aseptic technique.

8. Correct Answer: D

Rationale: Cytotoxic drug excreta require hazardous precautions for at least 48 hours post-infusion; use double chemotherapy-rated gloves and an impermeable disposable gown. Never crush oral chemo (B). Gloves are required beyond 12 hours (A). Pregnant caregivers should avoid handling (C).

9. Correct Answer: A

Rationale: Hypokalemia potentiates digoxin toxicity. Normal HR (B), therapeutic digoxin level (C), and normal renal function (D) do not increase risk.

10. Correct Answer: C

Rationale: Dose = 18 units/kg/hr × 70 kg = 1,260 units/hr. Concentration = 25,000 units/250 mL = 100 units/mL. Rate = 1,260 ÷ 100 = 12.6 ≈ 13 mL/hr.

6.2.7 Reduction of Risk Potential

Question 1: A nurse receives a STAT lab report for a postoperative client showing a serum potassium of 6.8 mEq/L. The client is currently on a med-surg unit and denies chest pain. Which action should the nurse take first to reduce risk of complications?

[A] Initiate continuous cardiac monitoring and assess for dysrhythmias
[B] Repeat the blood draw to verify the result before taking any action
[C] Administer sodium polystyrene sulfonate (kayexalate) if available on the unit
[D] Place the client on a potassium-restricted diet and encourage oral fluids

Question 2: A client 24 hours after total hip arthroplasty reports new calf discomfort. Which finding most strongly suggests development of a deep vein thrombosis (DVT)?

[A] Unilateral calf warmth, tenderness, and increased circumference compared with the other leg
[B] Bilateral +1 pitting edema at the ankles by the end of the day
[C] Cool, pale foot with capillary refill less than 2 seconds
[D] Ecchymosis around the surgical site

Question 3: You are monitoring a client with a traumatic brain injury. Which new assessment finding is the highest priority to report immediately?

[A] Decline in GCS from 15 to 13 with new-onset projectile vomiting
[B] Oral temperature increase from 98.6°F (37°C) to 100.2°F (37.9°C)
[C] Headache rated 3/10 relieved with acetaminophen
[D] Blood pressure change from 130/80 mm Hg to 138/84 mm Hg

Question 4: A client with a new arteriovenous (AV) fistula for hemodialysis is learning fistula care. Which client statement indicates correct understanding?

[A] "I will use my fistula arm for blood draws so we don't have to poke the other arm."
[B] "It's okay to carry heavy grocery bags with my fistula arm as long as it doesn't hurt."
[C] "I should avoid blood pressure measurements and venipunctures in the fistula arm."
[D] "If I notice minor bleeding at the fistula site, I will apply a tight bandage overnight."

Question 5: A postoperative client suddenly becomes acutely short of breath with pleuritic chest pain and an SpO2 of 86% on 2 L nasal cannula. The client is tachycardic and anxious. Which action should the nurse take first?

[A] Notify the provider to request a STAT CT angiography
[B] Start a second large-bore IV for possible anticoagulation
[C] Position the client in high Fowler and encourage deep breathing only
[D] Elevate the head of bed and apply high-flow oxygen via nonrebreather mask

Question 6: The nurse is preparing to suction a client with a newly placed tracheostomy. Which action is most important to reduce the risk of hypoxemia during the procedure?

[A] Pre-oxygenate with 100% oxygen for 30–60 seconds before suctioning
[B] Instill 5 mL of sterile normal saline into the trach to loosen secretions
[C] Apply continuous suction while inserting the catheter to the measured depth
[D] Perform multiple rapid suction passes back-to-back to clear the airway quickly

Question 7: A client with type 1 diabetes is scheduled for surgery at 0800 and has been NPO since midnight. At 0700, the capillary glucose is 62 mg/dL, and the client is drowsy and diaphoretic. What is the priority action?

[A] Proceed to surgery and treat hypoglycemia intraoperatively
[B] Administer the scheduled long-acting insulin to prevent perioperative hyperglycemia
[C] Document the finding and recheck the glucose in 30 minutes
[D] Administer IV dextrose per hypoglycemia protocol and notify the surgeon/anesthesia

Question 8: A client with septic shock remains hypotensive after a 30 mL/kg crystalloid bolus. Vitals: BP 84/50 mm Hg, HR 122/min, MAP 58 mm Hg, SpO_2 93% on 4 L NC, urine output 15 mL/hr. Which order should the nurse anticipate to achieve hemodynamic goals?

[A] Start nitroprusside infusion to reduce afterload
[B] Initiate norepinephrine and titrate to maintain MAP ≥ 65 mm Hg
[C] Restrict fluids and administer a diuretic for oliguria
[D] Obtain an arterial blood gas and withhold vasopressors until results return

Question 9: Four hours after a total thyroidectomy, a client reports numbness around the mouth and tingling in the fingertips. The nurse also notes a positive Chvostek sign. Which intervention is the priority?

[A] Encourage oral calcium carbonate tablets with water
[B] Increase the IV lactated Ringer's rate to 150 mL/hr
[C] Place the client in Trendelenburg position and reassess in 15 minutes
[D] Prepare to administer IV calcium gluconate as prescribed

Question 10: A client with a recent stroke has facial droop and dysarthria. Before administering scheduled oral medications, which action is most appropriate to reduce aspiration risk?

[A] Hold oral medications and request a speech-language pathology swallow evaluation
[B] Crush all medications and mix with thin liquids to facilitate swallowing
[C] Place the client supine to reduce fatigue during swallowing
[D] Offer small sips of water to assess the gag reflex at the bedside

ANSWERS

1. Correct Answer: A
Rationale: Severe hyperkalemia places the client at immediate risk for life-threatening dysrhythmias. Initiating continuous cardiac monitoring is the first priority to detect and respond to arrhythmias while additional actions (repeat labs, treatment orders) are arranged.

2. Correct Answer: A
Rationale: Unilateral calf warmth, tenderness, and increased circumference are classic signs of DVT. Bilateral ankle edema is common and nonspecific; cool pale foot suggests arterial insufficiency; ecchymosis near the incision is expected post-op.

3. Correct Answer: A
Rationale: A drop in GCS and projectile vomiting indicate rising intracranial pressure and possible herniation risk, requiring immediate provider notification and interventions. Mild fever, mild headache, and small BP changes are less urgent.

4. Correct Answer: C
Rationale: Protecting the AV fistula includes avoiding BP measurements, venipuncture, and IVs in the fistula arm to prevent thrombosis or damage. Heavy lifting and tight bandaging can compromise flow.

5. Correct Answer: D
Rationale: Suspected pulmonary embolism is a life-threatening emergency. The priority is to improve oxygenation—elevate HOB and apply high-flow oxygen—while further diagnostics and treatments are initiated.

6. Correct Answer: A
Rationale: Pre-oxygenation reduces the risk of hypoxemia during suctioning. Instilling saline is not recommended; suction should be applied on withdrawal only, and passes should be limited and spaced to allow reoxygenation.

7. Correct Answer: D
Rationale: This client is hypoglycemic and symptomatic. Treat immediately with IV dextrose (NPO) and notify the surgical team; surgery may need to be delayed. Administering long-acting insulin or delaying treatment increases risk.

8. Correct Answer: B
Rationale: After adequate fluid resuscitation, persistent hypotension in septic shock warrants a vasopressor. Norepinephrine is first-line to maintain MAP ≥ 65 mm Hg. Nitroprusside would worsen hypotension; delaying vasopressors is unsafe.

9. Correct Answer: D
Rationale: Post-thyroidectomy hypocalcemia from parathyroid injury is an airway risk (laryngospasm). IV calcium gluconate is the priority intervention. Oral calcium acts too slowly; fluids and positioning do not correct hypocalcemia.

10. Correct Answer: A
Rationale: Clients with stroke require a formal swallow evaluation before any oral intake. Crushing meds into thin liquids or bedside “sip tests” increases aspiration risk; supine positioning further impairs airway protection.

6.2.8 Physiological Adaptation

Question 1: A 72-year-old postoperative patient is increasingly confused, complains of headache and nausea, and has a serum sodium of 118 mEq/L. Which initial nursing action is the priority?

[A] Initiate seizure precautions, maintain patent IV access, and notify the provider of acute neurologic changes
[B] Encourage increased oral free water intake to correct perceived dehydration
[C] Begin a hypotonic IV infusion (0.45% NS) at 125 mL/hr without a new prescription
[D] Restrict dietary sodium to prevent further fluid retention

Question 2: A patient with chronic kidney disease presents with muscle weakness. ECG shows tall peaked T waves and a widened QRS; serum potassium is 6.9 mEq/L. What is the nurse's immediate priority action?

[A] Administer oral sodium polystyrene sulfonate to remove potassium via the GI tract
[B] Start 0.9% normal saline at 250 mL/hr to promote urinary potassium excretion
[C] Give 10 units IV regular insulin without dextrose to shift potassium intracellularly
[D] Administer IV calcium gluconate to stabilize cardiac membranes while preparing additional therapies

Question 3: A postoperative patient on continuous NG suction has the following ABG: pH 7.50, $PaCO_2$ 47 mm Hg, HCO_3^- 36 mEq/L. Which interpretation is most accurate?

[A] Respiratory alkalosis with partial metabolic compensation
[B] Respiratory acidosis without compensation
[C] Metabolic alkalosis with partial respiratory compensation
[D] Metabolic acidosis with complete compensation

Question 4: A patient receiving IV antibiotics develops sudden wheezing, stridor, generalized urticaria, and hypotension. Which action should the nurse take first?

[A] Elevate the head of the bed and apply high-flow oxygen via nonrebreather mask
[B] Stop the antibiotic infusion and keep the IV line patent with normal saline
[C] Start a rapid infusion of 1–2 L of 0.9% normal saline
[D] Administer intramuscular epinephrine 0.3–0.5 mg (1 mg/mL) to the anterolateral thigh

Question 5: A 69-year-old arrives with right-sided weakness and facial droop. Last-known-well was 1 hour ago. BP is 190/110 mm Hg; fingerstick glucose is 60 mg/dL. Head CT is pending. What is the priority action?

[A] Prepare to administer alteplase immediately given the narrow time window
[B] Rapidly lower blood pressure to <140/90 mm Hg with IV antihypertensive
[C] Administer 25 g of IV dextrose (D50) and reassess neurologic status
[D] Give aspirin 325 mg PO while awaiting neuroimaging

Question 6: A patient with a chest tube to suction for a pneumothorax becomes anxious and short of breath. The nurse notes the chest tube has become disconnected from the drainage system. What should the nurse do first?

[A] Clamp the chest tube near the patient to prevent air entry into the pleural space
[B] Immediately apply petroleum gauze over the insertion site to seal the chest wall
[C] Reconnect the tube to the drainage system after wiping with alcohol
[D] Place the distal end of the chest tube into sterile water 1–2 cm to create a temporary water seal

Question 7: A patient 2 hours post–abdominal surgery has a rapidly saturating dressing with bright red blood, HR 126/min, BP 86/50 mm Hg, and cool, clammy skin. Which action is the priority?

[A] Increase maintenance IV fluids and reassess in 15 minutes
[B] Apply firm direct pressure to the incision, call a rapid response, and prepare for possible transfusion
[C] Remove the dressing to directly visualize the incision before intervening further
[D] Place the patient in Trendelenburg and leave to notify the surgeon immediately

Question 8: A 64-year-old with COPD exacerbation has dyspnea, RR 28/min, and SpO2 84% on room air. An ABG yesterday showed chronic hypercapnia. Which oxygen strategy is most appropriate initially?

[A] Nonrebreather mask at 15 L/min targeting SpO2 >98%
[B] Nasal cannula at 1 L/min targeting SpO2 ≥95%
[C] Venturi mask delivering 28% FiO2, titrated to maintain SpO2 88–92%
[D] High-flow nasal cannula at 60 L/min with FiO2 100%

Question 9: A telemetry patient becomes unresponsive, pulseless, and apneic. The monitor shows coarse ventricular fibrillation. What is the next best action?

[A] Perform synchronized cardioversion at the highest energy setting
[B] Administer atropine 1 mg IV and reassess rhythm
[C] Obtain a 12-lead ECG to confirm the arrhythmia before treating
[D] Deliver an immediate unsynchronized defibrillation shock, then resume CPR for 2 minutes

Question 10: The nurse is teaching a patient with chronic systolic heart failure about home management. Which statement indicates correct understanding?

[A] "I will drink at least 3 liters of water daily so my kidneys stay flushed."
[B] "I can take ibuprofen for joint pain because it won't affect my heart failure."
[C] "If I feel better, I can stop my beta-blocker so my heart rate won't get too low."
[D] "I will weigh myself every morning and call the provider if I gain 3 lb in a day or 5 lb in a week."

ANSWERS

1. Correct Answer: A
Rationale: Severe hyponatremia increases risk for cerebral edema and seizures. Priority is patient safety: institute seizure precautions, maintain IV access, and notify the provider. Encouraging free water (B) worsens hyponatremia. Initiating hypotonic fluids without orders (C) is inappropriate and harmful. Sodium restriction (D) is not indicated and can worsen the problem.

2. Correct Answer: D
Rationale: With ECG changes from hyperkalemia, the first priority is IV calcium to stabilize myocardial cells and prevent lethal arrhythmias. Insulin (with dextrose) and other measures follow to shift or remove potassium. Kayexalate (A) acts slowly. Normal saline (B) won't promptly correct hyperkalemia. Giving insulin without dextrose (C) risks hypoglycemia.

3. Correct Answer: C
Rationale: pH is alkalemic; HCO_3^- is elevated, indicating a metabolic alkalosis. The elevated $PaCO_2$ reflects partial respiratory compensation. Respiratory alkalosis (A) would show low $PaCO_2$. Respiratory acidosis (B) has low pH with high $PaCO_2$. Metabolic acidosis (D) would show low pH and low HCO_3^-.

4. Correct Answer: D
Rationale: IM epinephrine is the first-line, life-saving treatment for anaphylaxis with airway compromise and hypotension. Oxygen (A), stopping the causative agent (B), and IV fluids (C) are important adjuncts but must not delay epinephrine.

5. Correct Answer: C
Rationale: Hypoglycemia can mimic or worsen stroke deficits and must be corrected immediately. Thrombolysis (A) requires exclusion of hemorrhage and BP ≤185/110 mm Hg; giving aspirin (D) before imaging is unsafe. Rapid aggressive BP lowering (B) can reduce cerebral perfusion; modest BP control is considered only to meet tPA criteria.

6. Correct Answer: D
Rationale: Submerging the distal chest tube in sterile water creates a temporary water seal to prevent air from entering the pleural space until the system is replaced. Clamping (A) risks tension pneumothorax. Petroleum gauze (B) is for accidental tube dislodgment from the chest. Reconnecting directly (C) delays establishing a seal and risks contamination and air entry.

7. Correct Answer: B
Rationale: Findings suggest acute postoperative hemorrhage and shock. Priority is to control external bleeding with direct pressure, activate rapid response, and prepare for resuscitation (IV access, type and cross, transfusion). Simply increasing fluids (A) delays definitive action. Removing the dressing (C) can disrupt clots; reinforce instead. Do not leave the patient (D).

8. Correct Answer: C
Rationale: In COPD with chronic hypercapnia, target SpO_2 is 88–92%. A Venturi mask delivers precise FiO_2 for controlled titration. Nonrebreather at high FiO_2 (A) and 100% HFNC (D) risk oxygen-induced hypercapnia. A 1 L/min cannula targeting ≥95% (B) sets an inappropriate saturation goal.

9. Correct Answer: D
Rationale: Pulseless VF requires immediate unsynchronized defibrillation followed by CPR for 2 minutes before rhythm check per ACLS. Synchronized cardioversion (A) is for unstable tachyarrhythmias with a pulse. Atropine (B) is for bradycardia. A 12-lead (C) should not delay defibrillation.

10. Correct Answer: D
Rationale: Daily weights with prompt reporting of rapid gains help detect fluid overload in heart failure. Fluid restriction is often needed; 3 L/day (A) may worsen volume status. NSAIDs (B) exacerbate fluid retention and reduce renal perfusion. Beta-blockers (C) should not be stopped abruptly; they improve outcomes in HFrEF.

6.3 Exam 3

6.3.1 Management of Care

Question 1: A client is scheduled for an urgent laparoscopic appendectomy. The provider has not yet discussed risks, benefits, and alternatives with the client, and the consent form is not signed. The client is about to receive the prescribed preoperative sedative. What is the nurse's best action?

[A] Witness the client's signature on the consent form since the procedure is urgent.
[B] Hold the sedative and notify the surgeon to obtain informed consent prior to medication administration.
[C] Administer the sedative now and obtain the signed consent when the client is relaxed.
[D] Explain the risks, benefits, and alternatives to obtain informed consent as the nurse.

Question 2: The charge nurse is prioritizing assessments at the start of the shift. Which client should the nurse assess first?

[A] A client with COPD on 2 L/min via nasal cannula with an oxygen saturation of 90% and a productive cough.
[B] A client 2 hours post-thyroidectomy with new-onset stridor and difficulty breathing.
[C] A client NPO for a procedure who reports thirst and mild anxiety.
[D] A client post–total hip arthroplasty with pain rated 8/10 requesting analgesia.

Question 3: Which task is appropriate for the RN to delegate to an experienced LPN/VN?

[A] Perform the initial assessment on a client who just arrived with chest pain.
[B] Provide initial teaching on anticoagulant therapy to a client with new-onset atrial fibrillation.
[C] Titrate an IV insulin infusion for a client in DKA following a protocol change.
[D] Perform a sterile dressing change on a stable postoperative day-3 abdominal surgical wound.

Question 4: The case manager is planning discharge for a client with advanced COPD who will require continuous home oxygen, nebulizer treatments, and frequent follow-up. Which action best promotes continuity of care?

[A] Arrange durable medical equipment delivery (oxygen concentrator, portable tanks), confirm home health nursing visits, and schedule pulmonology follow-up before discharge.
[B] Personally recheck all medication dosages with the bedside nurse before the client leaves.
[C] Delay interdisciplinary rounds until staffing improves tomorrow to ensure more team members can attend.
[D] Suggest the family purchase medications abroad to reduce cost and improve adherence.

Question 5: A competent adult client who is a Jehovah's Witness refuses a blood transfusion for symptomatic anemia after receiving information about risks and alternatives. What is the nurse's best action?

[A] Ask the client's family to persuade them to consent due to the severity of the anemia.
[B] Explain that without blood, the hospital could be liable and transfusion is necessary.
[C] Respect the refusal, verify understanding, document the decision, notify the provider, and explore acceptable alternatives (e.g., epoetin, iron, volume expanders).
[D] Request a court order to proceed with the transfusion given the clinical indication.

Question 6: Unit data show an increased rate of patient falls on the night shift over the past month. What should the nurse manager do first as part of a quality improvement process?

[A] Implement bed and chair alarms on every patient immediately.
[B] Place the primary night-shift nurse on a performance improvement plan for negligence.
[C] Conduct a focused chart review and root cause analysis to identify patterns and system factors contributing to the falls.
[D] Provide an urgent in-service on fall prevention and require staff to sign attendance sheets.

Question 7: A 21-year-old client is stable after a motor vehicle collision. The client's father calls the unit and asks for an update on the client's condition. The client has not given permission to share information. What is the nurse's best response?

[A] Decline to provide information without the client's consent and offer to obtain the client's permission to speak with the father.
[B] Provide a brief update because the caller is an immediate family member.
[C] Transfer the call to hospital security to handle the situation.
[D] Ask the physician to call the father since providers can disclose information to family.

Question 8: The charge nurse is making assignments for one RN, one LPN/VN, and one UAP on a medical-surgical unit. Which assignment is most appropriate?

[A] RN: POD-2 cholecystectomy—dressing change; LPN/VN: new pneumonia admission—initial assessment; UAP: feeding a stroke client before a swallow screen (unsafe).
[B] RN: stable heart failure on oral diuretics; LPN/VN: start/titrate IV antibiotics for new pneumonia (not within scope); UAP: manage NG tube to low intermittent suction (not within scope).
[C] RN: admit new CAP (initial assessment + IV antibiotics) and reinforce sodium-restricted diet teaching for stable HF; LPN/VN: POD-2 cholecystectomy (sterile dressing change + scheduled oral analgesics); UAP: assist feeding after a documented swallow screen with posted precautions and ambulate with a walker per RN plan.
[D] RN: routine care to stable HF only (underutilized); LPN/VN: complete pneumonia admission assessment (not within scope); UAP: irrigate NG tube and verify placement before meds (not within scope).

Question 9: Which client may legally provide their own informed consent for a procedure?

[A] A 16-year-old with a court order of emancipation for independent living.
[B] A 70-year-old with advanced dementia who appears calm and cooperative.
[C] A 45-year-old who received IV opioids 30 minutes ago for severe pain.
[D] A 25-year-old who does not speak English and declines an interpreter.

Question 10: The RN delegates routine vital signs during a blood transfusion to an experienced UAP per unit protocol after the first 15 minutes. One hour into the transfusion, the UAP reports a temperature of 38.6°C (101.5°F) and chills. What is the RN's priority action?

[A] Ask the UAP to recheck the temperature in 15 minutes to confirm the reading.
[B] Document the finding and continue the transfusion because a mild fever is expected.
[C] Give acetaminophen per PRN order and reassess in 30 minutes.
[D] Stop the transfusion immediately, maintain IV access with normal saline, assess the client, verify identification, and notify the provider and blood bank.

ANSWERS

1. Correct Answer: B

Rationale: Informed consent must be obtained by the provider before sedation, which can impair decision-making. The nurse should hold the sedative and notify the surgeon. A: Witnessing is improper when the provider has not explained. C: Consent after sedation is invalid. D: Nurses cannot obtain informed consent by providing the procedure's risks/benefits.

2. Correct Answer: B

Rationale: New-onset stridor and breathing difficulty post-thyroidectomy indicates potential airway compromise (edema/hematoma/hypocalcemia) requiring immediate assessment. A: COPD sat 90% may be baseline. C: Discomfort is not emergent. D: Pain is important but not life-threatening compared with airway obstruction.

3. Correct Answer: D

Rationale: LPN/VNs can perform sterile procedures and care for stable clients. A: Initial assessment requires RN. B: Initial teaching is an RN responsibility. C: IV titration for an unstable metabolic condition (DKA) and protocol change requires RN judgment.

4. Correct Answer: A

Rationale: Case management focuses on coordination of services to ensure safe transitions and continuity of care, including arranging DME, home services, and follow-up before discharge. B: Med checks are a bedside RN task; not the primary role of case management. C: Delaying rounds hinders coordination. D: Advising foreign medication purchases is unsafe and inappropriate.

5. Correct Answer: C

Rationale: Respect for autonomy requires honoring informed refusal. The nurse verifies understanding, documents, notifies the provider, and explores acceptable alternatives. A and B: Coercion violates patient rights. D: Courts are not used to override a competent adult's informed refusal.

6. Correct Answer: C

Rationale: QI begins with problem identification and analysis (e.g., chart review, RCA) to determine system contributors before selecting interventions. A and D: Implementing interventions without analysis risks inefficacy. B: Punitive action undermines a just culture and may not address system causes.

7. Correct Answer: A

Rationale: HIPAA requires patient authorization before disclosing PHI. Offer to obtain consent from the client. B and D: Family or provider status does not negate the need for consent. C: Security is not indicated.

8. Correct Answer: C

Rationale: The RN handles initial assessments and higher-acuity tasks; the LPN/VN manages stable, predictable clients with sterile procedures and oral meds; the UAP assists with ADLs/ambulation/feeding after RN sets the plan and safety (swallow screen) is confirmed. A, B, D include assignments beyond scope (e.g., LPN completing initial admission assessment, UAP managing NG tube or feeding before swallow clearance).

9. Correct Answer: A

Rationale: An emancipated minor can legally consent. B: Dementia implies lack of capacity; a surrogate is needed. C: Recent opioids impair capacity. D: Consent without an interpreter does not ensure understanding and is not valid.

10. Correct Answer: D

Rationale: Fever and chills suggest a transfusion reaction. The RN must stop the transfusion, maintain IV with NS, assess, verify patient/blood product, and notify the provider/blood bank. A: Delays care. B: Minimizes a potentially serious reaction. C: Treating fever without stopping the transfusion is unsafe.

6.3.2 Safety & Infection Prevention and Control

Question 1: The nurse is preparing to enter the room of a patient on droplet precautions to administer medications. Which sequence best reflects the correct order for donning personal protective equipment (PPE) to reduce the risk of self-contamination?

[A] Gloves, gown, mask, goggles
[B] Mask, gown, gloves, goggles
[C] Gown, mask, goggles or face shield, gloves
[D] Goggles, mask, gloves, gown

Question 2: A patient arrives in the ED with weight loss, night sweats, hemoptysis, and a positive TB screening. Which action is the priority?

[A] Place a surgical mask on the patient and move them to a negative-pressure room; staff don N95 respirators before entry
[B] Initiate droplet precautions and provide tissues and a trash can at the bedside
[C] Collect three morning sputum samples for AFB before moving the patient to isolation
[D] Put on a standard surgical mask and place the patient with a roommate who has influenza to conserve private rooms

Question 3: During a central line dressing change using surgical asepsis, which action by the nurse maintains a sterile field?

[A] Reaching over the sterile field to reposition the drape if it shifts
[B] Moistening sterile gloves with sterile saline if they feel tacky
[C] Opening the sterile package by unfolding the top flap away from the body first and keeping all sterile items above waist level
[D] Considering the entire surface of the sterile drape sterile, including the outer 1-inch border

Question 4: The provider orders bilateral soft wrist restraints for a confused patient pulling at IV lines after all alternatives have failed. Which nursing action is appropriate?

[A] Apply restraints as needed and obtain the provider's order within 24 hours; no additional monitoring is necessary
[B] Tie the restraints to the side rails for quick removal in case of emergency
[C] Secure restraints to the bed frame with a quick-release knot, allow two fingers under the restraint, and assess skin, circulation, toileting needs, and range of motion at least every 2 hours
[D] Keep the patient supine with all four side rails up to further prevent falls and device removal

Question 5: The nurse is caring for a patient with Clostridioides difficile-associated diarrhea. Which infection-control approach is most appropriate?

[A] Wear a mask only if the patient is coughing; use alcohol-based hand rub when leaving the room
[B] Place the patient in a negative-pressure room and use an N95 respirator for all care
[C] Don gown and gloves for every room entry, perform hand hygiene with soap and water after removing PPE, and use dedicated equipment and a sporicidal disinfectant for surfaces
[D] Cohort this patient with another patient with MRSA to conserve private rooms

Question 6: The nurse must transport a patient on droplet precautions for influenza to radiology. Which action is correct?

[A] Don an N95 respirator and route the patient via a negative-pressure corridor
[B] Place a surgical mask on the patient, ensure hand hygiene, and notify radiology of droplet precautions
[C] No mask is needed if transport time is under 10 minutes; wear gloves only
[D] Cover the patient completely with a clean sheet to prevent droplet spread; no mask is necessary

Question 7: A nurse is exiting the room of a patient on airborne precautions. Which sequence for removing PPE minimizes self-contamination?

[A] Gown, gloves, mask, goggles; perform hand hygiene inside the room
[B] Gloves, face shield or goggles, gown, then remove the N95 respirator after leaving the patient room; perform hand hygiene
[C] Mask first to facilitate breathing, then gloves, goggles, gown; perform hand hygiene
[D] Gloves, gown, mask, goggles; then perform hand hygiene outside the room

Question 8: A cytotoxic chemotherapy solution spills on the floor outside the medication room. What is the nurse's immediate action?

[A] Wipe the spill with paper towels and discard them in a red biohazard bag
[B] Call housekeeping and continue medication administration until they arrive
[C] Place absorbent pads on the spill and remove gloves to prevent contamination
[D] Isolate the area, don chemotherapy-tested PPE, and clean the spill using the facility's chemo spill kit per the Safety Data Sheet (SDS), then report per policy

Question 9: The nurse discovers a small fire in a patient's trash can. Following the RACE protocol, which sequence is correct?

[A] Activate the alarm, then assess which patients need to be rescued, open doors for ventilation, and wait for the fire department
[B] Attempt to extinguish the fire first, then call the alarm, then remove patients if the fire spreads
[C] Remove oxygen from the wall outlets throughout the unit, then attempt to extinguish
[D] Remove the patient from immediate danger, activate the alarm, close doors to contain smoke, then use a fire extinguisher if safe

Question 10: Which practice best reduces alarm fatigue while maintaining patient safety on a telemetry unit?

[A] Set alarm thresholds to the widest allowable limits to minimize nuisance alarms
[B] Customize alarm parameters to the patient's condition, verify proper sensor placement, ensure alarms are audible, and respond promptly with escalation per policy
[C] Silence frequent alarms for up to 15 minutes while the nurse is in the room to prevent disturbing the patient
[D] Share a single pulse oximeter probe among multiple patients to reduce the number of devices alarming

ANSWERS

1. Correct Answer: C
Rationale: Donning sequence is gown, mask/respirator, goggles/face shield, then gloves. This order minimizes contamination of clean areas during donning.

2. Correct Answer: A
Rationale: Suspected pulmonary TB requires source control (surgical mask on the patient) and immediate airborne isolation in a negative-pressure room; staff must wear N95 respirators.

3. Correct Answer: C
Rationale: Surgical asepsis requires opening the sterile pack away from the body first, keeping items above waist level, and maintaining a sterile field. The 1-inch border is considered contaminated.

4. Correct Answer: C
Rationale: Safe restraint use includes securing to the bed frame with a quick-release knot, allowing two fingers under the restraint, and providing/documenting frequent assessments and care at least every 2 hours.

5. Correct Answer: C
Rationale: C. difficile requires contact precautions with gown and gloves, soap-and-water hand hygiene (alcohol is ineffective against spores), dedicated equipment, and sporicidal (bleach) surface disinfection.

6. Correct Answer: B
Rationale: For droplet precautions, place a surgical mask on the patient during transport and notify receiving departments. N95 and negative-pressure are not required for influenza.

7. Correct Answer: B
Rationale: Doffing order to reduce self-contamination: gloves, face shield/goggles, gown, then respirator after exiting the room, followed by hand hygiene.

8. Correct Answer: D
Rationale: Hazardous drug spills require isolating the area, donning chemo-tested PPE, and using the chemo spill kit per the SDS, followed by reporting/exposure procedures.

9. Correct Answer: D
Rationale: RACE: Rescue those in danger, Activate alarm, Contain by closing doors, Extinguish if safe. The sequence prioritizes life safety and containment.

10. Correct Answer: B
Rationale: Alarm safety focuses on individualized parameters, correct sensor placement, ensuring audible alarms, prompt response, and escalation—actions that reduce false alarms without compromising safety.

6.3.3 Health Promotion & Maintenance

Question 1: A parent of a 5-month-old asks about starting complementary foods. Which response by the nurse indicates correct guidance to promote safe nutrition and development?

[A] Start pureed solids at 3 months so the baby sleeps through the night; offer mixed foods to increase variety quickly.
[B] Wait until about 6 months, when the infant has good head/neck control and can sit with support; begin with single-ingredient, iron-fortified foods and introduce one new food every 3–5 days.
[C] Add honey to cereal to reduce the risk of allergies in the first year.
[D] Start cow's milk now to ensure adequate calcium and vitamin D intake.

Question 2: A client in her first trimester asks about the prenatal visit schedule. Which plan reflects evidence-based prenatal care for an uncomplicated pregnancy?

[A] Visits every 4 weeks until 28 weeks, every 2 weeks from 28–36 weeks, and weekly from 36 weeks until delivery; include screening for gestational diabetes at 24–28 weeks and group B streptococcus at 35–37 weeks.
[B] Monthly visits until 36 weeks, then weekly until delivery; no specific lab screening is needed if asymptomatic.
[C] No visits are necessary during the first trimester if the client feels well; begin visits at 20 weeks.
[D] Telehealth visits only unless complications occur, to minimize clinic exposure during pregnancy.

Question 3: A nurse teaches new parents strategies to reduce the risk of sudden infant death syndrome (SIDS). Which instruction is most appropriate?

[A] Place the infant to sleep prone with a rolled blanket to prevent reflux and choking.
[B] Use side-lying with a commercial sleep positioner to keep the infant from rolling.
[C] Place the infant supine on a firm mattress in an empty crib; room-share (not bed-share), avoid soft bedding and loose items, and consider a pacifier at sleep time.
[D] Bed-share with the infant so you can monitor breathing throughout the night.

Question 4: A 24-year-old with no history of abnormal results asks about cervical cancer screening. What should the nurse recommend?

[A] Primary high-risk HPV testing alone every 5 years starting at age 21.
[B] Cytology with high-risk HPV co-testing every 5 years beginning at age 21.
[C] Annual Papanicolaou (Pap) testing starting at age 21.
[D] Cytology (Pap test) alone every 3 years from age 21 to 29, with follow-up based on results.

Question 5: A pregnant client smokes 10 cigarettes/day. Which intervention best reflects first-line, evidence-based smoking cessation care in pregnancy?

[A] Start varenicline and bupropion together immediately and set a quit date.
[B] Advise cutting down to five cigarettes/day to minimize withdrawal and avoid quitting abruptly.
[C] Recommend e-cigarettes as a safer alternative to combustible cigarettes during pregnancy.
[D] Provide brief behavioral counseling (5 A's), set a quit date, connect to a quitline; consider nicotine replacement only if counseling alone fails and after risk–benefit discussion.

Question 6: A client at 28 weeks' gestation asks which vaccines are safe and recommended during pregnancy. Which action should the nurse take?

[A] Administer the measles–mumps–rubella (MMR) vaccine now to ensure maternal immunity.
[B] Administer Tdap between 27–36 weeks in this and every pregnancy, regardless of prior Tdap status, to enhance passive antibody transfer to the newborn.
[C] Provide the live attenuated intranasal influenza vaccine if it is flu season.
[D] Begin the HPV vaccine series now to reduce cervical cancer risk.

Question 7: During a 12-month well-child visit, which developmental finding should the nurse expect?

[A] Uses 2–3 word sentences and has a 20-word vocabulary.
[B] Copies a circle and rides a tricycle with supervision.
[C] Hops on one foot and ties shoelaces.
[D] Pulls to stand and cruises; may take a few independent steps; uses a pincer grasp; says "mama/dada" specifically and 1–2 additional words; follows simple one-step commands.

Question 8: A 46-year-old adult with average colorectal cancer risk asks about screening. What should the nurse recommend?

[A] Begin screening now at age 45; options include annual FIT, FIT–DNA every 1–3 years, or colonoscopy every 10 years if results are normal.
[B] Begin screening at age 50 unless symptoms occur earlier.
[C] Delay screening until age 55 if there is no family history or symptoms.
[D] Use stool DNA testing every 5 years only; colonoscopy is no longer recommended.

Question 9: A client 10 days postpartum calls the clinic. Which report requires immediate evaluation?

[A] Lochia serosa that is pink-brown and small-to-moderate in amount.
[B] Breast engorgement and firm, tender breasts on day 3 postpartum.
[C] Mild perineal pain controlled with ibuprofen following a second-degree laceration.
[D] Severe headache with visual changes and right upper quadrant/epigastric pain.

Question 10: A healthy 55-year-old had chickenpox as a child and shingles at age 50. What is the best immunization advice now?

[A] No vaccine is needed because prior infection confers lifelong immunity.
[B] Receive the recombinant zoster vaccine (RZV, Shingrix) in 2 doses 2–6 months apart, regardless of prior varicella or shingles history.
[C] Receive a single dose of the live zoster vaccine (Zostavax), which is preferred for those with prior shingles.
[D] Delay vaccination until age 65 to align with Medicare coverage.

ANSWERS

1. Correct Answer: B
Rationale: Solids should begin around 6 months when infants have good head control and can sit with support; start with single-ingredient, iron-fortified foods, introducing one new food every 3–5 days. Honey (risk of botulism), early cow's milk (risk of anemia and imbalance of nutrients), and starting solids at 3 months are contraindicated.

2. Correct Answer: A
Rationale: Standard prenatal care is every 4 weeks to 28 weeks, every 2 weeks to 36 weeks, then weekly; include GDM screening at 24–28 weeks and GBS at 35–37 weeks. The other options omit needed care or inappropriately reduce visit frequency.

3. Correct Answer: C
Rationale: Supine positioning on a firm surface in an empty crib, room-sharing without bed-sharing, and avoiding soft objects reduce SIDS. Prone/side positioning, sleep positioners, and bed-sharing increase risk.

4. Correct Answer: D
Rationale: For ages 21–29, cytology alone every 3 years is recommended for average-risk individuals. Primary HPV testing and co-testing are not standard before age 30, and annual Pap testing is not indicated without risk factors.

5. Correct Answer: D
Rationale: First-line therapy in pregnancy is behavioral counseling with support and quitline referral; NRT may be considered only if counseling fails and after risk–benefit discussion. Varenicline/bupropion are not first-line in pregnancy; cutting down or switching to e-cigarettes is not recommended.

6. Correct Answer: B
Rationale: Tdap is recommended during each pregnancy at 27–36 weeks to optimize passive immunity for the newborn. Live vaccines (MMR, intranasal influenza) and HPV are contraindicated/not recommended during pregnancy.

7. Correct Answer: D
Rationale: At 12 months, expected milestones include pulling to stand, cruising/early walking, mature pincer grasp, a few words with meaning, and following simple commands. The other options reflect abilities of older children (toddler/preschool ages).

8. Correct Answer: A
Rationale: Average-risk colorectal cancer screening begins at age 45. Options include annual FIT, FIT–DNA every 1–3 years, or colonoscopy every 10 years. Delaying to 50 or 55 is no longer recommended; colonoscopy remains a recommended option.

9. Correct Answer: D
Rationale: Severe headache with visual changes and RUQ/epigastric pain can indicate postpartum preeclampsia/HELLP and warrants urgent evaluation. Lochia serosa, transient engorgement, and mild perineal pain are expected postpartum findings.

10. Correct Answer: B
Rationale: Recombinant zoster vaccine (RZV, Shingrix) is recommended for immunocompetent adults ≥50 years in a 2-dose series regardless of prior varicella or shingles. Prior infection does not eliminate the need; live zoster vaccine is no longer preferred, and waiting until 65 is not advised.

6.3.4 Psychosocial Integrity

Question 1: A hospitalized client newly diagnosed with lymphoma says, "I'm terrified. I don't even know how I'm going to tell my kids." Which response by the nurse best demonstrates therapeutic communication?

[A] "You're feeling terrified and unsure how to share this with your children. Tell me more about what worries you most."
[B] "Just be honest with them; kids are resilient and will handle it better than you think."
[C] "Let's focus on your diet and discharge plan for now; you'll figure out how to tell them later."
[D] "Don't worry—everything will be fine once treatment starts."

Question 2: A college student reports frequent, intense anger after a breakup. He channels the energy into training for a mixed martial arts competition and states, "I feel calmer after practice." Which defense mechanism is he using?

[A] Denial
[B] Sublimation
[C] Projection
[D] Regression

Question 3: A client with major depressive disorder states, "I have a gun at home, and I plan to use it tonight when I'm alone." What is the nurse's priority action?

[A] Ask the client to sign a no-suicide contract and continue routine checks every 30 minutes.
[B] Encourage the client to verbalize feelings in a journal and schedule a therapy appointment.
[C] Initiate one-to-one observation, remove access to dangerous items, and notify the provider immediately.
[D] Arrange a family meeting to discuss support and discharge planning later today.

Question 4: A client with schizophrenia says, "The voices are telling me I deserve to be punished." Which response by the nurse is most therapeutic?

[A] "The voices aren't real. You need to ignore them."
[B] "I hear the voices too; they're not saying anything about punishment."
[C] "I don't hear the voices, but I can see this is scary. What are the voices saying right now?"
[D] "Go to your room until the voices stop, and try not to think about them."

Question 5: A client with chronic alcohol use presents with confusion, unsteady gait, and horizontal nystagmus. The provider prescribes IV thiamine, dextrose-containing fluids, and multivitamins. Which action should the nurse implement first?

[A] Start the dextrose-containing IV fluid to correct potential hypoglycemia.
[B] Administer naloxone to prevent respiratory depression.
[C] C. Administer IV thiamine before dextrose infusion.
[D] D. Draw serum ammonia levels prior to giving any medications.

Question 6: A pregnant client presents with bruising on her upper arms. Her partner insists on remaining in the exam room and answers questions for her. What is the nurse's most appropriate action?

[A] Document the partner's responses and proceed quickly to reduce stress.
[B] Request that the partner step out to conduct a private assessment and use nonjudgmental screening questions.
[C] Call hospital security and the police to remove the partner immediately.
[D] Confront the partner about suspected abuse and demand an explanation.

Question 7: A family member at the bedside of a dying client says, "If you give more morphine, you'll kill them." Which response by the nurse best supports end-of-life care?

[A] "We can stop the morphine if you prefer. It's your decision."
[B] "Morphine won't stop breathing unless the dose is huge, so there's nothing to worry about."
[C] "The doctor ordered this, so we have to give it."
[D] "Morphine is given to ease pain and breathing distress. We titrate carefully to comfort, not to hasten death."

Question 8: A widowed client joins a grief support group two weeks after her spouse's death. She says after the first session, "I didn't realize others feel the same waves of guilt and anger." Which therapeutic factor of group therapy does this most clearly illustrate?

[A] Catharsis
[B] Cohesiveness
[C] Universality
[D] Interpersonal learning

Question 9: Following a residential fire, multiple evacuees arrive at a community shelter. One adult appears anxious, disoriented, and repeatedly asks, "What am I supposed to do?" What is the nurse's priority action using Psychological First Aid principles?

[A] Facilitate a group debriefing to process emotions immediately.
[B] Obtain a detailed trauma history to inform counseling referrals.
[C] Encourage the client to express feelings for as long as needed.
[D] Provide calm, direct assistance to meet basic needs and ensure immediate safety (e.g., water, warmth, contact family).

Question 10: A client newly prescribed an SSRI for major depressive disorder asks when to expect improvement. Which response by the nurse is most accurate?

[A] "Some improvement may be noticed in 1–2 weeks, but full therapeutic effects often take 4–6 weeks."
[B] "You should feel completely better in 2–3 days; if not, the medication isn't working."
[C] "These medications work immediately, but side effects delay your awareness of improvement."
[D] "You'll need to take this for at least a year before any mood improvement is likely."

ANSWERS

1. Correct Answer: A
Rationale: Reflecting feelings and inviting elaboration are therapeutic and client-centered. B gives advice, C changes the subject, and D offers false reassurance—each is nontherapeutic.

2. Correct Answer: B
Rationale: Sublimation channels unacceptable impulses (anger/aggression) into socially acceptable activities (athletics). Denial (A) refuses reality, projection (C) attributes feelings to others, and regression (D) reverts to earlier behaviors.

3. Correct Answer: C
Rationale: A specific plan and means indicate imminent risk; priority is continuous observation, environmental safety, and provider notification. A no-suicide contract (A) is insufficient. B and D are supportive but not immediate safety measures.

4. Correct Answer: C
Rationale: Acknowledging the client's experience without validating the hallucination and assessing content promotes safety and trust. A argues about reality, B colludes with the hallucination, and D isolates and dismisses concerns.

5. Correct Answer: C
Rationale: In suspected Wernicke encephalopathy, thiamine must be given before glucose to prevent precipitating or worsening neurologic injury. Dextrose first (A) can exacerbate deficiency. Naloxone (B) treats opioid overdose, not alcohol-related encephalopathy. Ammonia level (D) is not the priority.

6. Correct Answer: B
Rationale: Best practice is to ensure privacy, use nonjudgmental IPV screening, and assess safety. A ignores client autonomy, C may not be legally appropriate and escalates risk, and D is confrontational and unsafe.

7. Correct Answer: D
Rationale: This response educates about the palliative intent of opioids and reassures regarding careful titration, aligning with ethical end-of-life care. A abandons symptom management, B provides false reassurance, and C is authoritarian.

8. Correct Answer: C
Rationale: Universality is recognizing that one is not alone in experiences and feelings. Catharsis (A) is emotional release, cohesiveness (B) is group bonding, and interpersonal learning (D) involves feedback and social skill development.

9. Correct Answer: D
Rationale: Psychological First Aid emphasizes safety, stabilization, and practical assistance first. Immediatedebriefing (A) and prolonged emotional ventilation (C) can be harmful acutely. Detailed trauma histories (B) are not a priority in the initial phase.

10. Correct Answer: A
Rationale: SSRIs commonly show partial improvement in 1–2 weeks with full effect in 4–6 weeks. B and C are inaccurate; D overstates the timeline for mood response.

6.3.5 Basic Care & Comfort

Question 1: A nurse is caring for a patient receiving continuous enteral tube feedings via a nasogastric tube. Which positioning intervention is most appropriate to reduce the risk for aspiration pneumonia?

[A] Place the patient in a supine position during the feeding to promote gastric emptying.
[B] Elevate the head of the bed 30–45 degrees during the feeding and for at least 30–60 minutes afterward.
[C] Position the patient in Trendelenburg during the feeding to minimize reflux.
[D] Place the patient in a right lateral position with the head flat to promote peristalsis.

Question 2: The nurse is teaching a nursing assistant about performing passive range-of-motion (ROM) exercises for a patient with complete left-sided paralysis. Which instruction is most accurate?

[A] Support the joint above and below, move each joint slowly to the point of resistance without pain, and repeat 5–10 times, 2–3 times daily.
[B] Move each joint until the patient reports mild pain to maintain flexibility and prevent stiffness.
[C] Perform ROM exercises only once weekly to prevent fatigue and joint inflammation.
[D] Focus only on the unaffected side to prevent injury; the affected side should remain immobilized.

Question 3: A patient with a long-term indwelling urinary catheter is at risk for catheter-associated urinary tract infection (CAUTI). Which nursing action is most effective for prevention?

[A] Irrigate the catheter every shift with sterile saline to prevent obstruction.
[B] Replace the catheter routinely every 48 hours to prevent biofilm formation.
[C] Obtain urine specimens from the drainage bag spout to minimize contamination.
[D] Maintain a closed drainage system, keep the collection bag below bladder level, secure the catheter, and perform routine perineal hygiene.

Question 4: The nurse provides discharge teaching to a patient with a new ileostomy. Which statement indicates correct understanding about diet and hydration to reduce complications?

[A] "I will take a laxative daily and add raw high-fiber vegetables early on to prevent obstruction."
[B] "I will drink 8–10 cups of fluid daily, add extra salt, avoid high-fiber foods like popcorn and nuts initially, chew thoroughly, and reintroduce foods gradually."
[C] "I should restrict fluids and sodium to reduce my ostomy output."
[D] "I will avoid all fruits and vegetables permanently to keep my output minimal."

Question 5: An older adult hospitalized for pneumonia reports difficulty sleeping in the hospital. Which nursing intervention is the best initial approach to promote sleep and rest?

[A] Implement a sleep-promotion bundle that clusters care to allow at least 90 minutes of uninterrupted sleep, reduces nighttime noise and light, and avoids nonessential overnight vital signs.
[B] Encourage long daytime naps to reduce fatigue during the night.
[C] Increase nighttime lighting to reduce fall risk and facilitate observation.
[D] Schedule hourly rounding with vital sign checks overnight to ensure safety.

Question 6: The nurse is selecting a comfort intervention for several patients. For which patient is cold therapy most appropriate?

[A] A patient with a new ankle sprain requesting a heating pad for pain relief.
[B] A patient with peripheral arterial disease and a pale, cool foot needing vasodilation.
[C] A patient with an acutely sprained ankle with edema in the first 24–48 hours, using a barrier and limiting application to 20 minutes at a time.
[D] A patient with diabetic neuropathy requesting an ice pack directly on the skin for foot pain.

Question 7: A patient with end-stage COPD in home hospice reports severe dyspnea and anxiety. The SpO2 is 88% on 2 L/min nasal cannula. The family asks what can be done now. What is the nurse's priority action consistent with palliative care principles?

[A] Immediately increase oxygen to 6 L/min and coach the patient to perform deep breathing exercises.
[B] Place the patient supine to conserve energy while reassessing respiratory rate.
[C] Administer the prescribed low-dose opioid for dyspnea, position the patient upright, and use a cool fan for nonpharmacologic relief.
[D] Call the provider to discuss intubation and mechanical ventilation for respiratory failure.

Question 8: The nurse performs oral care for an unconscious patient who is NPO. Which action is safest and most appropriate?

[A] Place the patient supine and use foam swabs soaked in water to aggressively cleanse the oral cavity.
[B] Brush vigorously even if the platelet count is low, as plaque removal takes priority over bleeding risk.
[C] Position the patient laterally with the head turned to the side, use a suction toothbrush or Yankauer, avoid excessive fluid, and apply water-based moisturizer to the lips.
[D] Use lemon-glycerin swabs frequently to stimulate saliva and freshen the mouth.

Question 9: A nurse inserts a nasogastric tube for enteral feeding in an adult patient. What is the most reliable method to verify initial placement before starting the feeding?

[A] Obtain radiographic confirmation and verify provider interpretation before initiating feedings.
[B] Inject air into the tube and auscultate a "whoosh" sound over the epigastrium.
[C] Check the gastric residual volume and proceed if more than 50 mL is aspirated.
[D] Confirm that the external tube length matches the expected insertion depth and begin feeding.

Question 10: The nurse is developing a bowel training program for a patient with a neurogenic bowel after a spinal cord injury. Which intervention is most effective to promote regular bowel elimination?

[A] Administer a stimulant laxative at bedtime and offer toileting on awakening to prevent nocturnal bowel movements.
[B] Schedule toileting 20–30 minutes after breakfast daily, offer a warm beverage, provide privacy and foot support, and use gentle abdominal massage to leverage the gastrocolic reflex.
[C] Instruct the patient to delay responding to the urge to defecate until afternoon to strengthen sphincter control.
[D] Perform digital disimpaction daily regardless of stool consistency to maintain regularity.

ANSWERS

1. Correct Answer: B

Rationale: Elevating the head of the bed 30–45 degrees during and after enteral feeding reduces reflux and aspiration risk. Supine and Trendelenburg positions increase aspiration risk; lateral with head flat is inadequate.

2. Correct Answer: A

Rationale: Passive ROM involves supporting the joint, moving slowly to the point of resistance without pain, and repeating 5–10 times 2–3 times/day. Moving into pain, infrequency, or immobilizing the affected side is inappropriate.

3. Correct Answer: D

Rationale: CAUTI prevention includes a closed system, dependent drainage, catheter securement, and routine perineal hygiene. Routine irrigation, sampling from the bag, and scheduled replacements are not recommended.

4. Correct Answer: B

Rationale: Ileostomy patients require adequate fluids and salt, thorough chewing, gradual food reintroduction, and initial avoidance of high-fiber/obstructive foods. Fluid/salt restriction and routine laxatives are unsafe; permanent avoidance of produce is unnecessary.

5. Correct Answer: A

Rationale: Clustering care to allow uninterrupted sleep, along with environmental modifications, is the most effective initial strategy. Long daytime naps, bright lights at night, and hourly overnight checks worsen sleep.

6. Correct Answer: C

Rationale: Cold therapy reduces pain and swelling in acute musculoskeletal injuries, applied with a barrier and time limits. Heat on a new sprain, cold on ischemic tissue, or direct ice on neuropathic skin are unsafe.

7. Correct Answer: C

Rationale: In palliative care, low-dose opioids effectively relieve dyspnea; upright positioning and a fan add nonpharmacologic relief. Escalating oxygen or invasive ventilation may not align with comfort goals.

8. Correct Answer: C

Rationale: Lateral positioning with suctioned oral care minimizes aspiration risk; avoid excessive fluids. Vigor, supine positioning, and lemon-glycerin swabs (drying) are inappropriate, especially with bleeding risk.

9. Correct Answer: A

Rationale: Radiographic confirmation is the gold standard for initial feeding tube placement. Air auscultation, residual checks, and external length are unreliable for initial verification.

10. Correct Answer: B

Rationale: Bowel programs leverage the gastrocolic reflex by scheduling toileting shortly after meals with supportive measures. Routine stimulant use at night, urge suppression, and daily disimpaction are inappropriate or invasive.

6.3.6 Pharmacological & Parenteral Therapies

Question 1: The nurse prepares to administer morphine sulfate 2 mg IV q2h PRN for severe pain. The client states, "I'm allergic to morphine; it made my throat swell before." The EMR shows "no known drug allergies," and the vial supplied is morphine 2 mg/mL. Which action demonstrates adherence to the rights of medication administration and client safety?

[A] Administer the medication after verifying two identifiers since the EMR lists no allergies.
[B] Ask an assistive personnel to remain with the client while you administer a test dose to assess tolerance.
[C] Document the client's statement and administer a reduced dose while monitoring closely.
[D] Withhold the medication; assess the reaction details, update the allergy record, and notify the provider and pharmacy for an alternative.

Question 2: The nurse provides discharge teaching for a client prescribed the monoamine oxidase inhibitor (MAOI) phenelzine for depression. Which statement indicates a need for further teaching?

[A] "I will check with my provider before taking any over-the-counter cold medicines."
[B] "I can enjoy aged cheeses and cured meats as long as I limit portions."
[C] "I'll wear a medical alert bracelet stating I take an MAOI."
[D] "I will report severe headaches or palpitations immediately."

Question 3: The provider prescribes 1,000 mL of 0.9% NS IV to infuse over 8 hours using gravity tubing with a drop factor of 15 gtt/mL. What is the correct flow rate in gtt/min?

[A] 31 gtt/min
[B] 21 gtt/min
[C] 39 gtt/min
[D] 47 gtt/min

Question 4: Fifteen minutes after initiation of a packed red blood cell (PRBC) transfusion, the client reports chills and back pain and has a temperature of 38.9°C (102.0°F). What is the nurse's priority action?

[A] Notify the provider and obtain a urine sample.
[B] Slow the transfusion rate and reassess in 10 minutes.
[C] Stop the transfusion immediately and maintain IV access with normal saline using new tubing.
[D] Administer acetaminophen and continue the transfusion if symptoms improve.

Question 5: While changing the administration set on a central venous catheter, the client suddenly develops dyspnea, chest pain, and a sense of impending doom. The nurse suspects a venous air embolism. What is the priority action?

[A] Clamp the catheter, place the client in left lateral Trendelenburg, and administer 100% oxygen.
[B] Place the client in high Fowler position and encourage deep breathing.
[C] Start rapid infusion of 0.9% NS and notify the provider.
[D] Obtain a stat chest x-ray before changing client position.

Question 6: A client receiving a continuous IV heparin infusion for a pulmonary embolism has an aPTT of 98 seconds. The control value at the facility is 30 seconds. Which action should the nurse take?

[A] Continue the infusion; the result is within the therapeutic range.
[B] Hold the infusion and notify the provider; prepare to administer protamine sulfate per protocol.
[C] Increase the infusion rate by 2 units/kg/hr per nomogram.
[D] Administer vitamin K as ordered to reduce bleeding risk.

Question 7: The nurse teaches a client about mixing NPH insulin with regular insulin for subcutaneous injection. Which statement by the client indicates correct understanding?

[A] "I will mix insulin glargine with regular insulin in the same syringe to reduce injections."
[B] "I should rotate sites by sticking to one quadrant to reduce variability."
[C] "I will draw up the regular insulin first, then the NPH insulin."
[D] "I will vigorously shake the NPH vial to resuspend the insulin."

Question 8: A client receiving total parenteral nutrition (TPN) via a central line finishes the current bag, and the next bag is not yet available from pharmacy. What should the nurse hang to prevent complications while waiting?

[A] 0.9% sodium chloride at the same rate as TPN
[B] 5% dextrose in water (D5W) at half the TPN rate
[C] 10% dextrose in water (D10W) at the prescribed TPN rate
[D] Lactated Ringer's solution at keep-vein-open (KVO) rate

Question 9: A postoperative client using a morphine PCA is drowsy with a respiratory rate of 6/min, oxygen saturation of 86% on room air, and pinpoint pupils. What is the nurse's priority action?

[A] Administer naloxone per protocol and reassess respirations.
[B] Encourage coughing and deep breathing exercises.
[C] Increase the IV fluid rate and apply 2 L/min oxygen via nasal cannula.
[D] Decrease the PCA dose and continue to monitor sedation level.

Question 10: During infusion of a vesicant chemotherapy agent through a newly placed peripheral IV, the client reports burning and the nurse notes swelling and blanching at the site. What is the best initial nursing action?

[A] Remove the IV catheter and apply a warm compress, then notify the provider.
[B] Elevate the extremity and resume infusion at a slower rate.
[C] Stop the infusion, leave the catheter in place, aspirate residual drug, and notify the provider for antidote administration per protocol.
[D] Flush the IV site with normal saline to dilute the medication.

ANSWERS

1. Correct Answer: D
Rationale: The nurse must honor the client's reported allergy, clarify the reaction (right assessment), update the allergy list (right documentation), and notify the provider/pharmacy for an alternative (right medication). Administering a "test dose" or giving despite the history violates safety principles and the rights of medication administration.

2. Correct Answer: B
Rationale: Tyramine-rich foods (aged cheeses, cured meats) are contraindicated with MAOIs due to risk of hypertensive crisis. OTC cold meds (often containing sympathomimetics) also require caution (A is appropriate teaching), medical alert identification is appropriate (C), and reporting severe headaches/palpitations is essential (D).

3. Correct Answer: A
Rationale: 1,000 mL over 8 hr = 125 mL/hr. Using 15 gtt/mL tubing: (125 mL/hr × 15 gtt/mL) / 60 = 31.25 ≈ 31 gtt/min. Other options miscalculate rate or rounding.

4. Correct Answer: C
Rationale: Suspected acute transfusion reaction requires stopping the transfusion immediately and maintaining IV access with normal saline using new tubing. Then notify the provider/blood bank and follow protocol (specimens, etc.). Slowing or continuing the transfusion is unsafe.

5. Correct Answer: A
Rationale: For suspected venous air embolism, clamp the catheter, position the client left lateral Trendelenburg to trap air in the right atrium, and administer 100% oxygen. High Fowler increases risk of air traveling; delaying positioning for imaging is unsafe.

6. Correct Answer: B
Rationale: Therapeutic aPTT for heparin is typically about 1.5–2.5 times control (≈45–75 sec if control is 30). An aPTT of 98 sec is supratherapeutic; hold or reduce per protocol and prepare protamine sulfate (antidote). Vitamin K reverses warfarin, not heparin.

7. Correct Answer: C
Rationale: When mixing insulins, draw up clear (regular) before cloudy (NPH) to prevent contaminating the short-acting insulin with protamine. Glargine should never be mixed (A incorrect). Sites should be rotated within and across regions to reduce lipodystrophy and variability (B incorrect). NPH should be gently rolled, not shaken (D incorrect).

8. Correct Answer: C
Rationale: If TPN is interrupted, hang D10W at the same rate to prevent rebound hypoglycemia due to sudden dextrose cessation. Normal saline, LR, or D5W do not provide sufficient dextrose replacement.

9. Correct Answer: A
Rationale: This is opioid-induced respiratory depression. Priority is to administer naloxone per protocol to reverse respiratory depression and then reassess. Supplemental oxygen alone does not address the underlying opioid effect; adjusting PCA without reversal is unsafe.

10. Correct Answer: C
Rationale: With suspected vesicant extravasation, stop the infusion, leave the catheter in place for aspiration of drug and potential antidote administration, and notify the provider/implement protocol. Removing the catheter immediately can prevent antidote delivery; flushing or continuing infusion worsens tissue injury.

6.3.7 Reduction of Risk Potential

Question 1: A client with chronic kidney disease has the following morning labs: potassium 6.3 mEq/L (3.5–5.0), creatinine 3.8 mg/dL (0.6–1.3), and peaked T waves on the cardiac monitor. Which action should the nurse take first to reduce risk of life-threatening complications?

[A] Place the client on continuous cardiac monitoring and assess for dysrhythmias while notifying the provider
[B] Restrict dietary potassium and educate the client to avoid high-potassium foods
[C] Prepare to administer IV furosemide as prescribed without further assessment
[D] Encourage intake of bananas and orange juice to prevent muscle cramps

Question 2: Ten hours after a subtotal thyroidectomy, a client reports tingling around the mouth and fingers, and the nurse elicits a positive Trousseau sign. Which action is the priority?

[A] Initiate seizure precautions and prepare to administer IV calcium gluconate per protocol
[B] Encourage vigorous coughing and deep breathing to clear secretions
[C] Lower the head of the bed and apply a nonrebreather mask at 15 L/min
[D] Administer IV insulin with dextrose to shift potassium intracellularly

Question 3: A client two days post–total hip arthroplasty reports calf discomfort. Which assessment finding most strongly suggests a deep vein thrombosis (DVT)?

[A] Unilateral calf warmth, erythema, and edema with a larger circumference than the opposite leg
[B] Dependent bilateral pitting edema of the ankles
[C] Cool, pale foot with absent dorsalis pedis pulse bilaterally
[D] Pain on forced dorsiflexion of the foot (Homan sign) without other symptoms

Question 4: A client with an arteriovenous (AV) fistula in the left arm is scheduled for hemodialysis in one hour. Which pre-dialysis action is most appropriate?

[A] Administer scheduled antihypertensives and antibiotics to prevent intra-dialytic hypotension and infection
[B] Use the left arm to obtain blood samples and measure blood pressure to assess fistula function
[C] Verify a palpable thrill and audible bruit at the fistula and hold blood pressure–lowering medications until after dialysis
[D] Provide a high-protein, high-potassium meal to prevent catabolism during dialysis

Question 5: A client with a severe traumatic brain injury is being monitored in the ICU. Which change requires the most immediate intervention as an early indicator of impending brain herniation?

[A] Temperature increase from 99.0°F (37.2°C) to 101.3°F (38.5°C)
[B] Urine output decrease from 60 mL/hr to 20 mL/hr
[C] Blood pressure drop from 130/80 to 100/60 with heart rate 110
[D] Systolic blood pressure rising with widening pulse pressure, heart rate decreasing, and irregular respirations

Question 6: A client with a recent stroke is receiving continuous enteral nutrition via nasogastric tube. Which nursing action best reduces the risk of aspiration?

[A] Maintain head-of-bed elevation at 30–45 degrees during feeding and for at least 30–60 minutes after, and verify tube placement per policy
[B] Lay the client flat during bolus feeds to improve comfort and prevent reflux
[C] Clamp the tube during coughing episodes to prevent regurgitation
[D] Use 30 mL of tap water to confirm tube placement instead of pH or x-ray verification

Question 7: A postoperative client receiving an insulin infusion for tight glycemic control suddenly becomes pale and anxious. Which assessment finding most strongly indicates hypoglycemia requiring rapid treatment?

[A] Increased thirst and frequent urination
[B] Deep, rapid respirations with abdominal pain
[C] Fruity breath odor and lethargy
[D] Diaphoresis, tremors, tachycardia, and confusion

Question 8: The nurse reviews lab results for a 68-year-old on postoperative day 1 after abdominal surgery. Which result requires immediate follow-up to reduce risk of dysrhythmias?

[A] Sodium 134 mEq/L (135–145)
[B] Potassium 2.9 mEq/L (3.5–5.0)
[C] Hemoglobin 10.8 g/dL (12–16)
[D] Calcium 8.5 mg/dL (8.6–10.2)

Question 9: The nurse teaches a client and caregiver about home tracheostomy care. Which statement indicates correct understanding and reduces risk of airway emergencies?

[A] "I'll clean the inner cannula daily with full-strength hydrogen peroxide to prevent infection."
[B] "I'll cut 4x4 gauze to fit around the tube so it lies flat against the skin."
[C] "I can change the tracheostomy ties by myself as long as I'm careful."
[D] "I will keep two spare trach tubes (same size and one size smaller), the obturator, and suction equipment at the bedside at all times."

Question 10: A client is postoperative day 1 after a bowel resection. Which trend should alert the nurse to potential clinical deterioration requiring rapid reassessment before it becomes an emergency?

[A] Heart rate rising from 84 to 112/min and respiratory rate from 16 to 24/min with stable blood pressure
[B] Oral temperature increasing from 98.6°F (37.0°C) to 99.5°F (37.5°C)
[C] Reports incisional pain increasing from 4/10 to 6/10 after coughing
[D] Oxygen saturation stable at 95% on room air

ANSWERS

1. Correct Answer: A
Rationale: Hyperkalemia with ECG changes is cardiotoxic. Immediate continuous cardiac monitoring and assessment for dysrhythmias is the first priority while notifying the provider for definitive treatment. Dietary restriction (B) is not urgent. Administering diuretics (C) may be part of treatment but monitoring comes first. D worsens hyperkalemia.

2. Correct Answer: A
Rationale: Perioral tingling and positive Trousseau indicate hypocalcemia, a known post-thyroidectomy complication that can progress to laryngospasm/seizures. Preparing to give IV calcium and instituting seizure precautions is priority. B and C do not treat hypocalcemia; D addresses hyperkalemia, not present.

3. Correct Answer: A
Rationale: Unilateral warmth, erythema, and edema with increased calf circumference are classic for DVT. Bilateral edema (B) suggests systemic fluid issues. Absent bilateral pulses (C) indicates arterial insufficiency, not DVT. Homan's sign (D) is unreliable and no longer recommended.

4. Correct Answer: C
Rationale: Assessing for thrill/bruit confirms fistula patency; antihypertensives are often held pre-dialysis to reduce hypotension risk. A can precipitate hypotension. B risks fistula damage and is contraindicated. D encourages hyperkalemia and is inappropriate.

5. Correct Answer: D
Rationale: Cushing's triad—widened pulse pressure, bradycardia, and irregular respirations—signals increased intracranial pressure and impending herniation, requiring immediate intervention. Fever (A) and oliguria (B) are concerning but less immediately life-threatening. Hypotension/tachycardia (C) suggest shock, not classic ICP rise.

6. Correct Answer: A
Rationale: Elevating the HOB and verifying tube placement reduce aspiration risk. Supine positioning (B) increases aspiration risk. Clamping during cough (C) does not prevent aspiration and may increase pressure. Water instillation (D) is unsafe; use pH/x-ray per policy.

7. Correct Answer: D
Rationale: Diaphoresis, tremors, tachycardia, and confusion are hallmark signs of hypoglycemia requiring rapid glucose administration. A, B, and C are more consistent with hyperglycemia or DKA.

8. Correct Answer: B
Rationale: Hypokalemia (2.9 mEq/L) increases risk for ventricular dysrhythmias; it requires prompt correction. The other values are only slightly abnormal or expected post-op and are less urgent.

9. Correct Answer: D
Rationale: Keeping spare trach tubes (same size and smaller), the obturator, and suction available reduces risk during accidental decannulation or obstruction. Full-strength peroxide (A) can irritate tissue. Cutting gauze (B) risks lint aspiration; use pre-cut. Changing ties alone (C) is unsafe.

10. Correct Answer: A
Rationale: Unexplained tachycardia and increasing respiratory rate are early signs of deterioration (e.g., occult bleeding, hypovolemia, or sepsis) and typically precede hypotension. Mild fever (B), increased pain (C), and stable SpO2 (D) are less urgent in comparison.

6.3.8 Physiological Adaptation

Question 1: A client with serum sodium of 118 mEq/L is confused, has a headache, and reports nausea. Which priority nursing action is most appropriate?

[A] Initiate seizure precautions and prepare to administer 3% hypertonic saline per protocol
[B] Encourage oral free water intake to improve hydration
[C] Start 0.45% (half-normal) saline at 150 mL/hr
[D] Administer a thiazide diuretic to increase sodium concentration

Question 2: A client with end-stage renal disease presents with muscle weakness and ECG changes showing peaked T waves. Potassium is 7.1 mEq/L. What is the priority intervention?

[A] Administer sodium polystyrene sulfonate (Kayexalate)
[B] Give IV furosemide to promote potassium excretion
[C] Place the client on continuous cardiac monitoring
[D] Administer IV calcium gluconate to stabilize the cardiac membrane

Question 3: A client with diabetic ketoacidosis (DKA) is admitted. Which arterial blood gas (ABG) is most consistent with this condition?

[A] pH 7.52, PaCO2 30 mm Hg, HCO3– 25 mEq/L
[B] pH 7.46, PaCO2 48 mm Hg, HCO3– 31 mEq/L
[C] pH 7.25, PaCO2 28 mm Hg, HCO3– 16 mEq/L
[D] pH 7.34, PaCO2 55 mm Hg, HCO3– 28 mEq/L

Question 4: A client develops sudden wheezing, stridor, urticaria, and hypotension after receiving the first dose of an IV antibiotic. What is the nurse's priority action?

[A] Place the client in Trendelenburg and begin a rapid infusion of normal saline
[B] Administer IV diphenhydramine as prescribed
[C] Apply high-flow oxygen via nonrebreather mask and call the provider
[D] Administer intramuscular epinephrine immediately

Question 5: A client with acute decompensated heart failure has been receiving IV furosemide for 24 hours. Which assessment finding best indicates the therapy is effective?

[A] Blood pressure increases from 98/64 to 116/72 mm Hg with no change in weight
[B] Weight decreases by 1.5 kg (3.3 lb), crackles diminish, and SpO2 improves from 90% to 95%
[C] Urine output totals 200 mL over 8 hours and heart rate decreases from 112 to 92
[D] Fewer premature ventricular contractions after electrolyte replacement

Question 6: Two hours after abdominal surgery, a client becomes tachycardic (HR 128), hypotensive (BP 82/48), cool, pale, and diaphoretic. The abdominal dressing is saturated, and the drain output has turned bright red and increased rapidly. What is the priority nursing action?

[A] Assess the incision and under the client for bleeding, apply firm pressure/reinforce the dressing, activate the rapid response team, and prepare for fluid resuscitation
[B] Administer ondansetron for possible nausea due to opioids
[C] Notify the surgeon and await further instructions
[D] Increase the opioid dose for suspected uncontrolled pain

Question 7: Which nursing action is appropriate for a client with an arteriovenous (AV) fistula for hemodialysis in the left forearm?

[A] Obtain routine blood samples from the fistula to preserve peripheral veins
[B] Assess for a bruit and thrill each shift and avoid blood pressures/venipunctures in the fistula arm
[C] Use the fistula for IV antibiotic administration with a microbore filter
[D] Elevate the fistula arm on pillows continuously to reduce blood flow

Question 8: A client arrives to the ED with crushing substernal chest pain radiating to the jaw, diaphoresis, and nausea for 30 minutes. Orders are placed for oxygen, aspirin, nitroglycerin, morphine, ECG, and cardiac enzymes. Which intervention should the nurse implement first to reduce mortality?

[A] Administer high-intensity statin therapy
[B] Start a heparin infusion per protocol
[C] Administer chewable aspirin 325 mg immediately (after confirming no contraindications)
[D] Give sublingual nitroglycerin and reassess pain in 5 minutes

Question 9: A client with a chest tube to water-seal drainage after a lobectomy is being assessed. Which finding requires immediate intervention by the nurse?

[A] Tidaling (rise and fall) in the water-seal chamber with respirations
[B] Absence of tidaling in a client whose recent chest x-ray shows full lung re-expansion
[C] Gentle continuous bubbling in the suction control chamber while suction is applied
[D] Sudden output of 250 mL bright-red drainage in 1 hour accompanied by tachycardia and hypotension

Question 10: A hospitalized adult suddenly collapses. The client is unresponsive, pulseless, and the monitor shows ventricular tachycardia without a pulse. What is the next best action?

[A] Administer atropine 1 mg IV push
[B] Administer amiodarone 300 mg IV before defibrillation
[C] Perform synchronized cardioversion at 100 J
[D] Deliver an immediate unsynchronized defibrillation shock and resume CPR

ANSWERS

1. Correct Answer: A

Rationale: Severe symptomatic hyponatremia (Na <120) can cause cerebral edema and seizures; priority care includes seizure precautions and administration of hypertonic saline (3%) per protocol. Hypotonic fluids (C) and free water (B) worsen hyponatremia. Thiazides (D) can precipitate or worsen hyponatremia.

2. Correct Answer: D

Rationale: In life-threatening hyperkalemia with ECG changes, immediate stabilization of the myocardium with IV calcium gluconate is priority. Kayexalate (A) and loop diuretics (B) lower potassium more slowly. Cardiac monitoring (C) is essential but does not treat membrane instability.

3. Correct Answer: C

Rationale: DKA causes metabolic acidosis (low pH, low HCO_3^-) with respiratory compensation (low $PaCO_2$). Options A and B reflect alkalosis; D reflects respiratory acidosis with metabolic compensation.

4. Correct Answer: D

Rationale: Anaphylaxis is an airway/breathing/circulation emergency; intramuscular epinephrine is the first-line, life-saving treatment. Fluids (A), antihistamines (B), and oxygen (C) are adjuncts after epinephrine.

5. Correct Answer: B

Rationale: Effective diuresis in acute heart failure is indicated by reduced fluid overload: weight loss, diminished crackles, and improved oxygenation. A (BP rise) without decongestion is insufficient. C indicates oliguria. D addresses arrhythmias, not decongestion.

6. Correct Answer: A

Rationale: The client shows signs of postoperative hemorrhagic shock. Immediate assessment of the source, application of direct pressure/reinforcement, activation of rapid response, and preparation for resuscitation are priorities. D and B ignore the life-threatening cause. C delays time-critical interventions.

7. Correct Answer: B

Rationale: Proper AV fistula care includes assessing for patency (bruit/thrill) and protecting the access by avoiding BP/venipunctures in that arm. A and C risk thrombosis/infection. D continuous elevation can impede flow; the fistula needs adequate perfusion.

8. Correct Answer: C

Rationale: Early chewable aspirin reduces mortality by inhibiting platelet aggregation in acute MI and should be given immediately if no contraindications. Nitroglycerin (D) relieves pain but does not confer the same mortality benefit. Heparin (B) and statins (A) are important but not first to reduce immediate mortality.

9. Correct Answer: D

Rationale: Sudden large-volume bright-red drainage with instability suggests hemorrhage and requires immediate intervention. Tidaling (A) is expected; absent tidaling after re-expansion (B) can be normal. Gentle bubbling in the suction control chamber (C) is expected when suction is applied.

10. Correct Answer: D

Rationale: Pulseless VT/VF requires immediate unsynchronized defibrillation followed by high-quality CPR per ACLS. Atropine (A) is for bradycardia, not pulseless rhythms. Amiodarone (B) is given after defibrillation attempts/CPR. Synchronized cardioversion (C) is for perfusing, unstable tachyarrhythmias with a pulse.

ACCESS YOUR BONUS MATERIALS

You've made it to the end—well done! Preparing for the NCLEX-RN isn't just about memorizing facts, it's about mastering the mindset, strategies, and clinical judgment skills that matter most. To support you even further, we've created a set of exclusive bonuses just for readers like you.

Here's what's waiting for you:

- **NCLEX-RN Exam Simulator**
  Generate unlimited practice exams with a realistic simulator that mirrors actual test-day conditions and puts your skills to the test.
- **1,000+ Interactive Flashcards**
  Build recall with 1,000+ interactive flashcards that turn short study windows into focused practice and make each review session faster, smarter, and more effective.
- **Full Question Bank Download**
  Access 2,400+ NCLEX-style questions with detailed explanations—so you're not just guessing answers, you're learning the logic behind them.
- **The SYSTEM-14 Course**
  A focused 14-day program that shows you how to master flashcards and retain high-yield concepts with a proven memory system.
- **Mindshift Video Program**
  Shift your mindset with exclusive videos that teach exam-day strategies, stress management, and how to stay confident under pressure.

Access your bonus materials by scanning the QR code or visiting the link below.
When prompted, enter the access code found at the bottom of this page

https://tinyurl.com/prep-nclexrn

Your secret code is: **nclexrn1254**